PRAISE FOR *HIGH RELIABILITY ORGANIZATIONS: A*
FOR PATIENT SAFETY & QUA

"This book is more than a must-read handbook. Oster and Braaten have developed a rare resource that will serve as an ongoing reference for healthcare students and providers embracing the call for a radically new model of patient safety and quality. The authors have masterfully described critically important HRO concepts within a framework illuminated by examples of application to practice and considerations of assimilation across the care continuum. All providers within all healthcare settings seeking to understand and positively influence high reliability will find this handbook extraordinarily useful!"

–Mary Cathryn Sitterding, PhD, RN, CNS
Vice President, Patient Services
Cincinnati Children's Hospital Medical Center

"This book is focused on safe, quality care and is a great resource for nurses and nursing students. Each chapter offers excellent examples, case studies, tools, techniques, and real-world experiences that are easy to relate to within complex health systems. I particularly love the content on Just Culture, TeamSTEPPS, Root Cause Analysis, Failure Mode and Effects Analysis (FMEA), and the inclusion of robust improvement strategies. I plan to make this a required text for CNL and DNP students as they begin their immersion experiences to better understand systems and improve care delivery and population health. A must-read for improvement practitioners!"

–Linda Roussel, PhD, RN, NEA-BC, CNL, FAAN
DNP Program Director and CNL Coordinator
The University of Alabama at Birmingham, School of Nursing

"This pragmatic handbook is the first written for front-line staff: nurses at the 'sharp point of care' where high reliability principles must be practiced every day, every time care is delivered. The authors present material in a clear, concise framework, beginning with the groundbreaking conceptual work by Reason, Weick, and Sutcliffe and The Joint Commission's Chassin and Loeb. Application of high reliability tenets involving leadership, human behavior, process redesign, and technology enablement are enriched by clinical examples such as alarm safety, falls, and infection prevention. The handbook highlights the complex cultural and communication challenges among team members in the care continuum. I enthusiastically endorse this valuable new resource on high reliability toward the goal of zero preventable harm."

–Ann Scott Blouin, PhD, RN, FACHE
Executive Vice President, Customer Relations
The Joint Commission and National Patient Safety Foundation Board of Directors

HIGH RELIABILITY ORGANIZATIONS

A Healthcare Handbook for Patient Safety & Quality

Cynthia A. Oster, PhD, MBA, APRN, ACNS-BC, ANP
Jane S. Braaten, PhD, APRN, CNS, ANP, CPPS

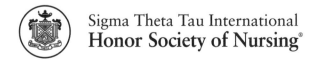

Sigma Theta Tau International
Honor Society of Nursing®

The Honor Society of Nursing, Sigma Theta Tau International (STTI) is a nonprofit organization founded in 1922 whose mission is to support the learning, knowledge, and professional development of nurses committed to making a difference in health worldwide. Members include practicing nurses, instructors, researchers, policymakers, entrepreneurs, and others. STTI has roughly 500 chapters located at 695 institutions of higher education throughout Armenia, Australia, Botswana, Brazil, Canada, Colombia, England, Ghana, Hong Kong, Japan, Kenya, Lebanon, Malawi, Mexico, the Netherlands, Pakistan, Portugal, Singapore, South Africa, South Korea, Swaziland, Sweden, Taiwan, Tanzania, Thailand, the United Kingdom, and the United States of America. More information about STTI can be found online at www.nursingsociety. org/about-stti.

Sigma Theta Tau International
550 West North Street
Indianapolis, IN, USA 46202

To order additional books, buy in bulk, or order for corporate use, contact Nursing Knowledge International at 888. NKI.4YOU (888.654.4968/US and Canada) or +1.317.634.8171 (outside US and Canada).

To request a review copy for course adoption, e-mail solutions@nursingknowledge.org or call 888.NKI.4YOU (888.654.4968/US and Canada) or +1.317.634.8171 (outside US and Canada).

To request author information, or for speaker or other media requests, contact Marketing, Honor Society of Nursing, Sigma Theta Tau International at 888.634.7575 (US and Canada) or +1.317.634.8171 (outside US and Canada).

ISBN:	9781940446387
EPUB ISBN:	9781940446394
PDF ISBN:	9781940446400
MOBI ISBN:	9781940446417

Library of Congress Cataloging-in-Publication data

Names: Oster, Cynthia, 1958- , editor. | Braaten, Jane, 1962- , editor. | Sigma Theta Tau International, issuing body.
Title: High reliability organizations : a healthcare handbook for patient safety & quality / Cynthia Oster, Jane Braaten.
Description: Indianapolis, IN : Sigma Theta Tau International, [2016] | Includes bibliographical references and index.
Identifiers: LCCN 2016004861| ISBN 9781940446387 (print : alk. paper) | ISBN 9781940446394 (epub) | ISBN 9781940446400 (PDF) | ISBN 9781940446417 (mobi)
Subjects: | MESH: Patient Safety--standards | Safety Management--organization & administration | Health Facility Administration | Health Facilities--standards | Quality of Health Care | Organizational Culture | United States

Classification: LCC RA971 | NLM WX 185 | DDC 362.1068--dc23 LC record available at http://lccn.loc.gov/2016004861

First Printing, 2016

Publisher: Dustin Sullivan	**Principal Book Editor:** Carla Hall
Acquisitions Editor: Emily Hatch	**Development and Project Editor:** Kate Shoup
Editorial Coordinator: Paula Jeffers	**Copy Editor:** Charlotte Kughen
Cover Designer: Michael Tanamachi	**Proofreader:** Todd Lothery
Interior Design/Page Layout: Rebecca Batchelor	**Indexer:** Joy Dean Lee

DEDICATION

This book is dedicated to the people on the front lines of healthcare who create and innovate to make high reliability a reality because they care.

ACKNOWLEDGMENTS

This text has come to fruition through the assistance, dedication, and support of many individuals. We would like to express our gratitude to the many colleagues, friends, and family members who saw us through this book. Thank you to all who provided support, talked things over, read, wrote, and encouraged us in spite of all the time it took us away from you. Each of you contributed to our success in ways too numerous to list.

We also wish to acknowledge and thank those at Sigma Theta Tau International for their guidance, creativity, and patience in making our vision a reality.

ABOUT THE AUTHORS

CYNTHIA A. OSTER, PHD, MBA, APRN, ACNS-BC, ANP

Cynthia A. Oster, PhD, MBA, APRN, ACNS-BC, ANP, is nurse scientist for Centura Health and a clinical nurse specialist for critical care and cardiovascular services at Porter Adventist Hospital in Denver, Colorado. With 35 years of experience, she has held research, clinical, educational, and administrative positions within and outside of Centura Health. Oster received her BSN from the University of Iowa, her MSN from the University of Nebraska Medical Center, and her PhD from the University of Colorado, College of Nursing. In addition, she earned an Adult Nurse Practitioner Certificate from Beth El College of Nursing in Colorado Springs, Colorado, and an MBA from the University of Colorado–Denver. Currently, she mentors novice researchers, facilitates the conduct of research, and facilitates the adoption of evidence-based practices in Centura Health. Oster is the principal investigator of several ongoing research studies in Centura Health and chairs the South Denver Evidence-Based Practice, Research and Innovation Council. Oster has presented at national and international meetings and has published in the areas of evidence-based practice and peer review. She is a member of Sigma Theta Tau International, the American Nurses Association, the American Association of Critical-Care Nurses, the National Association of Clinical Nurse Specialists, the American College of Healthcare Executives, and Beta Gamma Sigma.

JANE S. BRAATEN, PHD, APRN, CNS, ANP, CPPS

Jane S. Braaten, PhD, APRN, CNS, ANP, CPPS, is a patient safety manager and nurse scientist at Centura Health, Castle Rock Adventist Hospital in Castle Rock, Colorado. She has held positions within Centura Health as director of cardiology services, cardiac and intensive care clinical nurse specialist, cardiac nurse practitioner, and manager/charge RN/staff RN of intensive care and telemetry units. Braaten obtained her BSN from the Indiana University School of Nursing and holds degrees of Doctor of Philosophy, Clinical Nurse Specialist, and Adult Nurse Practitioner (certificate) from the University of Colorado, College of Nursing. She also is a Certified Professional in Patient Safety (CPPS). She has presented at national meetings and has published in the areas of hospital system barriers to rapid response team activation, quality improvement in telemetry, end-of-life care in the intensive care unit, leadership, and high reliability organizations and healthcare.

CONTRIBUTING AUTHORS

KELLY ALDRICH, DNP, RN-BC

Kelly Aldrich DNP, RN-BC, is an informatics nurse specialist and has served more than 25 years in healthcare clinical, leadership, and informatics roles. She graduated from the University of South Florida, Tampa, with a master of science in nursing healthcare systems leadership and nursing informatics degree in 2004. Following this, she obtained her doctorate of nursing degree in 2010, focused in educational informatics. The culmination of her work, titled "Putting Technology into Practice," has allowed for new innovations in technology to be appropriately blended into inpatient care environments. Aldrich is known as a visionary nursing informatics executive leader and is highly regarded for her innovative approach that provides a bridge between nursing practice and technology solutions. Her passion and dedication for a seamless, patient-centered care environment from an informatics lens has led to safer, more efficient, and more effective care environments.

GAIL E. ARMSTRONG, DNP, ACNS-BC, CNE

Gail E. Armstrong, DNP, ACNS-BC, CNE, was part of the University of Colorado Quality Safety and Education in Nursing (QSEN) pilot school team to update nursing curricula to reflect quality and safety trends. She continues her work with QSEN, focusing on prelicensure curriculum development, with an emphasis of threading the competencies and KSAs across learning settings. Along with her teaching, Armstrong is part of the faculty in a 12-month program for interdisciplinary clinical teams that focuses on health system leadership, organizational development, change management, and process improvement at the University of Colorado, College of Nursing.

AMY J. BARTON, PHD, RN, FAAN

Amy J. Barton, PhD, RN, FAAN, holds the Professor and Daniel and Janet Mordecai Endowed Chair in Rural Health Nursing and serves as associate dean for clinical and community affairs at the University of Colorado, College of Nursing. She is responsible for faculty practice and community partnerships. She provided the vision and strategic initiative to create Sheridan Health Services, a nurse-managed, federally qualified community health center serving low-income families. Her work in national quality and safety initiatives include the Quality and Safety Education for Nurses initiative and the Institute for Healthcare Improvement/Josiah Macy Jr. Foundation initiative, "Retooling for Quality and Safety." Barton is a member of the 2005 cohort of the Robert Wood Johnson Executive Nurse Fellows. She is chair of the Board of the

National Nursing Centers Consortium, is a Distinguished Practitioner in the National Academies of Practice, and holds fellowships in the Western Academy of Nursing and the American Academy of Nursing.

JEAN BECKEL, DNP, RN, MPH, CNML

Jean Beckel, DNP, RN, MPH, CNML, completed her doctor of nursing practice degree at the University of Pittsburgh, Pittsburgh, Pennsylvania; her master of public health degree at the University of Minnesota, Minneapolis, Minnesota; and her bachelor of science in nursing at the College of St. Teresa, Winona, Minnesota. She currently works as the Magnet® program director for Porter Adventist Hospital in Denver, Colorado and Parker Adventist Hospital in Parker, Colorado. She has 15 years of Magnet program director experience in two Magnet-designated hospitals. Beckel has been a Magnet Recognition Program® appraiser since 2007.

JULIE BENZ, DNP, RN, CNS-BC, CCRN

Julie Benz, DNP, RN, CNS-BC, CCRN, is a critical care nurse with more than 40 years of practice experience. For the last decade, Benz has been responsible for employment of the evidence base to acute coronary syndrome patient populations and the resuscitation products of Code Blue and Rapid Response at St. Anthony Hospital. Benz is a cardiovascular clinical nurse specialist with joint appointment to Regis University as assistant clinical professor, teaching undergraduate medical-surgical nursing. Her research interests include application of urban clinical practice guidelines to rural settings for STEMI patient care and the relationship between sleep apnea and Rapid Response or Code Blue events. She is active as a volunteer for the Colorado Heart Association and served as the nurse representative on a state of Colorado STEMI task force, appointed by Governor Hickenlooper. The task force developed legislation and reported to the Colorado legislature on methods to enhance STEMI outcomes in all areas of the state, both rural and urban.

NOREEN BERNARD, MS, RN, NEA-BC

Noreen Bernard, MS, RN, NEA-BC, is the vice president of professional resources for the Centura Health System, Colorado's largest healthcare organization and fourth-largest private employer. Bernard has been with Centura Health for more than 12 years and currently oversees the design and deployment of enterprise strategies and activities that promote professional development, knowledge management, staffing excellence, and clinical excellence on the part of Centura nurses and other healthcare personnel in all practice settings. Bernard is currently enrolled in a doctoral program for leadership and organization development. She holds a master of science degree from the University of Colorado with an emphasis on nursing administration and a bachelor of science in nursing degree from the University of Northern Colorado. She serves on multiple local and state education advisory boards and is president of the Colorado Hoopsters basketball club. She is also an active member of the American Organization of Nurse Executives and Denver Director for the Colorado Organization of Nurse Leaders.

KATHERINE BILYS, MBA, CPHQ

Katherine Bilys, MBA, CPHQ, is vice president of quality and performance improvement at a 346 licensed-bed acute care hospital in the Denver metropolitan area. She has been working with clinicians in the acute care setting since 2002 using a systems approach to improve patient outcomes and safety cultures.

LISA CAMPLESE, MBA, BSN, RN

Lisa Camplese, MBA, BSN, RN, is a seasoned healthcare executive with 28 years of experience in healthcare administration. A graduate of the Arkansas Medical Sciences Campus, Camplese is a bachelor's-prepared nurse and registered nurse practitioner. Camplese also has a master's in business administration from Brenau University, with an additional Health Services Administration certificate. Camplese joined Centura Health in 2006 as the vice president for clinical quality. Her responsibilities include content management for the building of evidence-based order sets for EMR, credentialing verification services, and quality, patient safety, and regulatory readiness for the system. Before working at Centura Health, Camplese served as chief operating officer, administrator, and quality executive in hospitals in Atlanta and Tucson.

NAN DAVIDSON, MA, RN, CNS-BC

Nan Davidson, MA, RN, CNS-BC, is a clinical nurse specialist for surgery services at Porter Adventist Hospital, Centura Health, and has extensive advanced practice nurse experience in the acute medical-surgical setting. Her career focus has been to implement evidence-based practice changes to improve perioperative care, pain management, and safety while on opioids at the hospital and system-wide level. Her work to implement progressive practice changes to enhance opioid safety has been featured at numerous regional and national conference presentations. Her research interests include establishing psychometrics for the Richmond Agitation-Sedation Scale (RASS) to prevent opioid-induced oversedation, patient safety, and satisfaction with pain.

SHERILYN DEAKINS, MS, RN, CPPS

Sherilyn Deakins, MS, RN, CPPS, has 30 years of experience as a nurse. Her diverse background includes clinical nursing experience in cardiac intensive care, nurse recruitment, human resources, new graduate RN program coordination, and management. Currently, her area of expertise and certification is in the field of patient safety.

ERIN DENHOLM, MSN, RN, RWJNEF

Erin Denholm, MSN, RN, RWJNEF, is president and CEO of Trinity Home Health Services. For 20 years she served Centura Health, most recently as SVP of clinical transformation. She is a Robert Wood Johnson Nurse Executive Fellow. She served on the CMS Innovation Center Advisory Council. She is a distinguished leader in healthcare, noted for her visionary commitment to transcend healthcare beyond hospital walls. In her last role for Centura Health, Denholm was responsible for clinical programming for population health. She pioneered the use of telehealth technology in reducing emergency department visits and adverse outcomes among heart failure patients in Colorado, and she led the successful legislative effort to make Colorado the first state in the country to provide Medicaid funding for telehealth services.

JANE ENGLEBRIGHT, PHD, RN, CENP, FAAN

Jane Englebright, PhD, RN, CENP, FAAN, provides professional leadership for facility chief nursing officers and approximately 80,000 nurses working in HCA hospitals, ambulatory surgery centers, and other sites of care. She leads HCA's CNO Council in driving excellence in nursing operations and outcomes, professional practice, and innovative leadership. Her professional title is chief nurse executive, patient safety officer, and senior vice president. Englebright founded HCA's industry-leading patient safety program in 2000. She has been a proponent of safety technology, leading several large-scale deployments across HCA. In 2014, Englebright chartered and implemented an AHRQ-listed patient safety organization to further accelerate HCA's patient safety programs. Englebright serves as the At-Large Nursing Representative to The Joint Commission's Board of Commissioners and chairs the Board of Advisors of the National Patient Safety Foundation. Englebright is vice-chair for the Expert Panel on Informatics and Technology for the American Academy of Nursing and is an adjunct faculty member at the Vanderbilt University School of Nursing.

GWENDOLYN CHERESE GODLOCK, MS-PSL, RN, CPHQ, CMSRN

Gwendolyn Cherese Godlock, MS-PSL, RN, CPHQ, CMSRN, began her military career as an enlisted soldier on December 1, 1987, and was promoted to the ranks of Sergeant First Class. On July 20, 2007, Captain (Retired) Godlock received her Commission as an Army Nurse Corps Officer. She retired from active duty Army as an Army Nurse Corps Officer on August 1, 2015, serving 27 years and 8 months and earning multiple awards and decorations. Her final position prior to military retirement was facility TeamSTEPPS master trainer project officer and department of nursing, patient safety officer, Brooke Army Medical Center, Ft. Sam Houston (San Antonio), Texas. She has a master of science degree in patient safety leadership from the University of Chicago at Illinois and a bachelor of science nursing degree from Hampton University. Godlock has earned the Certification Professional Healthcare Quality (CPHQ) and Certification Medical/Surgical Registered Nurse (CMSRN). Currently, she is a field representative–nurse surveyor for The Joint Commission (TJC), Oakbrook Terrace, Chicago, Illinois. She has two adult sons, Donte' and Dondre'.

DIANNA INGRAHAM, MS, RN, CNS

Dianna Ingraham, MS, RN, CNS, is currently employed as a clinical nurse specialist and chest pain coordinator for cardiovascular services at Centura Health, Littleton Adventist Hospital in Littleton, Colorado. She has 25 years of experience in nursing as a registered nurse with employment in a variety of clinical cardiovascular roles. Ingraham received her BSN from the University of Cincinnati and her MS from the University of California, San Francisco. Currently, her role as a cardiovascular clinical nurse specialist allows her to facilitate implementation of cardiovascular evidence-based practices in Littleton Adventist Hospital. Ingraham's additional role as a chest pain coordinator includes program management with process-improvement strategies related to care of the cardiovascular patient. She co-chairs the South Denver Evidence-Based Practice, Research and Innovation Council with Cynthia Oster and is a member of the American College of Cardiology Foundation as a Cardiovascular Team Section member.

ALMA JACKSON, PHD, RN, COHN-S

Alma Jackson, PhD, RN, COHN-S, is an associate professor of nursing at Loretto Heights School of Nursing, Regis University. Her primary teaching responsibilities include research and evidence-based practice courses in both master's and doctoral programs. In addition to working with nursing students to create change at the bedside, she also works with big data, serving on the board of the All Payers Claims Database. The APCD is governed by the Colorado Department of Health Care Policy and Finance and serves to increase transparency of medical costs and improve quality of care. Jackson is a certified occupational health nurse specialist and owner of Colorado Safety Works, Inc. She provides consulting services in and outside of the healthcare arena to promote workplace health and safety. Her clients range from 3M to Yellowstone. Through this work, she also developed a patent on a cushion that decreases shock and vibration to eliminate back injuries for drivers of heavy machinery. This won an award from the National Safety Council. Jackson is a well-known speaker at the American Association of Occupational Health Nurses, National Ergonomics Conference, and American Society of Safety Engineers.

FRANCES C. KELLY, MSN, RNC-OB, NEA-BC, CPHQ

Frances C. Kelly, MSN, RNC-OB, NEA-BC, CPHQ, is an obstetric nurse with 30 years of experience, having held numerous direct care, educational, and leadership positions in acute care hospitals. She has focused primarily on the care of low- and high-risk obstetric patients and their newborns, and has led moderate and large delivery volume women's and children's services. In her most recent role as director of quality and safety for a newly opened women's hospital that is part of a large, academic, free-standing children's hospital in the Texas Medical Center in Houston, Texas, Kelly has had the opportunity to partner with nursing, physician, and quality and safety experts to develop and implement a comprehensive obstetric/gynecologic quality and safety program. During the short 3 years this new women's hospital has been open, there has been a significant increase in both the volume of deliveries as well as the acuity of the patients, while there has been a statistically significant downward trend in the rate of obstetric adverse events. She also coaches and mentors advanced quality improvement teams, focusing on projects such as reducing the rate of surgical site infections among obstetric patients, increasing patient perception of readiness to participate in reducing risk of surgical site infection, and facilitating timely maternal discharges. Kelly is a member of the Association of Women's Health, Obstetric, and Neonatal Nurses (AWHONN) and certified as an inpatient obstetrics nurse (RNC-OB), an advanced nursing executive (NEA-BC), and a professional in healthcare quality (CPHQ). She has presented nationally on safety related topics and those relevant to the practice of obstetric nursing. Kelly is currently a doctoral student at the University of Texas Health Science Center at Houston's School of Nursing.

CYNTHIA R. LATNEY, MSN, RN, NE-BC

Cynthia R. Latney, MSN, RN, NE-BC, is the chief nursing officer (CNO) and vice president of patient care services for Penrose St. Francis Health Services (PSFHS), a 522-bed Magnet-recognized community health system. She also serves as the group CNO for Centura Health south state region organizations. Latney has 28 years of experience in many nursing leadership positions. She has previously held positions at the Hospital Corporation of America (CNO, VP, and director of critical care) and Methodist Hospital in Houston, Texas (director and manager). A strong transformational leader, she influences the hospital's strategic direction and ensures that nursing's goals and initiatives are aligned to advance patient care and organizational success. She is a member of the American Organization of Nurse Executives (AONE), Colorado Organization of Nurse Leaders (CONL), American Nurses Association (ANA), and American College of Healthcare Executives (ACHE), and a past president-elect of the American Association of Critical-Care Nurses–Dallas Chapter. In addition, she has been a board member of the Community College of Aurora Foundation and of the Community College of Aurora Council. Latney has a bachelor of science degree in nursing, a master's degree in healthcare administration, and is currently pursuing her PhD in healthcare administration. She is a board certified nurse executive.

APRYL SHENAE LEWIS, MSN, RN, CCTN

Apryl Shenae Lewis, MSN, RN, CCTN, has been practicing nursing since 1997 and worked in solid organ transplant for more than 16 years. She has most recently worked in hospital leadership for 9 years in the role of clinical nurse specialist and now nurse coordinator for patient safety and quality. Her work experience includes two major commercial insurance carriers as well as past work in home discharge planning for home infusion, parenteral nutrition, and home care services. She has twice served as president of the local chapter of the International Transplant Nurses Society.

MARY BETH FLYNN MAKIC, PHD, RN, CNS, CCNS, FAAN, FNAP

Mary Beth Flynn Makic, PhD, RN, CNS, CCNS, FAAN, FNAP, is a recognized critical care expert focusing on the translation of evidence-based practice to improve patient outcomes. She has focused her body of work on the reduction of hospital-acquired pressure ulcers, catheter-associated urinary tract infections, and improved bathing practices. She is recognized as an expert in critical care nursing practice, specifically in the fields of burn and trauma.

REBECCA S. MILTNER, PHD, RN, CNL, NEA-BC

Rebecca S. (Suzie) Miltner, PhD, RN, CNL, NEA-BC, is an assistant professor at the University of Alabama at Birmingham (UAB) School of Nursing and a nurse scientist at the Birmingham VA Medical Center. She completed a BSN from the Medical College of Georgia; an MS in nursing at the University of Wisconsin, Madison; and a PhD in nursing at the University of Maryland, Baltimore, Maryland. She completed a post-doctoral fellowship with the VA National Quality Scholars Program as well as an executive fellowship in patient safety at Virginia Commonwealth University. She has extensive clinical and leadership experience in military, private, and VA acute care settings, as well as experience in nursing education in both academic and organizational settings. Her research areas of interest are the quality of nursing care in acute care settings, practice variation in bedside nursing, and the science of quality measurement. She teaches in the nursing administration and doctor of nursing practice graduate programs at the UAB School of Nursing.

JULIANNE MORATH, MS, RN, CPPS

Julianne Morath, MS, RN, CPPS, is the inaugural recipient of the John Eisenberg Award for Individual Lifetime Achievement in Patient Safety and is president/CEO of the Hospital Quality Institute (HQI), a collaboration of the California Hospital Association and the regional associations. She is a founding and current member of the Lucian Leape Institute of the National Patient Safety Foundation and completed a term with the Board of Commissioners of The Joint Commission this year. Morath is a distinguished advisor to the National Patient Safety Foundation, past member of the National Quality Forum Best Practices Committee, and member of the Advisory Board to the Association for the Advancement of Medical Instrumentation (AAMI). She was appointed fellow to the Salzburg Seminar on Medical Errors. Morath serves on the Board of Directors of the Virginia Mason Medical Center and Health System. She was named by Becker Hospital Review as one of the top 50 experts leading patient safety this year. Morath has more than 3 decades of executive and academic experience in healthcare. Her work is distinguished through translating research into practice and building cultures of safety and excellence. Before joining the Hospital Quality Institute, Morath served as chief quality and patient safety officer for Vanderbilt University Medical Center. Her work as chief operating officer of Children's Hospitals and Clinics of Minnesota has been recognized in HBS case studies and featured in USNWR. She is an author of *Do No Harm* and *The Quality Advantage*. She is frequently published and is a recognized presenter in the field of safety and quality.

CARRIE NEYERS, BSN, RN, CCRN

Carrie Neyers, BSN, RN, CCRN, currently practices as an ICU nurse at Porter Adventist Hospital in Denver, Colorado. Carrie has a bachelor of arts degree in integrative physiology from the University of Colorado and graduated *cum laude* from Denver School of Nursing. She began her nursing career in a step-down unit. Three years ago, she wanted to expand her nursing skill set and made the transition to critical care. She has served as chair for the ICU/Step-Down Nurse Practice Council and has championed pressure ulcer and CAUTI prevention on her unit for the last 4 years.

MICHELLE NORRIS, BSN, RN, CCRN

Michelle Norris, BSN, RN, CCRN, has been practicing as a registered nurse for 15 years, with the last 8 years in the ICU at Porter Adventist Hospital in Denver, Colorado. She graduated *magna cum laude* from the University of Nebraska Medical Center, College of Nursing at its Lincoln campus and was accepted into Sigma Theta Tau International Honor Society of Nursing, Gamma Pi-at-Large chapter. During the last 5 years at Porter Adventist Hospital, she has been honored to hold the titles of pressure ulcer prevention (PUP) champion and catheter-associated urinary tract infection (CAUTI) prevention champion, and she is proud to be a part of a team that strives to keep patients safe. She looks forward to finding new ways to reduce harm in the ICU patient population.

KRISTEN A. OSTER, MS, APRN, ACNS-BC, CNOR, CNS-CP

Kristen A. Oster, MS, APRN, ACNS-BC, CNOR, CNS-CP, is an assistant nurse manager for the ENT, skull base, head/neck, and neuro surgery service line in perioperative services at Porter Adventist Hospital, Denver, Colorado. She received a bachelor of science degree in biology and education from Dennison University in Granville, Ohio. Hearing the call to nursing, Kristen earned a Bachelor of Science degree in nursing in the accelerated program at Regis University, Denver, Colorado. She holds a master of science in nursing degree—clinical nurse specialist focus in adult and geriatric acute care—from the University of Colorado, Denver. Kristen is a member of the Association of periOperative Registered Nurses.

PATRICIA A. PATRICIAN, PHD, RN, FAAN

Patricia A. Patrician, PhD, RN, FAAN, joined the University of Alabama at Birmingham faculty in August 2008, after a 26-year career in the U.S. Army Nurse Corps, where she held clinical, administrative, educational, and research positions. Her final position prior to military retirement was chief, department of nursing science, Academy of Health Sciences, Ft. Sam Houston (San Antonio), Texas. At UAB, she teaches in the PhD program and supervises PhD students. She conducts research on nurse staffing, the nursing practice environment, and patient and nurse quality and safety outcomes. In addition, she is a senior nurse scholar/faculty in the VA Quality Scholars (VAQS) fellowship program, an interprofessional pre- and post-doctoral program that focuses on the science of quality improvement. She is a scientist at the Center for Outcomes and Effectiveness Research and Education and a scholar at the Lister Hill Center for Health Policy at UAB.

JOANNE PHILLIPS, DNP, RN, CPPS

JoAnne Phillips, DNP, RN, CPPS, has a broad background in nursing. Her clinical background is in surgical critical care and trauma, where she has worked as a clinical nurse and clinical nurse specialist. In 2003, JoAnne began her career in patient safety as the clinical nurse specialist for patient safety. JoAnne is a 2008 fellow of the National Patient Safety Foundation and is a Certified Professional in Patient Safety from the National Patient Safety Foundation. JoAnne recently completed her doctorate in nursing practice degree at Vanderbilt University. In her current role, she is the manager of quality and patient safety for Penn Homecare and Hospice, part of the University of Pennsylvania Health System.

SHARON SABLES-BAUS, PHD, MPA, RN, PCNS-BC, CPPS

Sharon Sables-Baus, PhD, MPA, RN, PCNS-BC, CPPS, teaches both undergraduate- and graduate-level classes, including classes in the DNP program. Her work aims to promote the best research evidence and integrate or transform it into practice, targeting in particular neurodevelopmental health outcomes of hospitalized neonates and infants. Sables-Baus' research has explored ways to decrease neurodevelopmental morbidity and to optimize evidence-based caregiving practices that affect neurodevelopmental outcomes. Emblematic of this program of research, Sables-Baus was a part of team that conducted a longitudinal study of neonates born with congenital heart defects requiring 3-stage surgical. Furthermore, Sables-Baus chaired a national committee tasked with developing evidence-based, infant-driven, oral-feeding guidelines for hospitalized neonates. This work was presented at a national conference in October 2015. In her role as a scientist at Children's Hospital Colorado, Sables-Baus' focus is on safety science, including work on high reliability organizations. She was recently awarded a $25,000 grant from Clinical and Operational Effectiveness and Patient Safety (COEPS) Small Grants Program at Children's Hospital Colorado for a study entitled "Improving Effectiveness of the Target Zero (TZ) Safety Coach Program."

KERRY A. SEMBERA, MSN, RN, CCRN

Kerry A. Sembera, MSN, RN, CCRN, started her nursing career with Texas Children's Hospital in 2001. The first 6 years she spent in the PICU as a preceptor, charge nurse, and transport nurse; after that, Sembera joined the heart center to work in the CVICU. After graduating with her MSN in 2008, she started as a clinical specialist of the heart center. Her formal job title at Texas Children's Hospital is heart center clinical liaison. In the role of clinical specialist, Kerry serves as an educational resource for the patient, family, and healthcare professionals. She facilitates the acquisition of knowledge through formal and informal teaching and coordinates learning activities as needed. She is passionate about simulation and encourages the participation of simulation exercises almost daily in her current role.

BELINDA SHAW, DNP, RN, NE-BC, CEN

Belinda Shaw, DNP, RN, NE-BC, CEN, earned her BSN at Creighton University College of Nursing in Omaha, Nebraska. She completed her MSN and DNP through the Rueckert-Hartman College for Health Professions at Regis University in Denver, Colorado. Her expertise and clinical certification is in emergency department nursing and nursing leadership. In her current role as an associate chief nursing officer at Porter Adventist Hospital, her responsibilities include the emergency department, critical care, oncology, Heart Institute, palliative care, dialysis, and clinical informatics. Shaw incorporated her interest in resilience into her DNP research that explored the relationship between teamwork training with the Agency for Healthcare Research and Quality (AHRQ) TeamSTEPPS curriculum and resilience.

GWEN SHERWOOD, PHD, RN, FAAN, ANEF

Gwen Sherwood, PhD, RN, FAAN, ANEF, has a distinguished record in advancing nursing education locally and globally. Professor and Associate Dean for Strategic and Global Initiatives at the University of North Carolina at Chapel Hill School of Nursing, her work focuses on transforming healthcare environments by improving quality and safety through expanding relational capacity of healthcare providers and developing reflective practice. Her studies have examined patient satisfaction with pain management outcomes, teamwork as a variable in patient safety, and pedagogical approaches for integrating quality and safety. She was co-investigator for the award-winning Robert Wood Johnson–funded Quality and Safety

Education for Nurses (QSEN) project to transform curricula to prepare nurses for working in and leading quality and safety in redesigned healthcare. Widely published, she is co-editor of an AJN book of the year, *Quality and Safety Education: A Competency Approach for Nurses*, and three books related to reflective practice. She served as vice president of Sigma Theta Tau International Honor Society of Nursing and is past president of the International Association for Human Caring.

CONNIE VALDEZ, PHARMD, MSED, BCPS

Connie Valdez, PharmD, MSEd, BCPS, is an associate professor at the University of Colorado Skaggs School of Pharmacy and Pharmaceutical Sciences. She received her bachelor of science (pharmacy) degree and her doctorate of pharmacy degree from the University of Colorado and her master of science in education from the University of Southern California. She completed an ambulatory care/managed care residency with Centura Health. She completed a fellowship in teaching and learning and a fellowship in educational leadership from the Keck School of Medicine. Before joining the faculty at the University of Colorado, she practiced as an ambulatory care clinical specialist at Gates Exempla Community Health Center and University of Colorado Hospital. She joined the University of Colorado in November 2002 and currently has a clinical practice at the Denver Indian Health and Family Medicine clinic and the Sheridan Health Services clinic.

KELLY D. WALLIN, MS, RN, CHSE

Kelly D. Wallin, MS, RN, CHSE, is a pediatric nurse with more than 30 years of experience in a variety of clinical, educational, and leadership positions in pediatric healthcare. Her clinical background is in pediatric critical care with an emphasis on cardiac care and congenital heart surgery. In addition to patient-care roles, she has also served in a number of leadership, educator, and clinical specialist roles for these areas. Her quality/patient safety experience has included participation as a member as well as leader for a number of patient-safety and quality-improvement project teams, and she is a graduate of the Intermountain Healthcare Advanced Training Program in Healthcare Delivery Improvement. She is a Certified Healthcare Simulation Educator (CHSE) and currently serves as the operational director for the healthcare simulation center at Texas Children's Hospital. Wallin is dedicated to supporting the use of healthcare simulation in innovative ways to meet educational, quality/patient safety, and research goals.

TABLE OF CONTENTS

PART 1 THE NEED FOR A NEW MODEL OF PATIENT SAFETY AND QUALITY 1

1 THE NEED FOR A PARADIGM SHIFT IN HEALTHCARE CULTURE: OLD VERSUS NEW 3

Cynthia R. Latney, MSN, RN, NE-BC

2 CURRENT PATIENT SAFETY DRIVERS 25

Gwen Sherwood, PhD, RN, FAAN, ANEF and Gail E. Armstrong, DNP, ACNS-BC, CNE

PART 3 HRO CONCEPTS AND APPLICATION TO PRACTICE: RELUCTANCE TO SIMPLIFY 111

7 ROOT CAUSE ANALYSIS: A TOOL FOR HIGH RELIABILITY IN A COMPLEX ENVIRONMENT 113

Jane S. Braaten, PhD, APRN, CNS, ANP, CPPS

8 JUST CULTURE AND THE IMPACT ON HIGH RELIABILITY 139

Patricia A. Patrician, PhD, RN, FAAN, Gwendolyn Cherese Godlock, MS-PSL, RN, CPHQ, CMSRN, Apryl Shenae Lewis, MSN, RN, CCTN, Rebecca S. Miltner, PhD, RN, CNL, NEA-BC

PART 4 HRO CONCEPTS AND APPLICATION TO PRACTICE: SENSITIVITY TO OPERATIONS........................ 157

9 ALARM SAFETY: WORKING SOLUTIONS.................................159

JoAnne Phillips, DNP, RN, CPPS

APPENDIXES

FOREWORD

Estimates now suggest that 400,000 people die needlessly each year as a result of healthcare error (James, 2014). While the Agency for Healthcare Research and Quality (AHRQ, 2013) has reported some progress, with fewer deaths from hospital-acquired infections and falls, much work remains to be done to reach zero harm. One approach to reducing harm has been to institute high reliability into healthcare. Reliability is consistent performance according to a set of specifications or standards. In the case of healthcare, reliability is consistently high performance over a long period of time. Becoming a high reliability organization (HRO) is now a top leadership mandate, and while support must emanate from the board and top leadership, HRO development must permeate an entire organization. Generally, three elements are necessary: leadership commitment, a culture of safety, and continuous quality improvement processes. Much of the literature on HROs stresses the importance of top leadership. However, when all three elements are considered, it is obvious that HRO development must be threaded throughout the warp and weft of the organization—up and down and all across.

Leadership incorporates the governing body, medical staff, management, and nursing leaders. Each and every person in these groups must be knowledgeable about what constitutes high-quality, safe, and efficient care for people and their families—and needs to practice this commitment on a daily basis. In an HRO, each of these people knows the organization's progress on the path to zero harm and promotes an open, questioning, and participative practice with all who work in the organization. A safety culture is one that has a relentless focus on delivering safe care, where front-line nurses and others feel comfortable reporting near-misses and actual errors. Furthermore, where a Just Culture is in place, people do not fear retribution for reporting vulnerabilities in the system. A continuous focus on quality improvement means all people in an organization are knowledgeable about quality indicators in their particular areas and their progress in meeting target outcomes.

What has been missing from most of the literature has been a clear direction of how to spread HRO components across a healthcare organization (HCO). The focus of nurses and other healthcare providers has often been on the delivery of care, i.e., "how" to provide optimal care to people and their families. That is important. But what is also needed is equal attention to our *systems* of care delivery and safe working environments for people who are working in these highly complex systems. What has been needed is a book that explains the concepts of high reliability and HROs, provides examples of what the concepts would look like in everyday practice, and describes the information and tools nurses and other healthcare providers need for the organization to become an HRO. This text delivers on all three components.

High Reliability Organizations: A Healthcare Handbook for Patient Safety & Quality comprehensively describes how to infuse the knowledge, skills, and attitudes (KSAs) of an HRO into the fabric of an organization from the boardroom to the front lines of care, including patients and their families. The book is based on the premise that while a quest for high reliability must start in the boardroom, it must also be part of every person's focus. This takes more than a class or a checklist. The text challenges the nurse to move away from scripted protocols and practices and rituals to a focus on questioning: "Is this the most current practice?" "Is this the safest way to do this?" "What are possible 'errors waiting to happen' that we can prevent?"

The various chapters tease apart the multiple facets of HROs and apply the standards to every-day components of care. Chapter content blends leadership approaches with front-line clinician application. Multiple contemporary practice applications exist, such as Chapter 17 on use of HRO principles to improve pain management and Chapter 18 on pediatric patient safety.

Editors Cynthia Oster and Jane Braaten provide clear information on how to develop HROs so they facilitate safe passage for patients and families and guidance in moving toward zero harm. They make the business and quality case for active nursing engagement in reorienting an HCO to be as focused on safety and quality as it is on finances. Most importantly, the authors make a case for expanding the nursing focus from delivering quality care to also being accountable for helping build safe systems of care. Thus, they powerfully redefine and expand the role and responsibility of the professional nurse. This is critically important—not just for nurses, but also for our patients and their families.

–Jane Barnsteiner, PhD, RN, FAAN

REFERENCES

AHRQ. (2013). 2013 annual hospital-acquired condition rate and estimates. Retrieved from http://www.ahrq.gov/professionals/quality-patient-safety/pfp/hacrate2013.html

James, J. T. (2014). A new, evidence-based estimate of patient harms associated with hospital care. *Journal of Patient Safety*, *9*(3)122-128.

INTRODUCTION

There is a severe danger that blindness from tradition and practice will prevent proper exploitation of the potential of improvement actually present.

—Rasmussen, Pejtersen, and Schmidt, 1990

Patient safety and quality are of increasing importance to consumers, payers, providers, and organizations. As a large majority of the workforce, nurses are on the front line of the delivery and provision of safe and effective care. Although there is an abundance of new theory and research on the topics, the practical application of these concepts is challenging for the clinical nurse in practice. Furthermore, the current hospital environment of complexity, interdependent processes, and unpredictable conditions demands that new models and theories be applied to achieve outcomes. There is a need to bridge the gap between theory and practice to improve quality outcomes and patient safety in our current healthcare climate.

High reliability is not a new concept. These days, the term is used contagiously in healthcare organizations. Although high reliability is often discussed, and excitement and support grows, high reliability methods and science have still not been totally implemented into our healthcare culture. For example, although numerous efforts are undertaken to improve safety, we still have adverse events in hospitals and are not as reliable and safe as we desire to be (James, 2013). It seems that as soon as we begin to see an improvement, another issues arises. Emergent issues and unintended consequences of well-intentioned improvements seem to characterize healthcare today. It has been said that complexity leads to error, and that the best way to prevent error is to acknowledge complexity and to adapt or cope with it (Woods, Dekker, Cook, Johannesen, and Sarter, 2012). Acknowledgment of complexity entails accepting that perhaps we cannot control all factors and emergent situations that lead to outcomes. This is difficult for those in healthcare delivery systems to accept.

A gap is evident in the advancement of healthcare high reliability and might be explained by Thomas Kuhn's view of normal science and revolutionary paradigm shifts (1962). Kuhn argued that large shifts in thinking occur when current thinking and approaches become unacceptable because they do not solve current problems. Within hospitals, traditional thinking focusing on prediction, production, and control is common practice, although there is evidence that patient safety exists in a complex system that is dynamic, unpredictable, and emergent (Dekker, Cilliers, and Hofmyer, 2011; Effken, 2002). The thinking, however, is beginning to change. Many are realizing that solving patient-safety and quality problems requires a new approach. High reliability concepts provide the antidote to the traditional method, which is not effective in a highly complex environment.

So what is a highly reliable organization? High reliability organizations (HROs) are those organizations that are high-risk, dynamic, turbulent, and potentially hazardous, yet operate nearly error-free (Weick and Sutcliffe, 2007). Examples include aviation, nuclear engineering, defense operations, and acute care hospitals. HROs stay error-free by doing the following:

- Recognizing that small things that go wrong are often early warning signs of trouble
- Recognizing that these warning signs are red flags that provide insight into the health of the whole system
- Valuing near misses as indicators of early trouble and acting on them to prevent future failure
- Being innovative and creative and valuing input from all corners of the organization
- Recognizing the value of preparing for the unexpected and the unknown, as failures rarely occur if they are expected

This book elaborates on and gives practical examples of the following principles of HROs, as described by Weick and Sutcliffe (2007):

- **Preoccupation with failure:** HROs are preoccupied with all failures, especially small ones. Small things that go wrong are often early warning signals of deepening trouble and give insight into the health of the whole system. However, we have a tendency to ignore or overlook our failures (which suggests we are not competent) and focus on our successes (which suggests we are competent).

- **Reluctance to simplify:** HROs restrain their temptation to simplify through diverse checks and balances, adversarial reviews, and the cultivation of multiple perspectives.

- **Sensitivity to operations:** HROs make strong responses to weak signals (indications that something might be amiss). Everyone values organizing to maintain situational awareness.

- **Deference to expertise:** HROs shift decisions away from formal authority toward expertise and experience. Decision-making migrates to experts at all levels of the hierarchy during high-tempo times.

- **Commitment to resilience:** HROs pay close attention to their capability to improvise and act—without knowing in advance what will happen.

The current message in patient safety and quality literature is that we, in healthcare, need to strive to be highly reliable, meaning that we should be a system that detects and prevents errors from happening even though we operate in high-risk, emergent conditions. Most often, the conversation goes in the direction that healthcare should be similar to aviation. This message is not helpful to healthcare providers as they strive to understand what high reliability is and looks like in the healthcare field. This book addresses that gap by providing an understanding of HRO and the application of its concepts to clinical practice. Practical examples are provided that support each of the five concepts of HRO along with useful tools, measurements, and design strategies.

This book is meant to change current thinking by first highlighting challenges in our current healthcare system and our current process of addressing safety and quality and then suggesting HRO principles as an overarching framework for promoting a better model. This organizing framework expands reader knowledge and understanding by providing concrete examples that exemplify principles of HRO. The specific goals for writing this book are to do the following:

- Provide an overview of HRO science as an organizing framework for quality and patient safety

- Inform readers of the practical applications of HRO science, focusing on quality and patient safety

- Provide readers with knowledge and tools that can be applied to current quality and safety practice

We expect the primary audience of this text to be front-line nursing staff, nurses in adminis-tration, quality and patient safety professionals, advanced practice nurses, and nurse educators. The healthcare professional who purchases this book will do so with the desire to learn more about the application of HRO principles to patient safety and quality problems. This book is unique in that it uses HRO principles as an organizing framework for practical application. The intent of the editors is to provide a quality and patient safety book that is useful to professionals doing the work of healthcare. Although we do not intend this as a textbook, it could be used in graduate courses focused on patient safety or quality management in nursing, health services administration, or clinical programs.

The book is divided into seven parts with four appendixes:

- **Part 1, "The Need for a New Model of Patient Safety and Quality":** This part pro-vides the background of the current safety and quality climate. Chapter 1, "The Need for a Paradigm Shift in Healthcare Culture: Old Versus New," provides the rationale for a paradigm shift to a new model. Chapter 2, "Current Patient Safety Drivers," and Chapter 3, "Current Quality Drivers," review the current patient safety and quality drivers within our healthcare environment. Chapter 4, "Organizational Culture and the Journey to HRO," describes how the journey to high reliability is connected to organizational culture.

- **Parts 2–6, "HRO Concepts and Application to Practice":** These parts offer HRO con-cepts as a framework for the new model with examples. The first of these HRO concepts is that HROs have a preoccupation with failure. Chapter 5, "Using Failure Mode and Effects Analysis to Predict Failure," discusses how to use failure mode and effects analysis to predict failures. Chapter 6, "Close Calls and Near Misses: What's the Big Deal?" provides the reader with a review of close calls and near misses along with associated myths. The second of these HRO concepts is that HROs restrain the impulse to view events through a single lens and are reluctant to simplify. Chapter 7, "Root Cause Analysis: A Tool for High Reliability in a Complex Environment," presents how to use root cause analysis as a high reliability tool in a complex environment. Chapter 8, "Just Culture and the Impact on High Reliability," offers a discussion of how Just Culture affects high reliability. The third HRO concept is that HROs demonstrate sensitivity to operations by making strong responses to weak signs. Chapter 9, "Alarm Safety: Working Solutions," provides a discussion of working solutions for alarm safety. Chapter 10, "Innovative Technology, Standardization, and the Impact on High Reliability," explains how innovative technology and standardization affect high reliability. The fourth HRO concept is that HROs shift decision-making away from formal authority and apply deference to expertise. Chapter 11, "Interprofessional Collaboration," provides a discussion for interprofessional collaborative care and teamwork. Chapter 12, "Nurses Create Reliable Care by Advancing Patient Engagement," presents a discussion of nurses creating highly reliable care through patient engagement. The final HRO concept is that HROs have a commitment to resilience. Chapter 13, "Resilience: A Path to HRO," presents resilience as the path to high reliability. Chapter 14, "Building High Reliability Through Simulation," describes building high reliability through simulation. Chapter 15, "High Reliability Is Built with Resilience," expands on resilience and teamwork through the lens of emergency response teams. Chapter 16, "Sustaining a Culture of Safety: Strategies to Maintain the Gains," communicates strategies to sustain and maintain the gains in a resilient organization.

■ **Part 7, "Assimilation Into Practice Across the Continuum":** This part puts it all together and provides the reader with examples of how HRO concepts are assimilated into practice across the care continuum. Chapter 17, "The Use of HRO Concepts to Improve Pain Management and Safety," describes how a clinical nurse specialist uses HRO concepts to improve pain management effectiveness and patient safety. Chapter 18, "Pediatric Patient Safety: Utilizing Safety Coaching as a Strategy Toward Zero Harm," describes how high reliability can be achieved in pediatric care through safety coaching. Chapter 19, "Applying High Reliability Principles Across a Large Healthcare System to Reduce Patient Falls," explains how a leader working with staff nurses applied HRO principles to reduce patient falls across a large healthcare system. Chapter 20, "Magnet Recognition Program® Model Component Synthesis with HRO," describes the synergy between high reliability and the Magnet Recognition Program®. Chapter 21, "Achieving HRO: The Role of the Bedside Scientist in Research," illustrates the role of the bedside scientist in achieving high reliability.

■ **Appendixes:** The appendixes provide real-world examples of HRO principles employed in a variety of patient care areas, including operating room, intensive care unit, emergency department, and home care settings.

Healthcare professionals are constantly seeking practical tools and descriptions of practices that will improve and enhance patient safety and quality outcomes. High reliability is a current goal for hospitals, and the principles are sound. However, there is little in the literature that discusses how to apply the principles at the front line of care to improve outcomes. This text hopefully addresses this gap by placing the need for high reliability concepts into our current climate in healthcare through illustrative discussion (theory and research) of each of the five concepts of HRO, along with a description of a current best practice and/or tool that applies to the model. The goal of this book is to stimulate organizations to embrace high reliability concepts while striving to improve the quality and safety of care delivered to patients and families. We all benefit from a safer healthcare environment.

REFERENCES

Dekker, S., Cilliers, P., and Hofmyer, J. (2011). The complexity of failure: Implications of complexity theory for safety investigations. *Safety Science, 49*(6), pp. 939–945.

Effken, J. A. (2002). Different lenses, improved outcomes: A new approach to the analysis and design of healthcare information systems. *International Journal of Medical Informatics, 65*(1), pp. 59–74.

James, J. T. (2013). A new, evidence-based estimate of patient harms associated with hospital care. *Journal of Patient Safety, 9*(3), pp. 122–128. doi: 10.1097/PTS.0b013e3182948a69

Kuhn, T. S. (1962). *The structure of scientific revolutions*. Chicago, IL: University of Chicago Press.

Rasmussen, J., Pejtersen, A. M., and Schmidt, K. (1990). *Taxonomy for cognitive work analysis*. Roskilde, Denmark: Riso National Laboratory.

Weick, K. and Sutcliffe, K. (2007). *Managing the unexpected: Resilient performance in an age of uncertainty*. San Francisco, CA: Jossey Bass.

Woods, D. D., Dekker, S., Cook, R., Johannesen, L., and Sarter, N. (2012). *Behind human error* (2nd ed.). Burlington, VT: Ashgate.

PART 1

THE NEED FOR A NEW MODEL OF PATIENT SAFETY AND QUALITY

THE NEED FOR A PARADIGM SHIFT IN HEALTHCARE CULTURE: OLD VERSUS NEW

Cynthia R. Latney, MSN, RN, NE-BC

In the United States, the healthcare industry has shifted from a mostly provider-controlled culture to a consumer-driven model. This has revealed the need to raise the bar on both quality and patient safety—in other words, on reliability. In healthcare, reliability means delivering failure-free health-related processes, procedures, or services in the required time. In this context, failure can result from not applying the appropriate evidence-based practice, failing to respond in a timely manner, or failing to practice patient-centeredness by including patient preference (Nolan, Resar, Haraden, and Griffin, 2004).

Because of the complex, fragmented, and imbalanced healthcare system in the United States, the nation's healthcare industry is struggling with how to respond to the growing demands of the government, private payers, and consumers. Each of these parties needs to see the value of each dollar that is spent.

> "The biggest challenge we have in healthcare is not just to find the few holes that are really still there after years and decades of work, but it is to deal with layers of deficiencies that are more like sieves than they are shields."
>
> —Dr. Mark R. Chassin

In addition, under the Affordable Care Act (ACA) (U.S. Department of Health and Human Services, 2014), health insurance exchanges now give patients the option to shop for and compare health plans. This has made patients more conscious and aware of the service and quality of care they receive. As a result of these shifts, demands on the healthcare system to improve value, accessibility, efficiency, cost, service, and quality are growing. These issues are causing tremendous strain, stress, and safety risks among healthcare organizations and systems. There is pressure on all fronts for organizations to identify sustainable strategies to meet the needs of consumers and create a more reliable healthcare system. Clearly, a paradigm shift in healthcare is in order.

The purpose of this chapter is to discuss the current drivers of healthcare and the current healthcare culture. In addition, this chapter discusses why the high reliability organization (HRO) framework is a viable solution to addressing the complexity of the healthcare system.

CURRENT DRIVERS: COST, COST, AND COST

The U.S. healthcare system is in a state of flux. Many forces play a role in how the healthcare system is viewed as a whole. In addition, there is growing pressure to approach the delivery of healthcare differently. There is no doubt that the gap between the actual cost of care and reimbursement is increasing. The cost of healthcare is growing at an alarming rate, and access to care continues to be a challenge for many.

The U.S. is viewed by many countries as a leading nation in the world—except in its fundamental approach to providing healthcare to its citizens. In the U.S., healthcare is one of many goods in a free-market economy that citizens are expected to provide for themselves (with the exception of emergency services and Medicare benefits for inpatient, hospice, and home health services) (Barton, 2009). Many barriers affect citizens' access to health services and have a direct impact on healthcare expenditures and health outcomes.

The U.S. consumes a higher percentage of its gross domestic product (GDP) for healthcare—17%, which is more than any other developed country (Rice et al., 2014). According to the World Health Organization (WHO, 2015), the per-capita total expenditure for healthcare by U.S. citizens in 2012 was $8,895. In comparison, in Canada, which is similar in size to the U.S. (though with a smaller population) and on the same continent, citizens spend $4,676 per capita (World Health Organization, 2015).

The cost of healthcare in the U.S. has not only strained the federal government, it has also affected state governments and the private sector as well. New quarterly health spending estimates from the U.S. Census Bureau (2015) showed that first-quarter 2015 spending was 7.3% higher than the first quarter of 2014. The increased coverage of the Affordable Care Act may be the cause of the increased usage of physicians and outpatient services and higher spending in hospitals. Along with the overutilization of diagnostic tests and procedures, healthcare providers experience challenges in encouraging consumers to become active participants in their health.

Other factors affect healthcare spending, too. The growth of the elderly population, prescription drug charges, and the rising cost of caring for a segment of the population suffering from chronic diseases make up a large portion of healthcare spending. Prescription drugs represent approximately 11% of the overall U.S. healthcare expenditure—a number that is expected to climb due to the expansion of healthcare coverage (Schumock et al., 2014). Lastly, the failure to manage chronic diseases has become a crisis in the U.S. and is draining the healthcare system. The most common and costly, yet preventable, health problems are heart disease, stroke, cancer, diabetes, and obesity. These conditions cost close to $800 billion (Centers for Disease Control and Prevention, 2015). According to the CDC (2015), approximately half of Americans have one or more chronic health conditions. All these key areas can take a toll on the government's and on private insurers' bottom lines.

A highly reliable healthcare industry can aid in bending the cost curve. A highly reliable healthcare environment is unique in that it embraces the use of standardized processes and procedures to provide efficient and effective care.

A PUSH FOR PERFORMANCE

Because of the enormous dollars spent on healthcare, and because quality outcomes are below the standards expected in a developed country, health insurance payers have begun to question the value their beneficiaries are receiving. Healthcare organizations are experiencing a shift away from fee-for-service to value-based payment models. Payment models such as pay-for-performance and at-risk models have become more common. An example of a pay-for-performance program is the Centers for Medicare and Medicaid Services (CMS) Value-Based Purchasing program (CMS, 2015a). This approach moves away from incentivizing solely for quantity and moves toward accountability for quality, efficiency, and cost management. Pay-for-performance models have defined measures and require data collection and public reporting. In an at-risk model, base payment is predicated on the estimated expected cost of care to treat a condition or patient population. Success is based on the ability to manage cost control and expenditures.

These new payment models are a step toward improving quality and services, but doing so does not come without challenges. One challenge is agreeing on how to define and measure quality in healthcare. How value is defined by CMS and other regulatory agencies does not always align with the definition used by physicians, healthcare organizations, and consumers. CMS and commercial payers view value-based payment as a solution to growing healthcare costs. However, there are conflicting views on what quality measures to use to achieve value and lower cost. Some private insurers follow the CMS lead, whereas others have developed their own measures (Birk, 2015). This misalignment has contributed to uncertainty and unpredictability in the healthcare delivery system, where the overwhelming cry from providers, payers, and consumers is for standardization, transparency, and consistency.

Another key driver that is shifting the culture of healthcare is consumers' growing demand that the healthcare delivery system demonstrate value. More and more, consumers are evaluating the healthcare services they receive. They're accessing public reporting quality measures to choose their health plans and healthcare facilities. In 2012, Keckly and Coughlin published their longitudinal study of consumers' perceptions of the healthcare delivery system between 2008 and 2012. The study revealed that the healthcare system's overall performance has increased. However, the system was seen as confusing, complex, costly, and wasteful. There was little confidence that the healthcare industry was prepared to deal with future care expenses. Consumers did have confidence in their primary care physicians, but not in hospitals or their health plans. The current state of healthcare has made little progress since 2012. Healthcare spending remains out of control, and the industry has made only small incremental gains on the quality front.

To summarize, one driver that is shifting the healthcare culture paradigm is the focus on healthcare quality. More and more, quality performance and expectations have moved to center stage. Public reporting of healthcare systems' and hospitals' quality performance is used by insurance payers, financial institutions, and consumers to make decisions about their healthcare and investment. Unfortunately, the added spotlight on quality performance has not reduced incidences of patient harm or deaths due to preventable harm events in healthcare systems and hospitals.

Many years have passed since the Institute of Medicine's (IOM's) report "To Err Is Human" (1999), which sparked the nation to reflect on the state of the healthcare delivery system. It called for action to change how healthcare was being delivered. Although many healthcare systems and hospitals have made tremendous changes that have resulted in improved quality of care and patient safety, as a whole, the healthcare system and hospitals continue to experience unstirring results in preventable harm adverse events (IOM, 2011). In the category of operations being performed on the wrong side of the patient's body or at the wrong site altogether, there are 50 incidents per week. Fires continue to break out in operating rooms. Thousands of patients experience hospital-acquired conditions, and harmful errors occur every year. Deaths even occur as a result of safety alarms—which go off several hundred times per day—being silenced or turned off (The Joint Commission, 2015a). Undoubtedly, more work is needed to raise patient safety to the top of the list of concerns for healthcare systems and hospitals.

The foundation of a high reliability organization (HRO) is to improve patient safety and quality performance through preventative strategies, robust process improvement programs, and the engagement of staff to speak up on safety concerns and participate in developing strategies to mitigate risks (Chassin, 2012).

HEALTHCARE REFORM

The history of healthcare reform in the U.S. dates back to 1965, when President Lyndon Johnson introduced legislation that enacted Medicare (LBJ Presidential Library, 2012). In the last decade, progress has been made in both affordability and accessibility to healthcare. On March 23, 2010, President Barack Obama signed the Patient Protection and Affordable Care Act (PPACA), colloquially known as Obamacare or the Affordable Care Act (ACA). On March 30, 2010, PPACA became law after it was amended by the Healthcare and Reconciliation Act of 2010 (U.S. Department of Health and Human Services, 2014). On June 28, 2012, 2 years after PPACA became law, the United States Supreme Court upheld the ACA. A key part of the ACA was an individual mandate to obtain health insurance or to pay a penalty (U.S. Department of Health and Human Services, 2014). Since the passage of PPACA, there has been an increase of 11 million U.S. citizens with healthcare coverage (Congressional Budget Office, 2015).

In addition to expanding healthcare insurance coverage, healthcare reform shifted the landscape and paradigm of healthcare from volume to value. This shift has placed pressure on providers—healthcare systems, hospitals, and leaders—to demonstrate quality and service (Wagner, 2014). For healthcare systems and hospitals to be successful in this new environment, they must take a different approach to quality and service.

VALUE-BASED PURCHASING

The financial structure of the U.S. healthcare system is far from universal. The government funds significant areas in healthcare to support the public health programs known as Medicare and Medicaid. The remainder of insurance purchasers are employers and private payers (CMS, 2011). Given the rising cost of care, the government and private purchasers of healthcare have become more involved in the process of paying for healthcare. These purchasing groups have begun to monitor and measure how their dollars are spent. They also have come to expect improved quality and better clinical outcomes and service. This is collectively known as *value-based purchasing* (VBP), which is a purchasing practice that aims to increase the value of a dollar spent on improving quality and managing expenditures (CMS, 2011).

In 2010, the VBP program was established as part of the ACA. The VBP is a way for CMS to hold healthcare systems and hospitals accountable and to incentivize the use of evidence-based practices. It aims to enhance the quality of care and health outcomes and to improve the experience of care and value to its Medicare beneficiaries across various care settings (CMS, 2011). Participating hospitals are paid not only for quantity of service, but inpatient service is paid based on quality of service. The VBP program is "funded by a 1.75% reduction from participating hospitals' base operating diagnosis-related groups (DRG) payments" (CMS, 2015a). Distribution of funds is based on a Total Performance Score (TPS), which is made up of quality performance measures. The approved set of measures are grouped in specific quality domains

(CMS, 2011). Over the past 3 years, the CMS has raised the bar in quality expectations (see Table 1.1). In fiscal year (FY) 2016, outcome measure will hold 40% of the weight of the total measures (CMS, 2015b).

TABLE 1.1   CLINICAL PROCESS OF CARE DOMAINS AND PERFORMANCE MEASURES

Fiscal Year	Domains	Sample Performance Measure
2013	Clinical Process of Care Domain	HF1–discharge instructions
	Patient Experience of Care Domain	Overall rating
2014	Clinical Process of Care Domain	SCIP-inf-2 prophylactic antibiotic selection for surgical patients
	Patient Experience of Care Domain	Nurse communication
	Outcome Domain	Central line bloodstream infection rate
2015	Clinical Process of Care Domain	AMI8–primary PCI received within 90 minutes of hospital arrival
	Patient Experience of Care Domain	Pain management
	Outcome Domain	

Adapted from CMS (2011 and 2015)

HROs view the measurement of performance as one of the key ingredients in evaluating the organization's efficiency and effectiveness (Sutcliffe, 2011). The measurement of CMS VBP clinical and process metrics demonstrates measuring compliance with evidence-based practices and supports the essence of the HRO. Many of the CMS measures possess complex process steps and potential failure points, which cause patient safety issues and affect the organization financially.

Improving the quality of care in a healthcare organization requires focus on processes and outcomes. To achieve the expected measures, an organizational process must be reliable, providing the right care to the right patient at the right time. HRO principles encompass effective quality improvement tools that assist teams in eliminating waste and defects in a process. They also encompass robust analytics. Research demonstrates that healthcare organizations that use comprehensive process-improvement tools improve quality of care (DuPree et al., 2009; Chassin, 2015).

HEALTHCARE REGULATION

Healthcare systems and hospitals are regulated by a broad range of regulatory bodies and programs from local, state, federal, and private organizations. All these agencies and programs set their own standards and measures. This can pose problems and sow confusion for those who provide care. Moreover, in some cases, the level of authority is not clearly defined. In addition to the federal regulatory bodies that provide oversight for healthcare systems and hospitals, physicians, and insurance companies are the coordinating bodies for the local and state agencies. On the private-sector side are organizations such as the American Medical Association and the Board of Nursing, which provide oversight of medical and nursing professionals, respectively. Supplemental government standards also exist, where the hospital industry can choose to supplement the state license through The Joint Commission (Field, 2008).

Despite these oversight challenges, the healthcare community, the private sector, and consumers would agree that regulatory agencies are essential to balancing the power of one agency over another. Also, these regulatory agencies aid in advocating for the safety of patients and employees in healthcare facilities and in holding providers, healthcare systems, and hospitals accountable for health outcomes. Founded in 1951, The Joint Commission is a leading not-for-profit organization that has certified more than 20,000 healthcare organizations and programs in the U.S. (The Joint Commission, 2015b). The Joint Commission's mission is to "continuously improve healthcare for the public, in collaboration with other stakeholders, by evaluating healthcare organizations and inspiring them to excel in providing safe and effective care of the highest quality and value" (The Joint Commission Center for Transforming Healthcare, 2015). For hospitals to achieve accreditation from The Joint Commission, they must consistently meet many standards. Recently, The Joint Commission has added to these standards the accountability of hospital leadership to assess the hospital's culture of safety. Collectively, only a relatively small percentage of health systems and hospitals across the country achieve top-quality honors from The Joint Commission. In 2014, approximately 36% of The Joint Commission–accredited hospitals were named "Top Performer on Key Quality Measured" (The Joint Commission, 2015b). Clearly, more than half the health systems and hospitals in the country have work to do in providing consistent care.

Although progress has been made in healthcare systems and hospitals, the chief medical officer of The Joint Commission, Ana Pujols McKee, states that there needs to be more focus on improvement processes and that building a high reliability safety culture is critical. Cultivating a culture of safety must start with senior leaders (Birk, 2015) of the healthcare system or hospital. Because of the incremental gains in safety improvement in hospitals as a result of the adoption of high reliability strategies and methodologies, The Joint Commission has become an advocate of the approach. The Joint Commission has developed a forum for best practices through the creation of The Joint Commission Center for Transforming Healthcare (Birk, 2015).

The HRO approach can help healthcare organizations design systems to aid in identifying unsafe conditions well before they lead to harm (Chassin, 2015). This is different from the current healthcare environment, which is more reactive to mistakes. Also, HROs recognize that all errors cannot be prevented and that safety can be derailed. In an HRO environment, there is a willingness to grant the team or individual the decision-making authority to address the safety risk.

COMPLEXITY

Depending on the field of study, complexity has various meanings. In healthcare systems, *complexity* is defined as the interrelatedness of components of a system. Complexity increases with the number of components, the number of relationships among them, and the uniqueness of these relationships (Kannampallil, Schauer, Cohen, and Patel, 2011). For instance, consider the difference in complexity between a community hospital and the Mayo Clinic health system. The Mayo Clinic has more components than a community hospital; therefore, it is more complex.

Complex systems create cognitive and physical challenges for internal and external individuals who interact with the system. Individuals internal to the system expend substantial cognitive effort in performing tasks or creating shortcuts. External users of the system are challenged with interacting with the system, and significant aspects of the system may be ignored (Kannampallil et al., 2011).

The current healthcare system has many components: hospitals, clinics, nursing homes, rehabilitation units, patient homes, patients, and families. These components add complexity for users and produce unintended consequences, such as adverse drug reactions, hospital-acquired infections, readmissions, and functional declines (Lipsitz, 2012). These complex issues make it difficult for an organization to achieve high reliability. Understanding the complexity of healthcare is central to improving quality and safety.

Serious events in healthcare organizations occur daily. These expose the failure of systems to provide a culture of safety for patients, staff, and providers as well as exposing ineffective communication. The complex nature of healthcare organizations contributes to myriad uncertainties that affect safety and quality of care. Teams that are well-versed in high reliability are more likely to address complex issues and recognize the most minor variance in expected outcomes (Wilson, Burke, Priest, and Salas, 2005).

Regulatory agencies are another layer of complexity that causes uncertainty and unpredictability for providers, caregivers, and healthcare leaders. With the conflicting views on quality and outcome measures, healthcare systems and hospitals are at risk of becoming complacent. The opposite can occur in hospitals that ignore warning signs to meet VBP and pay-for-performance measures (Lipsitz, 2012).

According to Lipsitz (2012), in complex systems, individual, self-organized behaviors naturally occur, such as the flocking of birds or the schooling of fish. This creates silos. The key to success is driving collective outcomes that are greater than the sum of their parts. However, this is difficult in the current health system due to silos and the lack of care coordination. Also, the fee-for-service payment model does not support this partnership. The 2013 IOM report, "Best Care at Lower Cost: The Path to Continuously Learning Health Care in America," states that to achieve a high level of quality of care at a lower cost, there must be commitment across the system to learn from each other.

CURRENT HEALTHCARE CULTURE

Designing and sustaining a safety culture, which is required in order to improve reliability, is inherently difficult in healthcare due to the complexity. It is often difficult to visualize what is meant by safety. Patients add another level of complexity with regard to safety because human diseases are different from person to person. The design of the healthcare delivery process in itself creates safety risks and barriers, for which staff must implement workarounds (Khatri, Brown, and Hicks, 2009). Understanding the culture of healthcare and the various branches that add to the complexity can assist with developing solutions to address these challenges.

Many agree that the lack of a culture of safety in a healthcare organization could be a key contributor to organizational accidents. An organization's culture can be viewed as what is valued, its beliefs, and the norms that determine how members interact and act toward patient care and safety. Dynamics of a safety culture can have a direct impact on how issues are detected, corrected, and understood. Therefore, organizations have begun to adopt mindfulness in their safety culture programs. The idea is that a higher level of mindfulness and individuals being more aware of their surroundings and actions can lead to fewer errors and incidents (Sutcliffe, 2011).

Building a culture of safety is essential in an HRO environment. Building a culture of safety requires the promotion of trust, reporting, and improvement. HROs balance learning and accountability through the implementation of a Just Culture, where discipline is equally applied across the system. There is a high sense of accountability with regard to adherence to safety measures and processes. Staff are expected to speak up when there is an error or problem. To learn from communication, there is a system to support ongoing feedback (Chassin, 2015).

REACTIVITY VERSUS PROACTIVITY

The approach an organization takes for managing risk and preventing potential harm to patients depends on the organization's approach to identifying and responding to patient safety issues. The approach used to manage and minimize risk varies from one healthcare system to another. More often than not, this approach is reactive rather than proactive. However, healthcare systems and hospitals should work to support a proactive approach to increasing patient safety and decreasing risk and exposure to liability. This is key in improving reliability.

When it comes to patient safety, what is the difference between being reactive and being proactive? A proactive approach involves an intentional effort to identify risks before events occur and to correct issues before they arise. A leader in a proactive organization takes ownership of identifying risks and causes of incidents instead of blaming circumstances, conditions, or conditioning. Such a leader's behavior is the result of a conscious choice based on values, not feelings (Covey, 1989). This approach in preventing injury and loss allows for the ability to educate staff and the organization as a whole. In contrast, a reactive approach involves reviewing an event after it occurs for potential causes and process errors. With this approach, the patient could experience poor health outcomes as a result of the incident. This could lead to a legal claim (Stewart, 2011). A leader in this type of environment would more likely blame the event on circumstances or patient condition (Covey, 1989).

Suppose an elderly patient received a severe second-degree burn from a heating pad, which was used to treat back pain. In a reactive organization, the patient would receive treatment for the burn—possibly even a skin graft—and would face a long recovery. In a proactive organization, however, the staff would have been educated on the appropriate steps to take to apply the heating pad and the risk of burning to the elderly population, thereby preventing the incident in the first place.

It takes commitment, time, support, and an effective process-improvement program to develop a proactive organization. Once the program is in place, the organization's learning capabilities and collaborative nature help to increase patient safety and decrease organizational exposure to liability (Stewart, 2011).

BLAME/NO BLAME TO ACCOUNTABILITY

In managing risk, it's important for an organization to have an understanding or philosophy of how providers, caregivers, and leaders are held accountable for their actions. It is human nature to demand answers for why an adverse event happens. There is often a strong need to blame someone for an error and hold that person accountable. With this approach, there is an assumption that the person chose to make the error instead of adopting a wrong procedure or process that was on hand at the time of the event. In 1999, Charles Perrow suggested that 60 to 80% of operating errors were in part a result of system errors or failures. In other words, the system—rather than a person—was at least in part to blame for the error. But most company leaders have found that a blaming culture does not foster an environment that brings safety issues to the surface. Organizations that pride themselves on creating a culture of safety routinely examine all aspects of the system after an adverse event. Applying a system approach to investigating an error or adverse event ensures there is no blame.

In healthcare that involves human activity and a reliance on technology, it is likely there could be a situation in which individuals experience a problematic interaction or conflict or incorrectly interpret the actions or words of another. It is also likely they will experience problems when interacting with technology.

HROs have transitioned from a culture of blame, in which an individual or group is seen as the reason for an error, to one that accepts that no organization is free from error and understands that identifying the cause of an error can both offer operational lessons and enhance organizational learning (Weick and Sutcliffe, 2001; Provera, Montefusco, and Canato, 2010). Blaming an individual or group can seriously hinder an organization's ability to learn from the experience. In a blaming environment, individuals who make errors usually are not willing to share this information with their colleagues or managers. Instead, they try to fix it themselves or cover it up. The no-blame approach can be an effective way of enhancing an organization's ability to learn.

Weick and Sutcliffe (2007) and Khatri, Brown, and Hicks (2009) describe a no-blame system as possessing several characteristics:

- Individuals are encouraged to report errors and near misses and are rewarded for doing so.
- A high level of trust and openness allows individuals to exchange opinions without feeling judgment.
- Purposeful organizational analysis takes place with individuals and groups who experience an error.
- Managers review and approve corrective action plans and communicate lessons learned throughout the organization.
- There is a learning culture, enabling healthcare organizations to elicit greater staff involvement.
- Human resources management is integrated in the performance-management process.

Organizations that adopt a no-blame approach commit to a culture in which employees are mindful of their surroundings. Also, in this type of culture, employees become willing to support continuous organizational improvement and to make decisions to strengthen the organization (Weick and Sutcliffe, 2006). This can enable organizations to focus on the right things and avoid wasting valuable time.

When transitioning to a blameless culture, a spirit of accountability must play a role in managing human error. Many successful organizations have found that incorporating a disciplinary system that explores the role each person played in an event can foster an environment of organizational learning. In the healthcare industry, this approach is called a *Just Culture* (Center for Patient Safety, 2015). A Just Culture is characterized by a supportive environment in which the healthcare system or hospital holds itself accountable for the system it designs and holds providers and caregivers accountable for the choices they make within that system. Four behavioral concepts are used to evaluate discipline and patient safety:

- Human error
- Negligence
- Intentional rule violation
- Reckless behavior

In this type of environment, the individual is coached on his or her risky behavior, and the organization learns through the process.

> Commercial airlines have led the way in adopting no-blame practices by developing an environment that promotes collaboration and respectful dialogue among pilots. The National Transportation Safety Board has removed the placement of blame from all events except in cases of criminal activity. Gathering information through various approaches—both formal and informal—is encouraged. Pilots and technicians are required to report any issues during operations, including their own errors. Investigations of errors are done systematically, and corrective measures are communicated to all personnel (Roberts, Bea, and Bartles, 2001).

HIGH RELIABILITY ORGANIZATION THEORY

Organizational and human factors play a role in all accidents and incidents that result in patient harm. HRO theory focuses on the social and organizational foundation of system safety and accident prevention (Sutcliffe, 2011). Reliability is viewed as a top priority. HRO theory also suggests human processes and relationships are the underpinning of an HRO and a culture of safety (Weick and Sutcliffe, 1999). HROs that operate in high-risk environments or have high exposure to liability and loss demonstrate fewer errors than non-HROs. This is achieved through a driven passion for safety that is realized by the pursuit of two approaches (Sutcliffe, 2011):

- **Prevention (anticipation):** This involves an attempt to anticipate or identify risks that may lead to unplanned events or occurrences and to then create processes and procedures to avoid them. An example might be proactively shadowing a telemetry monitor technician to observe the application of a telemetry box to a patient and the implementation of continuous monitoring. This example might also involve identifying potential risks of failures in processes to ensure the right patient is connected to the right telemetry box.

- **Resilience (containment):** HRO cannot be achieved by prevention alone. It also requires resilience (Wildavsky, 1988). The essence of resilience is the ability to maintain or regain a stable state in the presence of stress. Resilience involves three abilities. First is the ability to absorb strain and preserve function in spite of adversity. Second is the ability to bounce back from untoward events. Third is the ability to learn and grow from previous episodes of resilient action (Sutcliffe, 2011). An example of resiliency is the heparin medication error that occurred in a California hospital in 2007. Three infants received 1,000 times more heparin than intended when vials of 10,000 units per milliliter instead of 10 units per milliliter were used to flush the infants' vascular access catheters. This error made national news, which placed a spotlight on the hospital's process for resolving the error. Fortunately, the infants recovered from the event. This event not only affected California but also had an impact on the nation. To prevent future mistakes, the hospital stopped stocking heparin in pediatric units. Only saline is used to flush vascular access lines (Institute for Safe Medication Practices, 2007).

In addition, HRO theory suggests that HROs have an optimistic attitude and focus on internal organizational practices and culture. There is a fundamental belief that reliability is enhanced by rules and standards of practice, technical and social redundancies, teaching, and decision-making that migrates toward expertise (Chassin, 2012).

THE HISTORY AND BACKGROUND OF THE HRO PARADIGM

The initial concept of the HRO paradigm was introduced by a group of researchers at the University of California Berkeley: Todd La Porte, Gene Rochlin, and Karlene Roberts. These researchers examined the links among aircraft carriers, air traffic control, and nuclear power operations (Rochlin, La Porte, and Roberts, 1987; Weick, 1987). Their research found that these industries had similar characteristics, that errors could be minimized through education, and that failures could be avoided by implementing a process to manage complex work and technologies (Rochlin et al., 1987; Weick, 1987).

According to Chassin and Loeb (2013), high reliability science is the study of "organizations in industries like commercial aviation and nuclear power that operate under hazardous conditions while maintaining safety levels that are better than in healthcare" (p. 459). HROs seek to improve reliability and intervene to prevent errors and failures as well as to cope and recover quickly should errors become manifest (Sutcliffe, 2011). HROs are distinguished by their effective management of innately risky technologies through organizational control of both hazards and probability. The hallmark of an HRO is not that it is error-free, but that errors do not disable it. HROs proactively identify weaknesses in the system and use robust process-improvement strategies to address them. They design their reward and incentive systems to recognize the costs of failures as well as the benefits of reliability. They train their people to look for abnormalities, recognize gaps, and act. Their communication consistently shares the big picture of what the organization seeks to do. An important goal is to communicate across the organization in such a way that individuals understand how they fit into the big picture (Chassin and Loeb, 2013).

HRO PRINCIPLES

HROs are unique in their ability both to prevent mishaps and to manage them before they spread throughout the system, thus causing widespread failure. To achieve an HRO environment, an organization must master five principles. As shown in Table 1.2, these principles focus on the practices embedded in the entire organization.

TABLE 1.2 HRO ORGANIZATION PRINCIPLES AND DEFINITIONS

	Principle	Definition
Anticipation	Preoccupation with failure	This means operating with a heightened awareness of potential risks and near misses that may jeopardize safety. Organizations that adhere to this principle engage in proactive and preemptive analysis and discussion and conduct after-action reviews. Individuals actively search for system signals that something is behaving unexpectedly. There is an understanding that small problems can lead to larger problems. The organization is preoccupied with learning and it engages in a robust process-improvement program to re-evaluate and assess areas (Chassin and Loeb, 2013). Employees are trained to look for abnormalities, recognize defects, and act. This principle creates an organizational culture that every problem belongs to the operator until he or she fixes it or finds someone else to do so.
	Reluctance to simplify interpretations	This means deliberately questioning assumptions and received wisdom to create a more complete and nuanced picture of current situations. Each potential risk, small or large, is investigated with the same level of intensity. Staff feel open to ask questions and refrain from making assumptions. Understanding complexity goes beyond the capabilities of one individual. As such, a diverse team of experts (not a homogenous group of individuals) is brought together to make an assessment (Sutcliffe, 2011).
	Sensitivity to operations	This refers to ongoing interaction and sharing of information about current human and organizational factors to create an integrated big picture so that small adjustments can be made to prevent errors from accumulating. HROs develop systems and processes to communicate all risks across the organization. They also encourage employees to think about what is happening and how it might affect their areas. Communication is a major challenge for many organizations. Many believe that if there is an awareness of broad risks, one can identify and address small risks before they become a larger problem.
Containment	Commitment to resilience	This means developing capabilities to cope with, contain, and bounce back from mishaps that have already occurred before they worsen and cause more serious harm. HROs spend a disproportionate amount of money training people to recognize abnormalities. Still, they understand that unanticipated events do occur. HROs develop a capacity to cope with these events, built on a large pool of employees who learn firsthand from unexpected events and simulation.
	Deference to expertise	This principle holds that during high-tempo times (that is, when attempting to resolve a problem or crisis), decision-making migrates to the person or people with the most expertise with the problem at hand, regardless of authority or rank. In a traditional organization structure, decisions are made by upper management. HROs take a different approach. In HROs, decision-making authority is delegated to the expert in the area in which the problem has arisen (Sutcliffe, 2011). This approach improves the organization's ability to respond quickly to unexpected events.

Adapted from Sutcliffe (2011)

To support the five HRO principles, organizations must adopt a fundamental approach in how they communicate and how individuals interact. That means ensuring the following (Chassin, 2012; Chassin and Loeb, 2013; DuPree, 2014):

■ A free flow of information

■ A safe environment in which to speak up

■ Respectful interactions

 When employees feel safe, they will be more likely to report concerns and near misses.

THE INTRODUCTION OF HRO AS A NEW PARADIGM

Human errors are inevitable and are caused by complex factors. Accepting this allows for strategies that can positively affect decision-making and help individuals develop a clearer perception of risks. Ignoring the inevitability of human error will result in continual frustration over adverse events, poor performance, and reactionary measures that focus too heavily on the last person involved in the error. The focus should be on the cumulative effects of organizational breakdowns, flawed defenses, and system failures that allowed the event to occur (Birk, 2015).

Table 1.3 displays some areas where the healthcare industry is moving from an old paradigm to a new one that focuses on high reliability. Healthcare providers and organizations will need to become comfortable with the new pay-for-performance models and must lead change in the area of transparency. The number of reportable quality outcomes, which consumers and insurance payers use to make decisions regarding healthcare services, is growing. Private organizations such as *U.S. News and World Report* (2015), Healthgrades (2015), and the Leapfrog Group (2012) also rank hospitals and quality care outcomes.

TABLE 1.3   OLD PARADIGM VERSUS NEW PARADIGM

Old Paradigm	New Paradigm
Fee-for-service model	Value-based payment models
More is better	Cost-effective
Siloed	Leadership ownership
Lack of trust, blaming culture, root causes limited to adverse events	High level of trust in all clinical areas, Just Culture, near misses and unsafe conditions routinely assessed
Physician-focused	Consumer-focused

continues

TABLE 1.3 OLD PARADIGM VERSUS NEW PARADIGM (CONTINUED)

Old Paradigm	New Paradigm
Quality not identified as a strategic initiative	Quality top priority on the strategic plan
Regulations-focused	Alignment for HRO, goal of zero harm
Limited use of quality management tools and limited resources for training	Robust process improvement program and tools, organizational budget allocated for education and training
Physicians hold organization responsible for improvement initiatives	Physicians lead quality improvement initiatives
Quality agenda items scheduled near the end of the meeting	Board of trustees' commitment to high-reliability
Quality measures are limited to closed meetings	Quality measures visible internally and publicly

Adapted from Griffith, 2015, and Chassin and Loeb, 2013

There has been a shift from the perspective that more is better to the perspective that focuses on what is provided given the cost of care. Since the passing of the ACA, more accountability is placed on consumers to secure health insurance. Due to the various options and out-of-pocket expenses, consumers are pausing to evaluate the cost of healthcare. Healthcare systems and hospitals are responding to the consumers' need to understand the value of their healthcare experience by posting quality outcomes and the cost of procedures on their websites.

Healthcare systems and hospitals are redirecting their focus toward the needs of the consumers. There is growing evidence that partnering with consumers can lead to improvements in quality, outcomes, and cost-effectiveness. Consumers are those individuals who autonomously make decisions regarding their health (Mittler, Martsolf, Telenko, and Scanlon, 2013). They no longer make decisions merely on the word of their physician. Some consumers do their homework and actively participate with their physicians to make healthcare decisions.

Leaders play a role here. To create a culture of safety that focuses on managing risk, increased engagement by leaders is critical (Sutcliffe, 2011). Leaders must commit to creating an environment that encourages team members to speak up. Leaders must also be willing to provide the resources to create a culture of ongoing learning. In the HRO paradigm, quality is a top priority of the healthcare system and hospital's strategic plan. This occurs when:

- Measures are aligned with the performance goals of all staff.
- There is a commitment to zero-harm goal, starting with the board of trustees.
- There is full engagement with physicians.

■ The organizational budget includes resources to provide ongoing education, training, and quality-management tools, which are used for improvement and to redesign care processes (Chassin and Loeb, 2013).

APPLICATION TO HEALTHCARE

HROs have demonstrated success in minimizing errors by creating mindful environments where employees are trained to look for and report small problems that could lead to big ones. They view these small errors and close calls as learning opportunities; they correct them and share details about them across the organization (Chassin, 2012; Shabot, 2015). For the healthcare industry to make real progress in developing HROs, three things must occur:

■ **The leadership team must commit to a goal of zero harm:** If a healthcare organization wants the staff to follow HRO practices, it must start at the top. There must be alignment among the board of trustees, physicians, senior leaders, and department managers, all committed to completely eliminating patient harm.

■ **HRO principles must be integrated with the organization to develop a culture of safety:** Hospitals struggle with this the most. In 2009, The Joint Commission required hospitals to create a culture of safety. Although most healthcare systems hospitals have elected to perform annual safety culture surveys, they have not put much effort or resources toward making sustainable changes to strengthen the culture of safety.

■ **The organization must adopt a robust process improvement program to improve its quality of care and outcomes:** HROs do not specify which process improvement tools and methods to use, but change-management tools, Lean, and Six Sigma are the most widely used. These types of tools incorporate a systematic approach, eliminate waste in the process, and foster discipline in measuring outcomes (Chassin and Loeb, 2013; Sutcliffe, 2011).

WHY ARE HROS NEEDED?

There is overwhelming evidence that preventable patient harm and adverse events continue to occur in U.S. healthcare systems and hospitals. Trends in healthcare outcomes demonstrate that our healthcare system is struggling to deliver consistent and reliable quality care. The dynamics of healthcare are ever-changing, and the pace of this change has made the healthcare industry more difficult for consumers to understand and navigate. Healthcare providers and caregivers work in a complex system with many competing priorities and shrinking revenues. It is as if they are standing on two floating logs—one representing the fee-for-service environment and the other the value-based payment environment. Both of these environments require dedication and focus to be successful. As a result, less attention is directed toward creating HRO environments to drive quality, safety, and service.

Healthcare systems and hospitals have not established sustainable solutions to prevent patients from receiving hospital-acquired infections (HAIs). In 2011, the CDC reported that one in 25 patients in acute care hospitals in the U.S. experienced at least one HAI—an estimate of 772,000 total (2015). Worse, approximately 75,000 patients with HAIs died during their hospitalization. Medical errors are a major killer in the U.S., third only to heart disease and cancer, claiming more than 400,000 lives (James, 2013).

In addition to HAIs, there are other preventable risks in the healthcare environment that could be improved by the adoption of HRO principles. For example, healthcare workers routinely face serious safety and health hazards in the workplace. These hazards may include blood-borne pathogens, biological hazards, chemical and drug exposures, ergonomic hazards from lifting patients, and workplace violence, to name a few (Occupational Safety and Health Administration, 2015). According to the Bureau of Labor Statistics, in 2011, there were more injury and illness cases in healthcare than in any other industry (2014).

BENEFITS TO PATIENT OUTCOMES, FINANCIALS, SAFETY, AND THE WORK ENVIRONMENT

In the healthcare industry, the benefits of integrating HRO principles and practices are significant. HRO phenomena are mainly present in large systems that would benefit greatly from anticipating unexpected events to prevent large system failures (La Porte, 1996). Equally, healthcare systems and hospitals have the potential risk of experiencing large system failures. These risks may include financial and human loss, negative impact on the workforce, or a loss of confidence and trust among members of the community, which could have a devastating effect on any health system or hospital.

In embracing HRO practices, health systems and hospitals gain a culture with a strong sense of mission and commitment to reliability in operations and capacity. Organizations that have adopted HRO practices have seen improvement in organizational effectiveness, efficiency, and culture, as well as in customer satisfaction and documentation (The Joint Commission Center for Transforming Healthcare, 2015). Such organizations foster and value safety, quality, and management accountability. They also gain a workforce that is highly skilled, knowledgeable, and engaged in the solutions to make their practice and organization safe (Shabot, 2015). There is also benefit on the cost side. The U.S. spends significant amounts of money on treating HAIs and unnecessary procedures and diagnostic tests.

Between 2010 and 2013, a 9% decline in HAIs saved $12 billion in healthcare costs (CDC, 2015). A further decline in HAI incidence would have a positive financial impact on the healthcare budget, to be reallocated to health programs. As well, a collaborative environment and reward and recognition programs, which are both needed for HRO environments to be successful, could have a positive impact on the work environment and employee turnover. Nurses thrive in environments that provide autonomy and allow for their empowerment, that offer a supportive leadership team, and that promote collegial relationships with their team, and evidence shows that satisfied nurses can have a positive impact on patient outcomes (Twigg and McCullough, 2014).

SUMMARY

The current healthcare system is complex and is burdened with inefficiencies. Overwhelming economic and quality barriers hinder progress in improving quality, safety, and service. The dynamics of the healthcare system are shifting such that HRO is a viable approach to creating a reliable healthcare system for providers, caregivers, and consumers. Evidence suggests that HRO principles create environments that are mindful of anticipating unexpected events and resilient in responding quickly to minimize exposure. In addition, the use of incident reviews in HROs builds institutional knowledge.

Many organizations outside of healthcare have achieved HRO status and have sustained their results over long periods of time (Chassin and Loeb, 2011). Although many healthcare organizations are on the path to adopting HRO principles—and an elite few are close to becoming HROs—we know for sure that the road to an HRO starts and ends with leadership.

KEY POINTS

- The current healthcare culture and trends demand a highly reliable healthcare delivery system.

- Adverse events have significant human and economic costs.

- High reliability organizations (HROs) create a culture of safety and help employees to remain alert for the smallest signal of a risk to the organization.

- Healthcare systems and hospitals that anticipate risks and manage unexpected events create a sustainable culture of safety.

- Leaders can build a set of capabilities to respond to adverse events and foster organizational learning.

- Only leaders can build a Just Culture that counteracts the blame game.

■ A robust process improvement approach—a combination of Lean, Six Sigma, and change-management tools—is foundational to creating an HRO.

■ Highly reliable organizations view culture as a core value.

REFERENCES

Barton, P. L. (2009). *Understanding the U.S. health services system* (4th ed.). Chicago, IL: Health Administration Press.

Birk, S. (2015). Accelerating the adoption of a safety culture. *The Joint Commission.* Retrieved from http://www.jointcommission.org/assets/1/18/Healthcare_Executive_McKee_032015.pdf

Bureau of Labor Statistics. (2014). Employer-reported workplace injuries and illness. Retrieved from http://www.bls.gov/news.release/pdf/osh.pdf

Center for Patient Safety. (2015). Just culture. Retrieved from http://www.centerforpatientsafety.org/just-culture/

Centers for Disease Control and Prevention. (2015). Chronic diseases: The leading causes of death and disability in the United States. Retrieved from http://www.cdc.gov/chronicdisease/overview/index.htm

Centers for Medicare & Medicaid Services. (2011). Hospital valued-based purchasing program. Retrieved from https://www.cms.gov/Outreach-and-Education/Medicare-Learning-Network-MLN/MLNProducts/downloads/Hospital_VBPurchasing_Fact_Sheet_ICN907664.pdf

Centers for Medicare & Medicaid Services. (2015a). Hospital value-based purchasing. Retrieved from https://www.cms.gov/Medicare/Quality-Initiatives-Patient-Assessment-Instruments/hospital-value-based-purchasing/index.html?redirect=/hospital-value-based-purchasing/

Centers for Medicare & Medicaid Services. (2015b). Fiscal year (2016) results for CMS value-based purchasing program. Retrieved from https://www.cms.gov/Newsroom/MediaReleaseDatabase/Fact-sheets/2015-Fact-sheets-items/2015-10-26.html

Chassin, M. R. (2012). Health care and high reliability: A cautionary tale. 5th International HRO conference. Chicago, IL.

Chassin, M. R. (2015). High reliability in healthcare: Working toward zero harm. Retrieved from http://arabhealthmagazine.com/press-releases/2015/issue-4/high-reliability-in-healthcare-working-toward-zero-harm/

Chassin, M. R., and Loeb, J. M. (2011). The ongoing quality improvement journey: Next stop, high reliability. *Health Affairs, 30*(4), pp. 559–568.

Chassin, M. R., and Loeb, J. M. (2013). High-reliability health care: Getting there from here. *The Milbank Quarterly.* Retrieved from http://www.jointcommission.org/assets/1/6/Chassin_and_Loeb_0913_final.pdf

Congressional Budget Office. (2015). Budget and economic outlook 2015–2025. Retrieved from https://www.cbo.gov/publication/49892

Covey, S. (1989). *The 7 habits of highly effective people: Restoring the character ethic.* New York, NY: Simon & Schuster.

DuPree, E. S. (2014). Leading change: The high reliability journey. Hospital Executive Briefing. The Joint Commission. Retrieved from http://www.mha.org/keystone_center/symposium/2015/documents/using_high_reliability_to_improve_quality.pdf

DuPree, E., Martin, L., Anderson, R., Kathuria, N., Reich, D., Porter, C., and Chassin, M. R. (2009). Improving patient satisfaction with pain management using Six Sigma tools. *Joint Commission Journal on Quality and Patient Safety, 35*(7), pp. 343–350.

Field, R. I. (2008). Why is health care regulation so complex? *Pharmacy and Therapeutics, 33*(10), pp. 607–608.

Griffith, J. R. (2015). Understanding high-reliability organizations: Are Baldrige recipients models? *Journal of Healthcare Management, 60*(1), pp. 44–61.

Healthgrades. (2015). About us. Retrieved from http://www.healthgrades.com

Institute for Safe Medication Practices. (2007). Another heparin error: Learning from mistakes so we don't repeat them. Retrieved from https://www.ismp.org/newsletters/acutecare/articles/20071129.asp

Institute of Medicine. (1999). To err is human. Retrieved from http://iom.nationalacademies.org/Reports/1999/To-Err-is-Human-Building-A-Safer-Health-System.aspx

Institute of Medicine. (2011). The Richard and Hinda Rosenthel lecture 2011: New frontiers in patient safety. Retrieved from http://iom.nationalacademies.org/reports/2011/the-richard-and-hinda-rosenthal-lecture-2011-new-frontiers-in-patient-safety.aspx

Institute of Medicine. (2013). Best care at lower cost: The path to continuously learning health care in America. Retrieved from http://www.nap.edu/catalog/13444/best-care-at-lower-cost-the-path-to-continuously-learning

James, J. T. (2013). A new evidence-based element of patient harm associated with hospital care. *Journal of Patient Safety*, *9*(3), pp. 122–128.

The Joint Commission. (2015a). Sentinel event data 1995–3Q 2015. Retrieved from http://www.jointcommission.org/assets/1/18/General-Information_1995-3Q-2015.pdf

The Joint Commission. (2015b). About the joint commission. Retrieved from http://www.jointcommission.org/about_us/about_the_joint_commission_main.aspx

The Joint Commission Center for Transforming Healthcare. (2015). High reliability: The gold standard in health care. Retrieved from http://www.centerfortransforminghealthcare.org/hro_portal_main.aspx

Kannampallil, T. G., Schauer, G. F., Cohen, T., and Patel, V. L. (2011). Considering complexity in healthcare systems. *Journal of Biomedical Informatics*, *44*(6), 943–947.

Keckly, P. H., and Coughlin, S. (2012). *2012 survey of U.S. health care consumers: Five-year look back*. Washington, DC: Deloitte University Press.

Khatri, N., Brown, G. D., and Hicks, L. L. (2009). From a blame culture to a just culture in health care. *Healthcare Management Review*, *34* (4), pp. 312–322.

La Porte, T. R. (1996). High reliability organizations: Unlikely, demanding and at risk. *Journal of Contingencies and Crisis Management*, *4*(2), pp. 60–71.

The Leapfrog Group. (2012). How safe is your hospital? Retrieved from http://www.leapfroggroup.org/policy_leadership/leapfrog_news/4894464

LBJ Presidential Library. (2012). The 1965 Medicare amendment to the Social Security Act. Retrieved from http://www.lbjlibrary.org/press/the-1965-medicare-amendment-to-the-social-security-act

Lipsitz, L. (2012). Understanding health care as a complex system: The foundation for unintended consequences. *Journal of American Medical Association*, *308*(3), pp. 243–244.

Mittler, J. N., Martsolf, G. R., Telenko, S. J., and Scanlon, D. P. (2013). Making sense of "consumer engagement" initiatives to improve health and health care: A conceptual framework guide policy and practice. *The Milbank Quarterly*, *91*(1), pp. 37–77.

Nolan, T., Resar, R., Haraden, C., and Griffin, F. A. (2004). Improving the reliability of health care. IHI Innovation Series white paper. Boston, MA: Institute for Healthcare Improvement. Retrieved from http://www.ihi.org/resources/Pages/IHIWhitePapers/ImprovingtheReliabilityofHealthCare.aspx

Occupational Safety and Health Administration. (2015). Workplace violence. Retrieved from http://www.osha.gov

Perrow, C. (1999). *Normal accidents: Living with high-risk technologies*. (2nd ed.). Princeton, NJ: Princeton University Press.

Provera, B., Montefusco, A., and Canato, A. (2010). A "no blame" approach to organizational learning. *British Journal of Management*, *21*(4), pp. 1057–1074.

Rice, T., Unruh, L. Y., Rosenau, P., Barnes, A. J., Saltman, R. B., and van Ginneken, E. (2014). Challenges facing the United States of America in implementing universal coverage. *Bulletin of the World Health Organization*. Retrieved from http://www.who.int/bulletin/volumes/92/12/14-141762/en/

Roberts, K. H., Bea, R., and Bartles, D. L. (2001). Must accidents happen? Lessons from high-reliability organizations. *Academy of Management Perspectives*, *15*(3), pp. 70–78.

Rochlin, G. I., La Porte, T. R., and Roberts, K. H. (1987). The self-designing high-reliability organization: Aircraft carrier flight operations at sea. *Naval War College Review*, *40*(4), pp. 76–90.

Schumock, G. T., Li, E. C., Suda, K. J., Matusiak, L. M., Hunkler, R. J., Vermeulen, L. C., and Hoffman, J. M. (2014). National trends in prescription drug expenditures and projections for 2014. *American Journal of Health-System Pharmacy*, *71*(6), pp. 482–499.

Shabot, M. M. (2015). New tools for high reliability healthcare. *BMJ Quality and Safety*, *24*(7), pp. 423–424.

Stewart, A. (2011). Risk management: The reactive versus proactive struggle. *Journal of Nursing Law*, *14*(3), pp. 91–95.

Sutcliffe, K. M. (2011). High reliability organizations (HROs). *Best Practice & Research Clinical Anaesthesiology*, *25*(2), pp. 133–144.

Twigg, D., and McCullough, K. (2014). Nurse retention: A review of strategies to create and enhance positive practice environments in clinical settings. *International Journal of Nursing Studies, 51*(1), pp. 85–92.

U.S. Census Bureau. (2015). Annual and quarterly services. Retrieved from https://www.census.gov/services/index.html

U.S. Department of Health and Human Services. (2014). Key features of the Affordable Care Act. Retrieved from http://www.hhs.gov/healthcare/facts-and-features/key-features-of-aca/index.html

U.S. News and World Report. (2015). Best hospitals. Retrieved from http://health.usnews.com/best-hospitals

Vogus, T. J., Sutcliffe, K. M., and Weick, K. E. (2010). Doing no harm: Enabling, enacting, and elaborating a culture of safety. *Academy of Management Perspectives, 24*(6), pp. 60–77.

Wagner, K. (2014). Health care reform and leadership: Switching from volume to value. *Physician Leadership Journal, 1*(1), pp. 22–26.

Weick, K. E. (1987). Organizational culture as a source of high reliability. *California Management Review, 29*(2), pp. 112–127.

Weick, K. E., and Sutcliffe, K. M. (2001). *Managing the unexpected: Assuring high performance in an age of complexity.* San Francisco, CA: Jossey-Bass.

Weick, K. E., and Sutcliffe, K. M. (2006). Mindfulness and the quality of organizational attention. *Organization Science, 17*(4), pp. 514–524.

Weick, K. E., and Sutcliffe, K. M. (2007). *Managing the unexpected: Resilient performance in an age of uncertainty* (2nd ed.). San Francisco, CA: Jossey-Bass.

Wildavsky, A. B. (1988). *Searching for safety.* Piscataway, NJ: Transaction Publishers.

Wilson, K. A., Burke, C. S., Priest, H. A., and Salas, E. (2005). Promoting healthcare safety through training high reliability teams. *Quality & Safety in Healthcare, 14*(4), pp. 303–309.

World Health Organization. (2015). World health statistics 2014. Retrieved from http://www.who.int/mediacentre/news/releases/2014/world-health-statistics-2014/en/

CURRENT PATIENT SAFETY DRIVERS

Gwen Sherwood, PhD, RN, FAAN, ANEF

Gail E. Armstrong, DNP, ACNS-BC, CNE

The first tenet health professionals learn is, "First, do no harm." Prevention of patient harm has gained momentum across the world since it was incorporated into the title of the initial Institute of Medicine (IOM) report, "First Do No Harm," documenting the extent of patient harm in the United States (1999). Still, 15 years later, it's believed that more than 400,000 people die each year as a result of healthcare harm (James, 2013).

The increasing emergence of high reliability organizations (HROs) in healthcare is helping to reframe perspectives on patient harm by emphasizing drivers for patient safety that relate less to the individual and more to shared accountability across the system. A systems perspective with shared accountability ensures errors are analyzed through root cause analysis, resulting in changes that reduce the possibility of a repeat error.

The purpose of this chapter is to provide an overview of safety drivers that affect healthcare delivery systems and explore how HROs contribute to patient safety.

> " Primum non nocere. *(First, do no harm.)*
>
> —*Thomas Sydenham, MD* "

It's difficult to cite exact numbers of deaths due to healthcare harm because of the hidden nature of healthcare harm, varying definitions, and lack of standardized reporting within and across systems. Professionals underreport patient harm, also called patient care errors or preventable harm, because they fear punishment and blame or fail to recognize reportable events. There is no national repository for this information, and the emphasis on reportable events and parameters for reporting vary across organizations. At best, the number of deaths due to patient harm is a projection.

OVERVIEW OF PATIENT HARM

Patient harm is a broad term with multiple layers and perspectives. This makes it challenging to establish operational definitions and a common understanding among providers. Although it's inevitable that individuals will make mistakes, there is often a chain of events within the system during which potential mistakes could be detected and interrupted.

All providers are susceptible to mistakes, regardless of role or skill level. Understanding and appreciating the full spectrum of patient harm enables providers to work within the system to prevent patient harm, recognize potential gaps in the system of care delivery, and develop skills in harm prevention. Improving safety begins with a deeper understanding of patient harm.

UNDERSTANDING PATIENT HARM BEGINS WITH SAFETY

A commonly used definition of safety in nursing is from the groundbreaking Robert Wood Johnson Foundation–funded national initiative, "Quality and Safety Education for Nurses" (QSEN) (Cronenwett et al., 2007). This was in turn based on the 2003 Institute of Medicine report. This definition states that safety refers to minimizing risk of harm to patients and providers through both system effectiveness and individual performance (www.qsen.org). Patient safety is freedom from accidental harm at any point during care delivery (IOM, 1999). Patient or healthcare harm refers to the failure of a planned action to be completed as intended or the use of an incorrect plan that results in a gap in patient care that can harm the patient (Reason, 2000).

Errors that lead to patient harm occur throughout the system and can happen to anyone involved with patients. Incorporating a systems perspective, the National Patient Safety Foundation's Lucian Leape Institute (2014) defines healthcare errors as unintended healthcare outcomes caused by a defect in care delivery to a patient. Therefore, accountability for patient harm is shared across the system.

To prevent harm to patients, organizations must adopt operational systems and processes that minimize risk and maximize the prevention of errors before harm occurs. Safe care, in fact, means preventing harm to patients during the administration of care that is intended to help them. Preventable harm describes errors that could have been avoided through reasonable actions and decisions. An adverse event is when patients are harmed from care delivery or care management. Sentinel events are preventable patient deaths due to healthcare harm (Barnsteiner, 2012). Examples of situations in which both individual providers and the system may share accountability include the multiple ways to prevent wrong-site surgery, poorly orchestrated or lack of standardized handover procedures between providers or units, and managing the multilayered process of ordering and administering medications (Mitchell, 2008).

TYPOLOGY OF PATIENT HARM

Dekker (2011) distinguished two perspectives for identifying errors:

- **Errors as a human competence problem:** In this case, human error is identified as the cause of the problem. The error is the conclusion of the investigation, and the target for improvement is the personnel involved. With this perspective, the supposition is that healthcare is basically safe but needs protection from unreliable people.

- **Errors as a systems problem:** This perspective focuses on system gaps and considers errors as symptoms of larger system interruptions. In this case, the error is the starting point for deeper understanding and the improvement of processes. Meaningful intervention targets the system factors that contribute to the error. This perspective acknowledges that healthcare was not purposefully designed as a reliable or safe system.

Table 2.1 lists different types of patient harm. The multiple levels and types of patient harm listed help explain the concept of patient harm and illustrate the complexity in how errors are classified, investigated, and managed. The typology is an important part of analyzing patient harm whereby a trained team traces the event pathway, identifies the type of error according to these classifications, and determines what actions should follow for recovery and redesign. The typology is an important part of provider education and helping personnel to better understand what is reportable. The typology focuses on what happened more than who made the error. When failure or harm occurs, the first question should focus on why the failure occurred rather than who caused the failure—for example, where did the safeguards fail (Armstrong and Sherwood, 2012)?

TABLE 2.1 TYPOLOGY OF HEALTHCARE HARM

Error Classification	Defining Characteristics
Patterns of Error	
Latent	The "blunt" end. These arise from decisions that affect organizational policies, procedures, and allocation of resources.
Active	These occur at the interface of contact with the patient, called the "sharp" end.
Actions Defining Errors or Harm	
Commission	Doing the wrong thing
Omission	Not doing the right thing
Execution	Doing the right thing incorrectly or with an unintended result
Planning	Intended action incorrect
Error Classifications	
Normal human errors	Slips or lapses, often the result of being forgetful or distracted
At-risk behavior	Failure to recognize risk, reasonable expectations not met, outside reasonable expectations
Reckless conduct	Conscious disregard for rules, creates danger
Process Errors	
Diagnostic	Premature closure of diagnosis or assessment, perhaps causing treatment to be incorrect or delayed
Treatment	Incorrect care or failure to deliver care
Organizational or system	Management decisions, policies, procedures, workforce decisions
Technical	Equipment or other resource failure

Adapted from Reason (2000)

Accurately identifying the type of error helps providers identify how harm occurred and reevaluate processes and decisions to prevent future occurrences.

Reason (2000) lists three major classifications (refer to Table 2.1):

- Normal human errors that happen to even highly skilled providers
- At-risk behavior, in which reasonable expectations are not met
- Reckless conduct that ignores safety precautions

Other typology may classify errors as diagnostic errors from premature closure of diagnosis or assessment, organizational or system errors, treatment errors, or technical errors. Error events may also be explained as latent or active. A latent error can lead to an active error—for instance, when an incorrect look-alike or sound-alike medication is mistakenly delivered to the unit and is administered by the nurse. If the nurse recognizes and corrects the mistake, it is an error interruption.

Systems that track error interruption manifest a key characteristic of HRO organizations: They demonstrate a healthy preoccupation with failure. Understanding the system gaps that led to a near miss can prevent similar errors from recurring. The National Safety Council (n.d.) defines a near miss as an unplanned event that did not result in injury, illness, or damage but had the potential to do so.

Although a healthy preoccupation with failure is a positive attribute of a learning system, many healthcare providers resist using the word *failure* in identifying values. Thus, some systems, like University of Maryland Medical Center, use a reward system to incentivize providers to report near misses. Another example is the use of safety huddles at the start of the nursing shift, in which each nurse reports patients who are at high risk for things to go wrong.

Reason (2000) illustrated the adverse event trajectory using the analogy of Swiss cheese. Swiss cheese, recognized for its holes, helps explain how faults in the different layers of the system can lead to errors and demonstrates how numerous triggers can set up a sequence of events that may cause an error to occur (that is, to move from latent to active). There are various system triggers, such as incomplete or overly complicated procedures and policies, patient flow pressures, delegation authority, inadequate communication training, distractions, and use of universal tubal connections for different treatments (Barnsteiner, 2012). In most situations, multiple defenses arising from situational awareness and monitoring prevent errors, such as when someone recognizes the potential for tubal misconnections and prevents the error from happening. Still, situations occur in which multiple lapses align to allow patient harm, like lining up the holes in slices of Swiss cheese.

MANAGING PATIENT HARM: INDIVIDUAL BLAME VERSUS SHARED ACCOUNTABILITY

Historically, when an error or patient harm event occurred, the initial response was to establish blame by identifying the person who made the mistake and disciplining that person (Barnsteiner, 2012). In emerging models, however, instead of simply blaming an individual, the focus shifts to analyzing what happened in a patient harm event. Individuals who make mistakes are accountable, but the focus is on the adverse event trajectory—that is, what triggered the gaps in the Swiss cheese slices to line up. Replacing the emphasis on blame with a broader culture of safety is vital. It enables providers to safely report near misses and adverse events for analysis, which can lead to system redesign. A safety focus shifts from the individual to the prevention of future errors by learning from each harm event. With this system, the perspective shifts from the individual nurse as the only line of defense when it comes to preventing medication errors, patients from falling, or decubitus ulcers (Armstrong and Sherwood, 2012). Instead, it considers how to incorporate prevention into the system as a whole.

Transparency is a hallmark of safety. Information is shared across the organization and with patients and families. Patients and families have a right to the truth. This organizational philosophy and practice may be referred to as Just Culture (Boysen, 2013). As discussed later in this chapter, HROs have policies, processes, and training directed toward disclosing healthcare errors and significant near misses to patients and their families (Barnsteiner, 2012).

AN EXAMPLE OF BLAME ATTRIBUTION VERSUS SHARED SYSTEM ACCOUNTABILITY

A large academic medical center implemented a significant update to its electronic health record (EHR) platform. Within the first 2 days, the pharmacy noticed a significant increase in medication errors on one unit. Because the EHR update coincided with the arrival of new medical residents, it was initially assumed the errors were due to their inexperience. Indeed, two residents in particular were involved with 50% of the errors. The chief medical officer quickly blamed and reprimanded these residents and their supervising physicians.

However, medication ordering errors continued to increase. Further investigation revealed that the errors were in fact due to new EHR functions connected to the update. Specifically, the new version of the EHR featured an autofill function. When an ordering provider started typing the first letters of a medication, the autofill function would offer possibilities (similar to when one types a search term in Google). The EHR system was quickly updated to remove this dangerous "improvement," and attention was paid to mending collegial damage between the chief medical officer and residents.

Although blaming individuals may be instinctive and appear to be efficient in addressing errors, this approach often leads to an incomplete analysis, distrust among providers, and perpetuation of the problem.

THE HIGH COST OF PATIENT HARM

Patient harm is costly for patients and families, organizations, and the public. Calculating cost is complex, whether related to patients and families or for organizations and the systems they represent. In the end, the public, too, pays a high price in higher healthcare costs, poor quality, a lessening of trust in healthcare providers, and continued breaks in the system. Examining the high cost of patient harm adds to the imperative for systems to focus on the principles of HRO organizations.

Costs to Patients and Families

In addition to the cost of healthcare, patient harm causes patients and families to experience lost productivity and income with extended time away from jobs, the cost of travel between home and care delivery sites, added healthcare costs, and other expenses. In addition to these are the intangible costs, such as separation from family and loved ones, suffering and pain, the inconvenience of delayed healing and treatment, lower satisfaction with care, and loss of trust in providers and the system (Sherwood, 2012). These have no true dollar amount.

Economic Impact on Organizations

Costs to the organization or system include extended lengths of stay for patients that continue to tie up beds needed for other patients, additional or replacement treatments due to treatment and diagnostic errors, and other system failures. Medication errors or adverse drug events are among the most common types of error. A 2006 IOM report estimates that almost 2% of admissions experience a preventable adverse drug event. This increases hospital costs by $4,700 per admission and adds up to $2.8 million each year for a 700-bed hospital. Compounded nationally, the total is $2 billion annually. A review of Medicare data from 2006 to 2008 of more than 950,000 patient safety incidents revealed that related care cost $8.9 billion (HealthDay News, 2008). Most of these costs are due to additional healthcare costs when tests and treatments have to be repeated or when other care elements have to be added, requiring patients to extend their hospital stay and thus continue to occupy a much-needed bed. Payment systems focus on quality of care, and these occurrences affect hospital reimbursements when there is patient harm, such as no reimbursement for hospital-acquired infections.

Workforce Factors

Healthcare workers are affected by the quality and safety of care in the systems in which they work. Workers want to work in quality, safe organizations. When there is a lack of organizational support to provide the best care possible, they report loss of morale (which leads to disengagement) and lower satisfaction. To foster a quality-focused work environment, a 2004 IOM report issued three primary recommendations (Page, 2004):

- Provide a voice for nurses by positioning the chief nurse executive with a leadership role in organizational decision-making.

- Decrease stress and overloaded work assignments by applying evidence-based staffing models that improve patient outcomes and reduce staff fatigue.

- Provide a safe work environment by implementing safe patient-handling and other procedures that minimize injury and promote healthy work environments.

Other system and human factors affect quality of care and drive safety. Interruptions, multitasking, distractions, task fixation that limits environmental scanning, hierarchy and authority gradients, interpersonal and interprofessional relationships, and the lack of education about safety are among the multiple workforce-related drivers that contribute to patient harm.

THE IMPACT OF CULTURE ON SAFETY

Organizations are shaped by culture—that is, how members share values and attitudes, act and react, and communicate. Norms around safe practice, valuing safety, inclusion of the patient and family to protect safety, and how lapses in safety are addressed are core components of healthcare culture. Ensuring that safety goals and culture are aligned is a critical part of improving safety. It has been said that culture overshadows process; developing a strong organization through committed leadership and consistent mission, vision, values, and practices is an important part of the transformation toward an HRO organization.

ORGANIZATIONAL CULTURE

Organizational culture is determined by the collective values, beliefs, and norms held by those at all levels in the organization. Organizational culture is important when assessing an organization's capacity for change and agility in implementing new practices aimed at improvement (Bellot, 2011). Effective organizations are learning organizations capable of responding to internal and external pressures in a dynamic environment and achieving best outcomes.

Three elements help explain organizations (Schein, 2010):

- **Artifacts:** Artifacts are visible in the environment. They include dress codes, policies, procedures, structure, and work processes.

- **Values:** Values are reflected in the organization's mission, philosophy, goals, and strategic plans, and are in turn reflected in the behaviors and attitudes of members of the organization.

- **Assumptions:** Assumptions remain largely invisible. They are the undercurrents that represent the beliefs through which culture is lived, influencing attitudes and actions.

The interactions among these elements capture the whole of an organization's culture. Incongruence among the three elements creates dissonance within the organization and compromises reliability for achieving best outcomes.

Culture may be learned and reinforced as those in the organization observe behaviors of others that are tolerated, rewarded, or punished (Schein, 2010). Members observe behaviors—particularly of leaders—and believe, correctly or incorrectly, that this is how the organization operates.

For instance, enforcement of rules about dress becomes important in assessing safety culture, as some rules help prevent infection. When some members of the community are allowed to break the rules without consequences, others become confused. It raises uncertainty about the integrity of the commitment to stated goals, mission, and actions. Group members may lose focus and lose confidence in leadership, which may contribute to inefficiencies, poor quality, and low morale (Schein, 2010).

Culture and communication—a major component of safety culture—are intertwined such that culture is expressed through the social interactions of group members (Bellot, 2011). Communication, as discussed later in this chapter, is continuous as group members receive, interpret, and evaluate input among themselves, their leaders, and the organization itself. The manner in which organizations communicate, manage change processes, and resolve problems and conflict either contributes to sustainability or weakens the organization (Singer et al., 2009). The journey toward high reliability begins with examining organizational culture and the role of safety as a subculture.

SAFETY CULTURE

Safety culture is a subset of organizational culture. It is the basis for establishing a high degree of reliability. Safety culture is the complex product of individual and group values, attitudes, perceptions, competencies, and patterns of behavior. The organization's commitment to safety management is a primary driver for safety culture and is developed through the seven domains discussed in the following list (Sammer, Lykens, Singh, Mains, and Lackan, 2010). A positive safety culture demonstrates effective communication guided by mutual trust, shared perceptions of the importance of safety among all members and leadership, and confidence that error-preventing strategies will work. Safety culture acknowledges the complexity of system and human factors that influence safety through an interplay of leadership, policies, and front-line staff. Following are seven domains essential to safety culture (Sammer, Lykens, Singh, Mains, and Lackan, 2010).

- **Leadership:** Reinforce safety as a priority by aligning decisions with vision and mission, fiscal and human capital, and personnel competencies.

- **Teamwork:** Collaborate, cooperate, and promote collegiality across the organization to foster relationships that are open, safe, respectful, transparent, and flexible.

- **Evidence-based:** Standardize care interventions to reduce variance to help achieve high reliability by helping eliminate breakdowns in work processes.

- **Communication:** Share information in multiple ways among those involved and encourage staff to speak up on behalf of patients.

- **Learning:** Engage in structured critical reflection as a change model that identifies what to do differently in the future, incorporating both experience and knowledge for individuals and the organization.

- **Just:** Recognize errors as system failures rather than focusing on individual blame.

- **Patient-centered:** Empower patients and families to participate actively in discussions about their care and ensure they are provided access to health information.

A safety culture involves the commitment and engagement of everyone, from the boardroom down (Wachter and Pronovost, 2009). It is founded on a non-punitive approach to patient harm. It emphasizes accountability, honesty, integrity, and mutual respect in a Just Culture. Accountability is a critical aspect of a culture of safety. Recognizing and acknowledging one's actions is a trademark of professional behavior. Staff across the organization are empowered to participate in an error-reporting system without fear of punitive action. Safety principles to eliminate hazards are a primary consideration in job design, equipment, working conditions, and simplifying and standardizing processes.

There are incentives for safety culture. The Joint Commission (2015) issues annual patient safety goals and has regulations that focus on safety, such as requiring a policy about civility among employees. Due to the increased focus on adverse outcomes, system gaps, quality improvement, and transparency of outcome data, there are stronger mandates by accrediting and payers for clinical agencies to implement safety culture. What used to be optional growth opportunities for healthcare systems are now becoming mandatory.

NURSES SHAPING ORGANIZATIONAL IMPROVEMENTS IN SAFETY

Nurses are a primary driver in developing safety culture because of their front-line presence with patients and families, their role in continuous assessment, and their skills in clinical decision-making. The Quality and Safety Education for Nurses (QSEN) (Cronenwett et al., 2007) project defined six competencies to prepare nurses to participate in and lead system redesign to improve safety and reduce patient harm. They are as follows:

- **Patient-centered care:** The patient and family are at the center of the decision-making process and understand the plan of care, which can prevent errors from occurring (Walton and Barnsteiner, 2012).

- **Evidence-based practice:** Clinicians use up-to-date science and consider clinical expertise and patient values to design a plan of care (Tracy and Barnsteiner, 2012).

■ **Teamwork and collaboration:** The healthcare team communicates and works together effectively with shared decision-making among professionals to achieve safe, high-quality care (Disch, 2012).

■ **Quality improvement:** Trending and analysis of data is provided to benchmark with comparable organizations and identify vulnerabilities in the system needing correction (Johnson, 2012).

■ **Informatics:** Clinicians use information and technology to communicate, access knowledge, and support decision-making to promote safe care (Warren, 2012).

■ **Safety:** Risk of harm to patients and providers is minimized through both system effectiveness and individual performance (Barnsteiner, 2012).

 You can find more complete information about these competencies on the QSEN website (www.qsen.org).

These competencies are essential for all health professionals in the drive to reduce patient harm. The essential knowledge, skills, and attitudes help build a workforce focused on developing teamwork behaviors and new communication skills, implementing safety enhancements that reduce reliance on memory through electronic and technology applications, and recognizing risk factors to focus on prevention of harm. Applying principles of safety design to eliminate unsafe practices such as shortcuts, workarounds, and dangerous abbreviations are workforce skills for building highly reliable systems.

HIGH RELIABILITY ORGANIZATIONS

With increased appreciation for the complexity of healthcare systems, healthcare leaders have recently looked to other industries, such as aviation and nuclear energy, where high-stakes errors are a concern due to complexity and risk. Identifying common system approaches in these industries has led healthcare leaders to increasingly apply attributes of HRO organizations. For example, like aviation, healthcare delivery systems are complex, with multiple interacting human factors. There are numerous threats to patient safety. High-impact errors can occur at all interfaces of care delivery. The lack of standardized processes and inherently complex operations contribute to the high number of unintended adverse and sentinel events in healthcare delivery systems, as first revealed in the 1999 IOM report. Patients should not be caught at the intersection of poorly designed processes and ineffective organizational culture. The principles learned from HROs offer a model to reduce obstacles to create a safe system that improves patient outcomes.

HROS AND SAFETY CULTURE

HROs manage work that involves hazardous environments (for example, nuclear power plants and air traffic control agencies) with a high possibility of error but actually experience low adverse events (Baker, Day, and Salas, 2006; AHRQ, 2008). Near misses are treated as opportunities to improve by examining gaps and correcting design flaws. In complex work environments, different team members may have critical information at different times. Each is empowered to speak up regardless of rank. HROs concentrate on standardizing processes across multiple system components so that results are predictable, thus improving reliability.

To examine the impact of how HROs are transformed, we must consider how systems operate and create culture. Systems are a set of interdependent components that interact to achieve a common goal. For example, a hospital is a system composed of service lines such as medical, cardiovascular, etc.; nursing care units; ancillary care departments; outpatient care clinics; the emergency department; and multiple others. The way these separate but dependent system components interact and work together is a significant factor in delivering high-quality, safe care. To achieve high reliability, organizational leaders must align quality and safety goals with the organization's mission and vision to develop processes that ensure these goals are addressed consistently throughout all areas and levels of the system. HROs focus on safety with mindful awareness of where the next error may occur (Barnsteiner, 2012). HROs monitor safety outcomes by systematically collecting data on sentinel events and near misses by reviewing according to standardized processes (AHRQ, 2008).

THE FIVE PRINCIPLES OF HROS

Five principles of HROs are as follows:

- **Sensitivity to operations:** Maintain situational awareness for quick notice of outliers or process anomalies to prevent larger consequences from errors.

- **Preoccupation with failure:** Focus on predicting and eliminating errors rather than being in the position of reacting to errors.

- **Reluctance to simplify:** Accept the complexity inherent in the system and seek multiple views and checks and balances.

- **Deference to expertise:** Cultivate a culture that shifts from authority to shared decision-making with those expert in the situation at hand.

- **Commitment to resilience:** Pay close attention to the organization's ability to quickly contain errors and return to functioning despite setbacks.

For more information, visit www.ahrq.gov.

In promoting a culture of safety, HROs foster a learning environment to ensure evidence-based care and promote positive working environments. Baker, Day, and Salas (2006) discuss how HROs implement a safety- and quality-centered culture, involve all levels of leadership and front-line personnel, align safety and quality efforts with the strategic plan, and promote continuous improvement. Employees are engaged in detecting high-risk situations, resources are dedicated to developing change, employees are empowered to act in dangerous situations, and the work environment is fair to employees (Page, 2004).

Reliability is expecting to get the same result each time an action occurs. Therefore, a reliable system seeks to have defect-free operations in spite of a high-risk environment (Riley, 2009). Healthcare organizations have reasons to seek reliability. Regulatory agencies are focusing on reduction in patient harm by linking hospital reimbursement to quality, safe care that may best be achieved through reliable processes and procedures (Schumann, 2012). Hospitals may be denied reimbursement for patient harms such as hospital-acquired infections (HAIs). Therefore, intense efforts must be made to follow handwashing procedures, adhere to evidence-based catheter insertion and care guidelines, and other evidence-based best practices.

NINE CRITICAL AREAS FOR IMPROVING SAFETY OUTCOMES

To facilitate the transformation of healthcare systems to achieve cultures of safety by integrating principles of HROs, the 2001 IOM report identified nine areas that are critical to improve safety outcomes and reliability. These areas provide a cross-reference for living the five principles of HROs described in the preceding section:

- **Apply user-centered design:** This makes it easier for the clinician to perform the right action. This includes alerts for patients who are at high risk for falls, labeling the correct body part prior to surgery, and a forcing function that makes the wrong choice impossible, such as tubing misconnection.

- **Avoid reliance on memory:** Standardize and simplify procedures and tasks, follow protocols and checklists, and take advantage of alarms and alerts.

- **Attend to work safety:** Manage work hours, workloads, staffing ratios, distractions, interruptions, and safe zones.

- **Avoid reliance on vigilance:** Use checklists, well-designed alarms, rotating staff, and breaks to lessen fatigue.

- **Implement training concepts for teams:** This fosters effective intra- and interprofessional communication and collaboration as well as teamwork behaviors.

■ **Involve patients in their care:** Include patients and their families in decisions about treatments, discharge planning, and education; share care plans; and hold rounds in patient rooms.

■ **Anticipate the unexpected:** Include front-line users in planning change and pilot testing before widespread implementation to identify vulnerabilities that may affect patient safety.

■ **Design for recovery:** Use simulation to practice and manage disaster situations.

■ **Improve access to accurate, timely information:** This includes decision-support tools, drug formularies, evidence-based standards, and patient records.

STEEEP

Since 2001, the IOM has provided healthcare delivery organizations with a road map to improve quality and safety using the STEEEP model (see Figure 2.1). STEEEP outlines performance measures to ensure care is as follows:

■ Safe   ■ Efficient

■ Timely   ■ Equitable

■ Effective   ■ Patient-centered

These aims provide the measures of quality and accountability that further align with the goals of high reliability and reimbursement regulations.

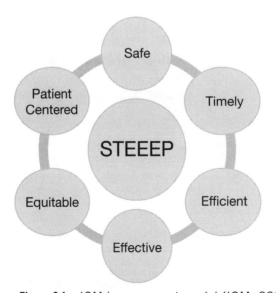

Figure 2.1   IOM improvement model (IOM, 2003).

DRIVERS FOR SAFETY IN HROS

With an increased capacity for tracking errors and system gaps across settings, system-focused improvements are increasingly important. Understanding healthcare systems as complex adaptive systems is the basis for transforming organizations as HROs. By examining the interplay of people, work processes, technology, and the environment, healthcare systems are beginning to integrate the science of human factors into their operations. HROs have increased attention to standardized processes, systematic reporting and review of patient harms, and provider education and training about safety.

This section examines seven current drivers for improving patient safety outcomes through HROs:

- Human factors
- Teamwork and collaboration
- Communication
- Handovers
- Medication administration
- Adverse event reporting systems

HUMAN FACTORS

Human factors are the science of defining the interrelationship among humans, the technology they use, and the environment in which they work (IOM, 1999). Adapted from engineering principles, human factors consider components of human-system interfaces; organizational, social, and physical environments; the nature of the work being done; individual characteristics; and aspects of performance (Henrickson, Dayton, Keyes, Carayon, and Hughes, 2008).

Human factors consider how the "human condition" influences how we do our work. The study of human factors may examine the challenge of doing multiple things at once, yet maintaining accuracy. Actions may be the result of mental models we develop from performing recurrent tasks that become well-developed habits, such as admitting a patient or administering an intramuscular injection. Human factors flip the paradigm to emphasize the anticipation and prevention of harm rather than reacting to harm. Fatigue, distraction, and interruptions affect cognitive abilities, which lessens the capacity to see error potential and problem-solve (Reason, 2000). To improve reliability and thus safety, systems can be designed to reduce the probability of errors or harm to patients or employees.

By focusing on system failures rather than human failures, systems can apply human factors to protect against human errors and to address needs of clinicians within the healthcare system. The very nature of nurses' work involves frequent interruptions, a high risk factor (Brixey et al., 2005). On average, nurses are interrupted 12 times per hour. Most interruptions (22%) occur while performing tasks critical to safety, such as administering medications (Trbovich, Prakash, Stewart, Trip, and Savage, 2010).

How can the application of human factors enable nurses to develop proactive approaches to deal with multitasking, distractions, fatigue, physical injury, and workload variability? Improving safety requires all team members, regardless of the role they play in a healthcare system, to work mindfully to recognize safety hazards. All must be mindful of the importance of interdependent system factors that affect safe care, yet recognize and report system demands on the clinical environment. In this way, human factors are also dependent on other safety drivers such as teamwork and collaboration, communication, and a systematic adverse event reporting system.

TEAMWORK AND COLLABORATION

The definition of teamwork and collaboration from the QSEN framework (refer to the section "Nurses Shaping Organizational Improvements in Safety" earlier in this chapter) focuses on developing the individual strengths of each team member to improve collective actions (Disch, 2012). Teamwork and collaboration are the basis for the interprofessional education competencies approved for all the major health professionals in 2011 by the Interprofessional Education Collaborative (IPEC). Healthcare professionals must achieve the knowledge, skills, and attitudes for the four competency domains that define interprofessional education. These domains are as follows:

- Knowing the roles and responsibilities of each team member
- Respecting the ethics and values for interprofessional practice
- Developing effective interprofessional communication
- Implementing effective approaches to teamwork and collaboration (IPEC, 2011)

Team refers to anyone who is involved in the care of a patient. Teams are flexible and dynamic, with members constantly shifting through the continuum of care. Teamwork behaviors define how team members work together to accomplish patient care. Patients engaged in their care become valuable team members and should be empowered with information and coaching to join in decisions about their care. Effectively working together is a key strategy for safe care.

Collaboration achieves a mutually satisfying solution, resulting in the best outcome. Collaboration begins with self-development based on emotional intelligence to monitor appropriate reactions and responses to team members. Collaboration is a win-win for everyone on the team, including patients and families. Collaboration is a process—a way of working together with commitment to a common mission. Developing an attitude of collaboration across the healthcare team to ensure safe coordination of care contributes to safe care. Teamwork and collaboration is the collective and shared environmental scanning and engagement of all team members (for example, patients, families, all disciplines, and staff) to maintain safety and prevent patient harm. In effective teams, leadership is shared and shifts to the provider most expert in the situation.

The aviation industry implemented crew resource management to emphasize the role of human factors in high-stress, high-risk work environments by improving teamwork (Oriol, 2006). The five domains of crew resource management (see Figure 2.2) can apply to both healthcare and aviation. Both environments are noted for high stress, complexity, the need for highly function-ing teams, the importance of accurate and precise communication, and a high cost of system failures. Crew resource management has improved team functioning in operating rooms, emer-gency departments, labor and delivery teams, and peri-operative teams (Salas, Wilson, Burke, and Wightman, 2006). For example, to manage distractions while administering medications, nurses applied crew resource management principles of aviation's sterile cockpit procedures in a unit-based project. The number of distractions and medication error rates reduced over time through the use of "Do Not Disturb" signs and the wearing of identifying orange vests while administering medications (Fore, Sculli, Albee, and Neily, 2013).

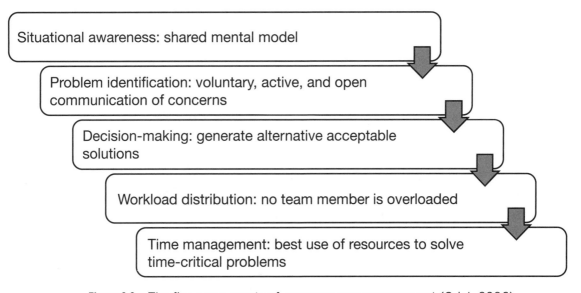

Figure 2.2   The five components of crew resource management (Oriol, 2006).

COMMUNICATION

Communication drives safe care. How well (or how poorly) healthcare professionals communicate and work together accounts for as much as 70% of healthcare errors (IOM, 1999). Ineffective communication, hierarchy, and disruptive behavior are challenges to patient safety but can be addressed through education and training. Cross-discipline communication is the foundation for smooth care coordination. Understanding the scope of responsibility and roles for all providers fosters effective communication and routing of critical information. Organizations must provide a safe environment in which anyone in the organization can speak up when safety is compromised (Armstrong and Sherwood, 2012). All team members must be taught skills in problem-solving, conflict resolution, and negotiation to help coordinate safe care across interprofessional teams (IPEC, 2011).

There are several approaches for effective healthcare communication such as using crew resource management (Oriol, 2006) or Team Strategies and Tools to Enhance Performance and Patient Safety (TeamSTEPPS), an evidence-based curriculum available from AHRQ (2008). Education and workplace training for all health professionals must include opportunities to learn and practice effective communication (IOM, 2003) for sharing critical information, solving problems, and resolving conflict. Standardized communication, discussed in the next section, can ensure safe handovers between providers or settings, provide clear direction in seeking and sharing information between providers, and instill collaborative behaviors for speaking up to prevent errors from occurring.

HANDOVERS

The Joint Commission International Center for Patient Safety defines *handover* (also known as *handoff*) as the real-time process of passing patient-specific information from one caregiver or team of caregivers to another to ensure continuity and safety of care (The Joint Commission, 2005). Handing over a patient from one nurse to another is a daily part of nursing practice and may occur at shift change, from one unit to another, discharge, or anytime there is a change in who has responsibility for the patient (Dayton and Henriksen, 2007; Riesenberg, Leitzsch, and Cunningham, 2010). Transitions in care and handovers are vulnerable points in healthcare. As high-risk activities, they require a standardized process built on effective communication (Dayton and Henriksen, 2007; Friesen, White, and Byers, 2008; Welsh, Flanagan, and Ebright, 2010). Standardized change of shift reporting checklists, communication between providers using SBAR (situation, background, assessment, and recommendation) (Disch, 2012), and safety huddles among front-line staff are evidence-based handover strategies that demonstrate improvements in patient safety (Gerke, Uffelman, and Chandler, 2010).

MEDICATION ADMINISTRATION

Safe medication administration is a team effort with carefully orchestrated interactions among physicians, pharmacists, and nurses. Nurses typically administer medications provided by pharmacists based on orders from physicians. The complex interactions are error-prone. Medication errors account for more than 7,000 deaths annually (IOM, 2006). Medication errors are the largest category of error. Inpatients are likely to experience at least one medication error per day. About 4% of patients experience a serious medical error during their hospitalization. At least 1.5 million preventable adverse drug events occur each year.

Applying advances in technology can help reduce medication errors. Examples include using system alerts for high-risk medications, alerts during administration to indicate a solution has infused, or warnings for sound-alike, look-alike medications. Other strategies include wearing an identifying vest while administering medications to help reduce interruptions and distractions and applying principles of mindfulness (Fore et al., 2013).

Redundant patient-identifying procedures may seem annoying, but they demonstrate how double-check practices ensure the correct patient receives the correct medication. Engaging patients and families as safety allies encourages them to speak up if they are unsure of the medications administered. They can help prevent medication errors by being empowered to ask questions. Transparency in sharing information about medication errors across the system helps prevent errors in other units, thus demonstrating the power of systematic reporting and reviewing both medication errors and critical near misses. Medication safety is an example of the interplay of the system and individual providers, of technology and human design, and of the application of human factors to create reliable medication administration procedures.

SYSTEMATIC PATIENT HARM REPORTING SYSTEM

This chapter has discussed the importance of speaking up about safety, particularly through a systematic patient harm reporting system. Safety depends on organizational support for a systematic patient harm reporting system within a safe environment to increase the capacity of every staff member to speak up about safety (Wolf and Hughes, 2008). Education and workplace training on patient harm and error reporting is the basis for improving care through learned experiences. Still, recent research suggests that physician underreporting may be as high as 96% (Harper and Helmreich, 2014).

Trained investigators may use root cause analysis (RCA) or failure mode and effects analysis (FMEA) to examine factors contributing to an adverse event or near miss (Johnson, 2012). RCA is typically performed after an event. FMEA, an evaluation process to identify failures, problems, or errors in a system, can be employed before errors occur. Using FMEA when a gap is identified allows for a redesign of the process to eliminate the risk. By examining all sentinel events to outline the action sequence leading up to the event, the factors that contributed to the event can be identified and studied. Using these systematic review processes and procedures is part of designing a more reliable, safe healthcare system.

 Resources to guide implementation of RCA and FMEA are available on the AHRQ website (http://www.ahrq.gov/professionals/quality-patient-safety/patient-safety-resources/index.html).

KEY RESOURCES

- **Agency for Healthcare Research and Quality:** http://www.ahrq.gov
- **Institute for Healthcare Improvement (IHI):** www.ihi.org
- **Institute for Safe Medication Practices (ISMP):** www.ismp.org
- **Institute of Medicine (IOM):** www.iom.edu
- **The Joint Commission:** www.jointcommission.org
- **Joint Commission Resources Quality and Safety Network:** http://www.jcrqsn.com
- **National Patient Safety Foundation:** http://www.npsf.org/
- **National Quality Forum:** http://www.qualityforum.org
- **Patient Safety Institute:** http://www.ptsafety.org
- **Quality and Safety Education for Nurses (QSEN):** www.qsen.org
- **Robert Wood Johnson Foundation Transforming Care at the Bedside Toolkit:** http://www.rwjf.org/pr/product.jsp?id=30051
- **TeamSTEPPS:** http://teamstepps.ahrq.gov
- **VA National Center for Patient Safety:** http://www.patientsafety.va.gov/

SUMMARY

The Institute of Medicine Roundtable on Value and Science-Driven Healthcare (IOM, n.d.) introduced the concept of a learning healthcare system as one that optimizes effective teamwork, communication, safety culture, and quality improvement. A learning healthcare system is defined as a system that aligns science, informatics, incentives, and culture to be able to approach operations for continuous improvement and innovation. Best practices are seamlessly embedded in caring for patients and families, who become active participants in all aspects of their care. New knowledge is reflectively captured as an integral byproduct of the work of the system. This is an ambitious goal for our healthcare system, but this framework is the basis for eventually bringing together all facets of improvement. The current drivers promoting safer systems and fewer adverse outcomes come out of their silos to achieve a connected, integrated approach through a synergistic adoption of reliability. By bringing together the guiding forces in healthcare, we can coalesce on common goals and shared outcomes for improvement. The mandate for safer, highly reliable systems is clear and is becoming stronger. Systems that work toward integrating high reliability practices will be best equipped to change outcomes so that we can expect the same effective results every time.

KEY POINTS

- Organizations that support safety culture provide opportunities for individuals to integrate the QSEN and IPEC competencies as part of system improvement.

- HROs focus on improvements through changing the way people interact and work together, coordinating care, and redesigning healthcare processes.

- Principles from HROs applied to key safety drivers (that is, human factors, teamwork and collaboration, communication, handovers, systematic adverse event reporting systems, and safe medication administration) reduce harm and improve patient outcomes.

- Applying a human factors framework to guide research in identifying and quantifying processes that lead to error will increase our understanding of the complexity of nurses' work in the acute care environment.

REFERENCES

Agency for Healthcare Research and Quality. (2008). Becoming a high reliability organization: Operational advice for hospital leaders. Retrieved from http://www.ahrq.gov/qual/hroadvice/hroadvice.pdf

Armstrong, G., and Sherwood, G. (2012). Patient safety. In J. F. Giddens (Ed.), *Concepts for nursing practice* (pp. 434–442). St. Louis, MO: Elsevier.

Baker, D. P., Day, R., and Salas, E. (2006). Teamwork as an essential component of high-reliability organizations. *Health Services Research*, *41*(4), pp. 1576–1598.

Barnsteiner, J. (2012). Safety. In G. Sherwood and J. Barnsteiner (Eds.), *Quality and safety in nursing: A competency approach to improving outcomes* (pp. 149–170). Hoboken, NJ: Wiley-Blackwell.

Bellot, J. (2011). Defining and assessing organizational culture. *Nursing Forum*, *46*(1), pp. 29–37. doi: 10.1111/j.1744-6198.2010.00207

Boysen, P. G. (2013). Just culture: A foundation for balanced accountability for patient safety. *The Ochsner Journal*, *13*(3), pp. 400–406.

Brixey, J. J., Robinson, D. J., Tang, Z., Johnson, T. R., Zhang, J., and Turley, J. P. (2005). Interruptions in workflow for RNs in a level one trauma center. AMIA Annual Symposium Proceedings, pp. 86–90.

Cronenwett, L., Sherwood, G., Barnsteiner, J., Disch, J., Johnson, J., Mitchell, P., Sullivan, D. T., and Warren, J. (2007). Quality and safety education for nurses. *Nursing outlook*, *55*(3), pp. 122–131.

Dayton, E., and Henriksen, K. (2007). Communication failure: Basic components, contributing factors, and the call for structure. *Joint Commission Journal on Quality and Patient Safety/Joint Commission Resources*, *33*(1), pp. 34–47.

Dekker, S. (2011). *Patient safety: A human factors approach*. Boca Raton, FL: CRC Press, Taylor and Francis Group.

Disch, J. (2012). Teamwork and collaboration. In G. Sherwood and J. Barnsteiner (Eds.), *Quality and safety in nursing: A competency approach to improving outcomes* (pp. 91–112). Hoboken, NJ: Wiley-Blackwell.

Fore, A. M., Sculli, G. L., Albee, D., and Neily, J. (2013). Improving patient safety using the sterile cockpit principle during medication administration: A collaborative, unit-based project. *Journal of Nursing Management, 21*(1), pp. 106–111.

Friesen, M. A., White, S. V., and Byers, J. F. (2008). Handoffs: Implications for nurses. In R. G. Hughes (Ed.), *Patient safety and quality: An evidence-based handbook for nurses* (pp. 2-285–2-333). Rockville, MD: Agency for Healthcare Research and Quality, Publication No. 08-0043.

Gerke, M. L., Uffelman, C., and Chandler, K. W. (2010). Safety huddles for a culture of safety. *Patient Safety and Quality Healthcare*, May/June, pp. 24–28.

Harper, M. L., and Helmreich, R. L. (2014). Identifying barriers to the success of a reporting system. In *Advances in patient safety*. Rockville, MD: Agency for Healthcare Research and Quality. Retrieved from http://www.ahrq.gov/professionals/quality-patient-safety/patient-safety-resources/resources/advances-in-patient-safety/index.html

HealthDay News. (2008). Medical errors costing U.S. billions. Retrieved from http://www.washingtonpost.com/wp-dyn/content/article/2008/04/08/AR2008040800957.html

Henrickson, K., Dayton, E., Keyes, M. A., Carayon, P., and Hughes, R. (2008). Understanding adverse events: A human factors framework. In R. G. Hughes (Ed.), *Patient safety and quality: An evidence-based handbook for nurses* (pp. 1-67–1-85). Rockville, MD: Agency for Healthcare Research and Quality (AHRQ), Publication No. 08-0043.

Institute of Medicine. (n.d.). Roundtable on value and science-driven health care. Retrieved from http://iom.nationalacademies.org/Activities/Quality/VSRT.aspx

Institute of Medicine. (1999). *To err is human: Building a safer health system*. Washington, DC: The National Academies Press.

Institute of Medicine. (2001). *Crossing the quality chasm: A new health system for the 21st century*. Washington, DC: The National Academies Press.

Institute of Medicine. (2003). *Health professions education: A bridge to quality*. Washington, DC: The National Academies Press.

Institute of Medicine. (2006). *Identifying and preventing medication errors*. Washington, DC: The National Academies Press.

Interprofessional Education Collaborative (IPEC) Expert Panel. (2011). *Core competencies for interprofessional collaborative practice: Report of an expert panel*. Washington, DC: Interprofessional Education Collaborative.

James, J. T. (2013). A new, evidence-based estimate of patient harms associated with hospital care. *Journal of Patient Safety, 9*(3), pp. 122–128. doi: 10.1097/PTS.0b013e3182948a69

Johnson, J. (2012). Quality improvement. In G. Sherwood and J. Barnsteiner (Eds.), *Quality and safety in nursing: A competency approach to improving outcomes* (pp. 113–132). Hoboken, NJ: Wiley-Blackwell.

The Joint Commission. (2015). National patient safety goals. Retrieved from http://www.jointcommission.org/standards_information/npsgs.aspx

The Joint Commission. (2005). Joint Commission International Center for Patient Safety offers new web site. *Joint Commission Perspectives, 25*(6), pp. 1–2(2).

Mitchell, P. (2008). Defining patient safety and quality care. In R. G. Hughes (Ed.), *Patient safety and quality: An evidence-based handbook for nurses* (pp. 1-1–1-6). Rockville, MD: Agency for Healthcare Research and Quality, Publication No. 08-0043.

National Patient Safety Foundation's Lucian Leape Institute. (2014). Safety is personal: Partnering with patients and families for the safest care. Boston, MA: National Patient Safety Foundation. Retrieved from http://www.npsf.org/?page=safetyispersonal

National Safety Council. (n.d.). Near miss reporting systems. Retrieved from http://www.nsc.org/WorkplaceTrainingDocuments/Near-Miss-Reporting-Systems.pdf

Oriol, M. D. (2006). Crew resource management: Applications in healthcare organizations. *Journal of Nursing Administration, 36*(9), pp. 402–406.

Page, A., Ed. (2004). Keeping patients safe: Transforming the work environment of nurses. Committee on the Work Environment for Nurses and Patient Safety. Washington, DC: The National Academies Press.

Reason, J. (2000). Human error: Models and management. *British Medical Journal, 320*(7237), pp. 768–770.

Riesenberg, L. A., Leitzsch, J., and Cunningham, J. M. (2010). Nursing handoffs: A systematic review of the literature. *American Journal of Nursing, 110*(4), 24–34.

Riley, W. (2009). High reliability and implications for nursing leaders. *Journal of Nursing Management, 17*(2), pp. 238–246. doi: 10.1111/j.1365-2834.2009.00971.x

Salas, E., Wilson, K. A., Burke, C. S., and Wightman, D. C. (2006). Does crew resource management training work? An update, an extension and some critical needs. *Human Factors, 48*(2), pp. 392–412.

Sammer, C., Lykens, K., Singh, K. P., Mains, D. A., and Lackan, N. A. (2010). What is patient safety culture? A review of the literature. *Journal of Nursing Scholarship, 42*(2), 156–165.

Schein, E. H. (2010). *Organizational culture and leadership.* San Francisco, CA: Josey-Bass.

Schumann, M. J. (2012). Policy implications driving national quality and safety initiatives. In G. Sherwood and J. Barnsteiner (Eds.), *Quality and safety in nursing: A competency approach to improving outcomes* (pp. 23–48). Hoboken, NJ: Wiley-Blackwell.

Sherwood, G. (2012). Driving forces for quality and safety: Changing mindsets to improve healthcare. In G. Sherwood and J. Barnsteiner (Eds.), *Quality and safety in nursing: A competency approach to improving outcomes* (pp. 3–21). Hoboken, NJ: Wiley-Blackwell.

Singer, S. J., Falwell, A., Gaba, D. M., Meterko, M., Rosen, A., Hartmann, C. W., and Baker, L. (2009). Identifying organizational cultures that promote patient safety. *Health Care Management Review, 34*(4), 300–311.

Tracy, M. F., and Barnsteiner, J. (2012). Evidence-based practice. In G. Sherwood and J. Barnsteiner (Eds.), *Quality and safety in nursing: A competency approach to improving outcomes* (pp. 133–148). Hoboken, NJ: Wiley-Blackwell.

Trbovich, P., Prakash, V., Stewart, J., Trip, K., and Savage, P. (2010). Interruptions during the delivery of high-risk medications. *Journal of Nursing Administration, 40*(5), pp. 211–218.

Wachter, R. M., and Pronovost, P. J. (2009). Balancing "no blame" with accountability in patient safety. *New England Journal of Medicine, 361*(14), pp. 1401–1406.

Walton, M. K., and Barnsteiner, J. (2012). Patient-centered care. In G. Sherwood and J. Barnsteiner (Eds.), *Quality and safety in nursing: A competency approach to improving outcomes* (pp. 67–90). Hoboken, NJ: Wiley-Blackwell.

Warren, J. (2012). Informatics. In G. Sherwood and J. Barnsteiner (Eds.), *Quality and safety in nursing: A competency approach to improving outcomes* (pp. 171–187). Hoboken, NJ: Wiley-Blackwell.

Welsh, C. A., Flanagan, M. E., and Ebright, P. (2010). Barriers and facilitators to nursing handoffs: Recommendations for redesign. *Nursing Outlook, 58*(3), pp. 148–154.

Wolf, Z. R., and Hughes, R. G. (2008). Error reporting and disclosure. In R. G. Hughes (Ed.), *Patient safety and quality: An evidence-based handbook for nurses* (pp. 2-333–2-379). Rockville, MD: Agency for Healthcare Research and Quality (AHRA), Publication No. 08-0043.

CHAPTER 3

CURRENT QUALITY DRIVERS

Mary Beth Flynn Makic, PhD, RN, CNS, CCNS, FAAN, FNAP

The healthcare community and the public became vividly aware of the issue of quality in healthcare with the Institute of Medicine's publication, "Crossing the Quality Chasm: A New Health System for the 21st Century" (2001). This seminal document challenged healthcare systems and professionals to critically examine the way care was provided in order to improve patient outcomes.

The report provided six critical elements that, if incorporated into daily patient care, could positively affect patient outcomes. These six elements suggest that care should be as follows (IOM, 2001):

- Safe
- Effective
- Patient-centered
- Timely
- Efficient
- Equitable

Current quality drivers for patient and healthcare outcomes continue to embrace these six tenets for consistent delivery of high-quality care. Today, the healthcare industry continues to strive to provide care that minimizes errors and

> Improvement begins with I.
>
> —*Arnold H. Glasow*

embraces current best evidence to achieve exceptional performance in quality, safety, and cost effectiveness (Melnyk, 2012; Harder and Marc, 2013).

Embracing key elements found within high reliability organizations (HROs) provides a framework for developing and sustaining a culture within healthcare organizations to deliver safe care that minimizes error (Melnyk, 2012). Nurses are critical to the success of the healthcare team in meeting the public's expectation of safe, high-quality care with every healthcare encounter.

DRIVERS OF QUALITY INDICATORS

Multiple dynamics define and drive current and future quality metrics. The drivers that influence quality metrics can be broadly categorized into four groups:

- Patient and population expectations

- Regulatory and accreditation quality metrics

- Financial efficiency

- Healthcare and hospital administration (Carayon, Xie, and Kianfar, 2013)

PATIENT AND POPULATION EXPECTATIONS

Public conversations about healthcare quality and the ability of patients to search for information about healthcare on the Internet have directly and indirectly influenced quality care expectations. Savvy consumers have numerous opportunities to search the Internet for healthcare information from the following sources:

- Government sources, such as https://www.nlm.nih.gov/medlineplus/, www.cdc.gov, www.medicare.gov/hospitalcompare/About/What-Is-HOS.html, etc.

- Private not-for profit sources, such as http://www.aarphealthcare.com, http://www.aha.org, etc.

- Healthcare-specific websites, such as http://www.mayoclinic.org, http://www.webmd.com, etc.

Media reports, such as those found at http://healthleadersmedia.com/Quality, may influence quality expectations. Additionally, social networking sites have been found to effect changes in health behaviors, but little is currently understood about the influence of social networks in driving quality metrics (Laranjo et al., 2015).

Patients seeking healthcare services expect quality care. Patient satisfaction with care is measured by healthcare organizations and is tied to reimbursement—for example, through Hospital Consumer Assessment of Healthcare Providers and Systems (HCAHPS) surveys. Early research found that public reporting of HCAHPS increased hospital transparency, improved consumer decision-making, and increased incentives for organizations that provided high-quality healthcare (Giordano, Elliott, Goldstein, Lehrman, and Spencer, 2010). A recent study found a positive association between organizations with high HCAHPS scores, high performance outcomes, and other Centers for Medicare and Medicaid Services (CMS) pay-for-performance programs (Doyle, Lennox, and Bell, 2013).

Information about hospital performance is obtained through a national, standardized HCAHPS survey. The survey consists of 32 items that explore patients' perceptions of their hospital experience and their level of satisfaction (HCAHPS Fact Sheet, 2015). The goal of HCAHPS is threefold:

- To obtain standardized, objective, meaningful information, allowing for the comparison of hospital experiences
- Public reporting of survey findings, providing incentives for hospitals to improve care
- Increased transparency of hospital care

Table 3.1 provides survey question domains to measure quality. Healthcare organizations actively use HCAHPS metrics to evaluate overall hospital performance. Patient satisfaction, which is largely influenced by quality of care, is a key driver for organizations, which strive to consistently achieve high quality outcomes.

TABLE 3.1   HCAHPS SURVEY QUESTION DOMAINS

Domain	Focus of Questions
Summary measure items	Providers' communication with patient
	Nurses' communication with patient
	Staff responsiveness to the patient's needs
	How well the patient's pain was managed
	How well the staff communicated with the patient about new medicines
	Whether key information was provided at discharge
	The patient's understanding of care needed after discharge

continues

TABLE 3.1   HCAHPS SURVEY QUESTION DOMAINS   (CONTINUED)

Domain	Focus of Questions
Individual items	Cleanliness of patient room
	Quietness of patient room
Global items	Overall hospital rating
	Would the patient recommend the hospital to family and friends

Adapted from HCAHPS (2015)

REGULATORY AND ACCREDITATION QUALITY METRICS

Individually and collaboratively, regulatory and accreditation agencies define and influence quality metrics for care. Organizations have long used regulatory and accreditation agencies to provide drivers for quality care metrics. The most notable agencies are The Joint Commission (TJC) and CMS. Both these organizations drive quality by publishing quality metrics, which healthcare agencies strive to meet or face financial consequences. TJC began publishing core measures in 1999 (TJC, 2015a), and in 2007, CMS instituted quality metrics for serious reportable events, frequently referred to as *never events*, beginning with wrong-site surgery. Both these agencies work independently and collaboratively to identify gaps in quality of care and to set standards for patient outcomes.

Another significant regulatory driver for improving quality care is the National Quality Forum (NQF). The NQF is an influential nonprofit organization that identifies gaps in healthcare and endorses evidence-based solutions to improve healthcare outcomes (National Quality Forum, n.d.). NQF coined the term *never event* in 2001 in reference to particularly shocking medical errors (such as wrong-site surgery) that should never occur. The list of adverse events recognizes care outcomes that are clearly identifiable and measurable and that can result in significant harm.

A nursing-specific accrediting agency that influences quality drivers is the American Nurses Credentialing Center (ANCC) Magnet Recognition Program® (ANCC, 2015). Organizations that want to be recognized as Magnet® hospitals need to demonstrate a culture of safety and quality in the delivery of evidence-based, patient-family–centered care (Swanson and Tidwell, 2011). Nursing-sensitive quality indicators have been identified as important metrics for hospitals to demonstrate the impact of nursing care excellence and outcomes (Montalvo, 2007).

KEY RESOURCES FOR REGULATORY AND ACCREDITATION QUALITY METRICS

- **The Joint Commission Patient Safety page:** http://www.jointcommission.org/topics/patient_safety.aspx
- **The Centers for Medicare and Medicaid Services Quality Measures page:** https://www.cms.gov/Medicare/Quality-Initiatives-Patient-Assessment-Instruments/QualityMeasures/index.html
- **The Joint Commission Core Measure Sets page:** http://www.jointcommission.org/core_measure_sets.aspx
- **The National Quality Forum Measuring Performance page:** http://www.qualityforum.org/Measuring_Performance/Measuring_Performance.aspx
- **The American Nurses Credentialing Center Magnet Recognition Program® page:** http://www.nursecredentialing.org/Magnet

FINANCIAL EFFICIENCY

Financial incentives are tied to several regulatory influences for quality care. For example, CMS does not reimburse an organization if an error in care occurs—especially if the error has been identified by CMS as a never event or preventable adverse patient outcome. Other CMS initiatives that result in reduced or denied payment are the Readmissions Reduction Program and the Hospital-Acquired Condition (HAC) Reduction Program. Hospitals with poor performance face financial penalties.

KEY RESOURCES FOR FINANCIAL EFFICIENCY

- **CMS Preventable Outcomes document:** http://downloads.cms.gov/cmsgov/archived-downloads/SMDL/downloads/SMD073108.pdf
- **CMS Readmissions Reduction Program page:** https://www.cms.gov/Medicare/medicare-fee-for-service-payment/acuteinpatientPPS/readmissions-reduction-program.html
- **CMS Hospital-Acquired Condition (HAC) Reduction Program page:** https://www.cms.gov/Medicare/Medicare-Fee-for-Service-Payment/AcuteInpatientPPS/HAC-Reduction-Program.html

The Affordable Care Act (ACA) has incorporated several pay-for-performance measures that, if unmet, result in reduced financial reimbursement. The Hospital Value-Based Purchasing (VBP) Program, which is part of the ACA, financially incentivizes organizations to deliver high-value quality care to Medicare recipients. Hospitals participating in the VBP Program are eligible for a variety of performance-based incentive payments from CMS—*if* they meet quality measurements in six areas (Blumenthal and Jena, 2013; CMS, 2015; Brooks, 2014):

■ Patient safety

■ Care coordination

■ Clinical process and outcomes

■ Population/community health

■ Efficiency and cost reduction

■ Patient/caregiver–centered experience

The HCAHPS survey provides essential outcome data used in calculating VBP incentives paid to hospitals. HCAHPS performance has driven up to 30% of a hospital's VBP score, affecting incentive payments (Blumenthal and Jena, 2013; Dempsey, Reilly, and Buhlman, 2014). Growing numbers of healthcare consumers who are Medicare patients are influencing organizations' need to improve the safety and quality of care as well as overall patient satisfaction. Similarly, insurance organizations provide reimbursement depending on high-quality care outcomes and the efficiency of resources used to achieve high, reliable results.

HEALTHCARE AND HOSPITAL ADMINISTRATION

The summative impact of patient expectations, regulatory guidelines, and reimbursement for services provided has shaped the quality lens of healthcare administrators and chief nursing officers. The financial structure of healthcare is increasingly tied to quality of care and patient satisfaction. Additionally, increasing transparency with regard to public reporting of quality patient care outcomes is an expected hospital performance norm (Epstein et al., 2014).

To meet external drivers for quality care, hospital administration critically evaluates performance and sets goals for quality care success. A critical element in meeting quality care goals is ensuring the environment and culture of the organization have the tools to meet patients' needs. The IOM report "Keeping Patients Safe: Transforming the Work Environment of Nurses" (2003) highlighted critical elements necessary to support nursing practice and empower nurses to provide consistently high-quality care. Transformational nurse leaders are instrumental in cultivating a culture within an organization that allows nurses to practice successfully, thereby positively affecting patient outcomes (Ferguson, 2015).

No single entity drives quality measures. Rather, it is the synergy of the different influences that define quality metrics for improving patient outcomes. Equally important is recognizing changes in evidence that inform healthcare practice interventions and decisions. The following sidebar provides websites of major quality organizations that can offer a deeper understanding of current quality drivers and potential processes for implementing successful strategies for achieving quality measure outcomes. Establishing a reliable and resilient culture fosters error-free care delivery, ultimately improving overall patient safety and quality. (Note that information on quality measures is dynamic and rapidly changing. Nursing leaders should frequently read information at reputable organization websites to continually improve the practice environment. Note, too, that the following is not meant to be an all-inclusive list.)

KEY RESOURCES FOR HEALTHCARE AND HOSPITAL ADMINISTRATION

- **AARP Healthcare & Insurance:** http://www.aarphealthcare.com
- **Agency for Healthcare Research and Quality:** http://www.ahrq.gov
- **American Hospital Association:** http://www.aha.org/
- **American Nurses Credentialing Center:** http://www.nursecredentialing.org/Magnet
- **American Organization of Nurse Executives:** http://www.aone.org/education/qualitysafetyresources.shtml
- **American Society for Healthcare Risk Management:** http://www.ashrm.org/
- **American Society for Quality:** http://asq.org/knowledge-center/index.html
- **Association for Patient Experience:** http://www.patient-experience.org/Home.aspx
- **Centers for Medicare and Medicaid Services Hospital-Acquired Condition (HAC) Reduction Program page:** https://www.cms.gov/Medicare/Medicare-Fee-for-Service-Payment/AcuteInpatientPPS/HAC-Reduction-Program.html
- **Centers for Medicare and Medicaid Services Quality Measures page:** https://www.cms.gov/Medicare/Quality-Initiatives-Patient-Assessment-Instruments/QualityMeasures/index.html
- **Choosing Wisely:** http://www.choosingwisely.org/
- **HealthLeaders Media:** http://healthleadersmedia.com/Quality
- **Institute for Healthcare Improvement:** http://www.ihi.org
- **Institute for Safe Medication Practices:** http://www.ismp.org
- **Johns Hopkins Medicine Armstrong Institute for Patient Safety and Quality:** http://www.hopkinsmedicine.org/armstrong_institute
- **The Joint Commission:** http://www.jointcommission.org/
- **Medicare.gov Hospital Compare:** https://www.medicare.gov/hospitalcompare/About/What-Is-HOS.html
- **National Association for Healthcare Quality:** http://www.nahq.org
- **National Patient Safety Foundation:** http://www.npsf.org/
- **National Quality Forum:** http://www.qualityforum.org

> ■ **Quality and Safety Education for Nurses Institute:** http://qsen.org
>
> ■ **Robert Wood Johnson Foundation:** http://www.rwjf.org/en.html

NURSING-SENSITIVE QUALITY DRIVERS

Evaluating the quality of nursing care dates back to Florence Nightingale, when she began measuring patient outcomes (Dossey, 2005; Montalvo, 2007). The 1990s brought a growing attention in healthcare to focusing on quality outcomes and costs of care.

The American Nurses Association (ANA) conducted a series of pilot studies to evaluate linkages between nursing staff and quality of care (Montalvo, 2007; ANA, 2000; Gallagher and Rowell, 2003). Evidence from this seminal work identified 10 nursing-sensitive indicators that could be used to evaluate the quality of patient care influenced by nursing practice. Nursing-sensitive measures identify care processes that are distinct to nursing practice; thus, the patient outcome can be directly influenced by nursing care (Montalvo, 2007; Gallagher and Rowell, 2003).

To begin to measure the impact of these identified nursing-sensitive indicators, the ANA established the National Database of Nursing Quality Indicators (NDNQI). Hospitals submit data to the NDNQI. Quarterly analysis is completed, providing a comparison of observed outcomes in a meaningful way, stratified by institutional and unit characteristics. Today, more than 2,000 U.S. hospitals participate in the NDNQI program (Press Ganey Solutions, 2015).

Benefits of submitting data to NDNQI include the following:

■ Unit-level data for focused quality improvement celebrations and opportunities

■ Unit-level data for refinement of care processes to reduce errors within unit processes and promote a safety culture

■ Benchmarking data with like hospitals and units

■ Providing a "voice" to nursing practice through nursing practice survey responses (Press Ganey Solutions, 2015)

Table 3.2 provides an overview of nurse-sensitive outcomes that may be analyzed and trended by participating units and NDNQI.

TABLE 3.2   NDNQI NURSE-SENSITIVE MEASURES

Nursing-sensitive measures reflect the structure, process, and outcome of nursing care.

Structure is influenced by the nursing skill mix, level of nurses' education and certification, and availability of nurses to provide care.

Process measures aspects of care related to assessment, interventions, education, communication, and decision-making. Nurses' job satisfaction is also a process indicator.

Outcomes relate to the impact nursing care had on the patient. There are improved outcomes when the quality of nursing care is higher.

NDNQI Core Measures

Nursing hours per patient day

Nursing staff skill mix

Falls and falls with injury

Hospital- and unit-acquired pressure ulcers

Pain assessment and interventions

Peripheral IV infiltration

Physical/sexual assault

Restraint prevalence

Nursing staff turnover

Healthcare-acquired infections

Catheter-associated urinary tract infection rate

Central line–associated bloodstream infection rate

RN education/certification

Ventilator-associated pneumonia

RN survey: practice and job satisfaction

Adapted from Press Ganey Solutions (2015); Gallagher and Rowell (2003); Montalvo (2007); American Sentinel University-Healthcare (2011)

By understanding nurse-sensitive measures, nursing leaders—both formal and informal—have an opportunity to positively affect care. For example, the individual nurse may be inspired to become certified, while the nurse manager may focus on adjusting staffing patterns to optimize the mix of licensed and unlicensed personnel to better meet patient care acuity and volume needs. A nurse who is passionate about pressure ulcer prevention may decide to champion a pressure ulcer prevention quality improvement project for his or her unit using data from NDNQI reports to trend the unit's success. Using nursing-sensitive measures provides a locus of ownership that allows for the recognition of potential errors and correction to prevent patient harm.

INTERFACE BETWEEN NURSING-SENSITIVE QUALITY INDICATORS AND CORE MEASURES

Several nursing-sensitive outcomes overlap with TJC- and CMS-identified quality metrics. For example, CMS focuses on the reduction or elimination of several hospital-acquired conditions, including catheter-associated urinary tract infections, central line–associated bloodstream infections, patient falls, hospital-acquired pressure ulcers, and ventilator-associated pneumonia. TJC also looks at hospital-acquired infections, as well as pain management, restraint use, and hand hygiene.

The interface between regulatory agency quality drivers and nursing-sensitive measures provides a unique opportunity to both collaborate with healthcare providers and identify the impact of nursing care on shared quality outcome measures. For example, efforts to reduce central-line bloodstream infections were brought to light with the success of the Keystone project, which implemented an interprofessional evidence-based approach to the central-line insertion process using a checklist (Agency for Healthcare Research and Quality, 2014). After the line is successfully placed, the focus turns to the nursing practice as it relates to the care of the central-line catheter as well as collaborative daily discussions between the nurse and healthcare provider regarding the ongoing need for the device. If a patient develops an infection associated with the central line, root cause analysis can focus on the collaborative care as well as nursing-specific care to identify opportunities for future error reduction. The central-line infection rates are then reported to both CMS and NDNQI, creating an intersection in the quality measure and the opportunity to look at the processes in place to prevent future errors from an interprofessional process and/or a nursing-focused process.

INTERFACE BETWEEN NURSING PRACTICE AND HCAHPS

During a hospital admission, nurses spend a significant amount of time with the patient and his or her family, influencing the overall patient experience (Dempsey et al., 2014). Patient satisfaction as captured on HCAHPS survey reports directly influences VBP and is tied to overall hospital quality and safety outcome measures, financial reimbursement, and national hospital performance ranking.

A study conducted by Press Ganey (2013) examined the predictive relationships of the HCAHPS survey question domains. The study found that several items clustered together, suggesting that each of these domains influences the others. The researchers likened the clustering to "follow the leader," providing a nice analogy for how nurse leaders who improve patient experience in one domain of the HCAHPS survey can positively influence other areas of patient satisfaction.

Analysis found that five HCAHPS dimensions consistently clustered together:

- Communication with nurses
- Responsiveness of hospital staff
- Pain management
- Communication about medicine
- Overall rating

Specifically, nurse communication influenced the remaining four areas of patient satisfaction. This suggests that improving nursing communication will likely improve the other dimensions of patient experience measured by the HCAHPS survey (Press Ganey, 2013).

Dempsey and colleagues (2014) outline how nurse leaders can create a culture that promotes improved nurse communication with patients, affecting overall patient safety and quality. Strategies put forth align well with key elements of HROs. Strategies found to improve nurse communication include the following:

- Training to improve patient experience
- Purposeful hourly rounding
- Bedside shift report
- Senior leader rounding
- Improving patient flow
- Nurse manager training

Developing strategies—and, more importantly, developing a culture that encourages and supports a nursing practice focused on communication and meeting the individual needs of each patient—will improve safety and overall patient experience.

EVIDENCE-BASED PRACTICE INFORMING QUALITY DRIVERS

The primary premise of EBP is for all healthcare professionals to know and apply current best evidence in daily care of patients to improve outcomes and reduce costs. Key elements of EBP align with principles of HROs:

- EBP provides a consistent body of knowledge that can be applied in the delivery of care, providing predictable and consistent outcomes.

- Adapting evidence to meet unique patient-specific needs allows for rapid adaptation by nurses to prevent patient harm.

- The effectiveness of the application of evidence in practice can be measured through patient outcomes (for example, absence of error) (Melnyk, 2012).

To illustrate, consider the evidence to prevent patient harm from infection. TJC continues to track hand-hygiene compliance as a quality outcome measure. Hand hygiene remains the most important intervention for the prevention of hospital-acquired infections and the spread of infections (TJC, 2015b). However, a Cochrane review found that healthcare workers continue to demonstrate poor compliance with hand hygiene, often citing barriers such as time and lack of access to hand-cleansing products (Gould, Moralejo, Drey, and Chudleigh, 2010). Applying principles of HROs to assist with the translation of evidence supporting hand hygiene would look something like this:

- Establish a no-tolerance policy for lack of hand hygiene such that everyone (healthcare provider, nurse, secretary, administrator, and family) is expected to wash hands upon entry and exit to a patient room. Evidence suggests hand hygiene improves when *all* individuals are expected to comply with the practice (Gould et al., 2010).

- Identify the optimal location for hand-cleansing products to allow for easy and effective hand hygiene. Engage supervisors and administration as needed to facilitate placement of hand-hygiene cleansing dispensers in optimal locations and numbers (Gandra and Ellison, 2014).

- If hand hygiene is missed, evaluate the barrier and make improvements to prevent future hand-hygiene omissions (TJC, 2015b).

- Engage all healthcare team members, patients, and families in meeting the hand-hygiene standard and encourage open feedback to continually improve processes to advance consistent compliance with hand-hygiene practice (Conway et al., 2014).

■ Train staff to be resistant to events in which hand hygiene may be omitted. For example, during an acute emergency, interventions or processes can be quickly put into place to expect hand hygiene be performed to reduce the risk to patients from the hand-hygiene omission (Gandra and Ellison, 2014).

Creating cultures that embrace EBP and HROs allows for consistent, high-quality practice that reduces the risk for patient harm. Individual responsibility and healthcare team collaboration in the process of care intersect in the application of EBP and HRO to consistently improve patient care quality outcomes. Linking EBP with patient outcomes and quality drivers supports a culture that empowers the healthcare worker to apply and adapt processes to prevent patient harm. Individuals and teams are responsible for creating the intersection between EBP and HROs to achieve high-quality patient care.

ACHIEVING EXCELLENCE IN CURRENT QUALITY OUTCOME DRIVERS

As patient errors continue to permeate healthcare practice, more quality drivers will be mandated. Establishing a workplace culture that supports safety and quality is essential to enabling nurses to deliver high-quality care that reduces error and prevents patient harm.

TJC has stated that a safety culture promotes trust and empowers staff to report errors, near misses, and risks to reduce errors and improve overall quality (TJC, 2014). Embracing the five key concepts of HROs provides a framework for cultivating and sustaining an environment that facilitates the delivery of safe, error-free, high-quality care.

Achieving quality outcomes requires both a team approach and individual accountability. As a team, healthcare workers need to feel fully informed; understand the vision for care; feel empowered to act on, report, and address potential errors; and trust each other's intentions in the provision of safe care (Melnyk, 2012; Hershey, 2015). Individually, the nurse should feel empowered to communicate when safety processes are compromised and implement corrective interventions.

Hospitals will continue to face demands to improve the quality and cost effectiveness of care (Owens and Koch, 2015). Ensuring a culture of safety through HRO structures will help achieve the goal of excellent care for every patient, every time.

SUMMARY

Multiple dynamics define and affect the delivery of high-quality patient care to every patient, every time. Quality drivers can be broadly categorized into four groups. In reality, however, all the quality drivers work together to improve the quality and safety of healthcare. Nurses are in an ideal position to lead practice- and process-improvement initiatives that improve patient care. When nurse leaders create cultures that encourage translation of current best evidence into practice as well as empower the bedside nurse to take actions to keep patients safe, the essence of an HRO culture can be achieved, positively affecting patient care.

KEY POINTS

- Delivery of high-quality, error-free care is an expectation.

- Multiple interrelated factors influence quality metrics to improve care, including patient/family expectations, regulatory and accrediting agencies, financial considerations, and healthcare administration and leadership.

- Nursing-sensitive quality indicators are outcome metrics that can be directly influenced by nursing practice to improve patient outcomes.

- Translation of current best evidence into daily practice is necessary to reduce patient harm.

- A culture supporting patient safety and quality is essential to improving patient outcomes.

- HROs provide a culture that supports individual healthcare workers to consistently provide safe, high-quality, efficient, error-free care.

REFERENCES

Agency for Healthcare Research and Quality. (2014). Central line insertion care team checklist. Retrieved from http://www.ahrq.gov/professionals/quality-patient-safety/patient-safety-resources/resources/cli-checklist/index.html

American Nurses Association. (2000). *Nurse staffing and patient outcomes*. Washington, DC: American Nurses Publishing.

American Sentinel University-Healthcare. (2011). What are nursing sensitive quality indicators anyway? Retrieved from http://www.americansentinel.edu/blog/2011/11/02/what-are-nursing-sensitive-quality-indicators-anyway/

Blumenthal, D., and Jena, A. B. (2013). Hospital valued-based purchasing. *Journal of Hospital Medicine, 8*(5), pp. 271–277.

Brooks, J. A. (2014). The new world of health care quality and measurement. *American Journal of Nursing, 114*(7), pp. 57–59.

Carayon, P., Xie, A., and Kianfar, S. (2013). Human factors and ergonomics as a patient safety practice. *BMJ Quality & Safety, 23*(3), pp. 196–205.

Centers for Medicare & Medicaid Services. (n.d.). Readmission reduction program. Retrieved from https://www.cms.gov/Medicare/medicare-fee-for-service-payment/acuteinpatientPPS/readmissions-reduction-program.html

Centers for Medicare & Medicaid Services. (2015). Hospital value based purchasing. Retrieved from https://www.cms.gov/Medicare/Quality-Initiatives-Patient-Assessment-Instruments/hospital-value-based-purchasing/index.html?redirect=/hospital-value-based-purchasing/

Conway, L. J., Riley, L., Saiman, L., Cohen, B., Alper, P., and Larson, E. L. (2014). Implementation and impact of an automated group monitoring and feedback system to promote hand hygiene among health care personnel. *Joint Commission Journal on Quality and Patient Safety, 40*(9), pp. 408–417.

Dempsey, C., Reilly, B., and Buhlman, N. (2014). Improving the patient experience: Real-world strategies for engaging nurses. *Journal of Nurse Administration, 44*(3), pp. 142–151.

Dossey, B. M., Selanders, L. C., Beck, D. M., and Attewell, A. (2005). *Florence Nightingale today: Healing, leadership, global action.* Silver Spring, MD: American Nurses Association.

Doyle, C., Lennox, L., and Bell, D. (2013). A systematic review of evidence on links between patient experience and clinical safety and effectiveness. *BMJ Open, 3*(1). doi:10.1136/bmjopen-2012-001570 3

Epstein, A. M., Jha, A. K., Orav, E. J., Liebman, D. L., Audet, A. J., Zezza, M. A., and Guterman, S. (2014). Analysis of early accountable care organizations defines patient, structural, cost, and quality of care characteristics. *HealthAffairs, 31*(1), pp. 95–102.

Ferguson, S. L. (2015). Transformational nurse leaders key to strengthening health systems worldwide. *Journal of Nursing Administration, 45*(7–8), pp. 351–353.

Gallagher, R. M., and Rowell, P. A. (2003). Claiming the future of nursing through nursing-sensitive quality indicators. *Nursing Administration Quarterly, 27*(4), pp. 273–284.

Gandra, S., and Ellison, R. T. (2014). Modern trends in infection control practices in intensive care units. *Journal of Intensive Care Medicine, 29*(6), pp. 11–26.

Giordano, L. A., Elliott, M. N., Goldstein, E., Lehrman, W. G., and Spencer, P. A. (2010). Development, implementation, and public reporting of the HCAHPS survey. *Medical Care Research and Review, 67*(1), pp. 27–37.

Glasgow, A. H. Arnold H. Glasgow. Daily Quote. Retrieved from http://www.dailyquote.eu/arnold_h_glasow

Gould, D. J., Moralejo, D., Drey, N., and Chudleigh, J. H. (2010). Interventions to improve hand hygiene compliance in patient care. *The Cochrane Database of Systematic Reviews,* (9). doi: 10.1002/14651858.CD005186.pub3

Harder, K. A., and Marc, D. (2013). Human factors issues in the intensive care unit. *AACN Advanced Critical Care, 24*(4), pp. 405–414.

Hershey, K. (2015). Culture of safety. *The Nursing Clinics of North America, 50*(1), pp. 139–152.

Hospital Consumer Assessment of Healthcare Providers and Systems. (2015). HCAHPS Fact Sheet. Retrieved from http://www.hcahpsonline.org/Files/HCAHPS_Fact_Sheet_June_2015.pdf

Institute of Medicine. (2001). *Crossing the quality chasm: A new healthcare system for the 21st century.* Washington, DC: The National Academies Press. Retrieved from http://www.nap.edu/openbook.php?record_id=10027

Institute of Medicine of the National Academies. (2003). *Keeping patients safe: Transforming the work environment of nurses.* Washington, DC: The National Academies Press. Retrieved from http://books.nap.edu/openbook.php?record_id=10851

The Joint Commission. (2015a). Core measure sets. Retrieved from http://www.jointcommission.org/core_measure_sets.aspx

The Joint Commission. (2015b). Hand hygiene. Retrieved from http://www.jointcommission.org/topics/hai_hand_hygiene.aspx

The Joint Commission. (2014). Patient safety and performance measurement fact sheets. Retrieved from http://www.jointcommission.org/about_us/patient_safety_fact_sheets.aspx

Laranjo, L., Arguel, A., Neves, A. L., Gallagher, A. M., Kaplan, R., Mortimer, N., and Lau, A. Y. S. (2015). The influence of social networking sites on health behavior change: A systematic review and meta-analysis. *Journal of the American Medical Informatics Association, 22*(1), pp. 243–256.

Melnyk, B. M. (2012). Achieving a high-reliability organization through implementation of the ARCC model for system-wide sustainability of evidence-based practice. *Nursing Administration Quarterly, 36*(2), pp. 127–135.

Montalvo, I. (2007). The National Database of Nursing Quality Indicators (NDNQI). *The Online Journal of Issues in Nursing, 12*(3). Retrieved from http://www.nursingworld.org/MainMenuCategories/ANAMarketplace/ANAPeriodicals/OJIN/TableofContents/Volume122007/No3Sept07/NursingQualityIndicators.html?css=print

National Quality Forum. (n.d.). Measuring performance. Retrieved from http://www.qualityforum.org/Measuring_Performance/Measuring_Performance.aspx

Owens, L. D., and Koch, R. W. (2015). Understanding quality patient care and the role of the practicing nurse. *Nursing Clinics of North America, 50*(1), pp. 33–43.

Page, A., Ed. (2004). *Keeping patients safe: Transforming the work environment of nurses.* Committee on the Work Environment for Nurses and Patient Safety. Washington, DC: The National Academies Press.

Press Ganey. (2015). Nursing quality: NDNQI. Retrieved from http://pressganey.com/ourSolutions/performance-and-advanced-analytics/clinical-business-performance/nursing-quality-ndnqi

Press Ganey. (2013). The rising tide measure: Communication with nurses. Retrieved from http://www.prnewswire.com/news-releases/press-ganey-study-finds-nurse-communication-a-rising-tide-measure-206406161.html

Swanson, J. W., and Tidwell, C. A. (2011). Improving the culture of patient safety through the Magnet journey. *Online Journal of Issues in Nursing, 16*(3). doi: 10.3912/OJIN.Vol16No03Man01

CHAPTER 4

ORGANIZATIONAL CULTURE AND THE JOURNEY TO HRO

Lisa Camplese, MBA, BSN, RN

The 1999 Institute of Medicine (IOM) report "To Err Is Human" invigorated healthcare organizations in their unrelenting pursuit of a safer environment for the delivery of patient care. After the report's initial aftershocks, leaders continued the quest to determine causes for medical errors. They launched many improvement efforts to win the confidence of the patients and families they served in their ability to provide safer healthcare.

Unfortunately, with the complexity of healthcare delivery, the pace at which this improvement has occurred has not been quick. Although there was a concerted effort to determine the cause of errors in healthcare environments, it quickly came to light that a cultural shift with regard to patient safety would be pivotal to moving organizations forward with meaningful and sustainable safety efforts. Edgar Schein, a noted leader in organizational culture, states that "Culture is an abstraction, yet the forces that are created in social and organizational situations deriving from culture are powerful. If we don't understand the operation of these forces, we become victim to them" (Schein, 2010, p. 7).

> "
> Culture can become a 'secret weapon' that makes extraordinary things happen.
>
> —Jon Katzenbach
> "

Due to the complexity of healthcare and its reliance on human performance and inputs, the path to safer care delivery was riddled with complications. There was an obvious need to address safety from many fronts, but addressing safety through culture change would prove to be vital. We must understand the forces that drive culture, such as leadership support, the promotion of a learning mentality, and the importance of a learning environment. We must also embrace the notion of reaching zero defects. When one measures and designs for zero, one invariably uncovers many different ideas, enabling innovation. Aiming for this higher level of performance will set the tone for the culture of the organization and the journey toward high reliability.

In a *Health Affairs* article published in 2013, Mark Chassin commented, "There can be no higher priority today for healthcare leaders than eliminating the barriers to a strong and vibrant culture of safety" (p. 1764). The U.S healthcare system is striving to create an environment in which zero preventable harm occurs. To achieve this, healthcare organizations have become more interested in high reliability principles and organizations that practice this disciplined approach. One of the central takeaways from these organizations is the importance of a culture of safety, where errors and dangerous conditions are reported with ease and freedom, accountability for adherence to safe practice is embraced, and communication among all team members regardless of rank or education is appreciated and respected. Weick and Sutcliffe (2007) refer to this cultural attitude as "collective mindfulness." This culture transformation means that everyone who works in an organization is acutely aware of safety and that failure in safe practice and procedures can lead to larger failures. They are designing for zero defects!

UNDERSTANDING ORGANIZATIONAL CULTURE

There is no singular correct definition of culture. However, the definition of organizational culture is not so elusive. Bellot (2011) traced the history of organizational culture research and found that most research is within corporate structures. Furthermore, she found consensus in the literature around five basic tenets of organization culture:

- It exists.
- It is ambiguous.
- It is unique and malleable.
- It is socially constructed and is the product of group interactions.
- It is adaptable to healthcare.

To understand a culture, one must first be aware of drivers of culture. Schein (2010) refers to these areas as "levels of culture." Schein identified three major areas that help to define or shape culture:

- **Artifacts:** These are processes and structures that are seen in the culture as well as behaviors that are observable. (Note that one may see ideologies and rationalizations within an organization that do not align with its artifacts.)

- **Espoused beliefs and values:** These include goals, values, and aspirations.

- **Basic underlying assumptions:** These are one's unconscious beliefs and values with respect to how an organization functions or those we simply assume are present.

Another key component is understanding the maturity of a culture or an organization. The maturation of an organizational culture measures the ability of that organization to tolerate change and adopt new practices. Measuring the maturity of the organization provides insight into the sustainability of new ideas and concepts. This helps to determine a starting point for aligning efforts to address a particular project within a culture and also provides a basic assessment of an organization's readiness to change (Chassin and Loeb, 2013).

In 1990, Rousseau, an anthropological scholar, upheld that organizations were cultures in themselves. Other researchers (Cameron and Quinn, 2006) have embraced the idea that culture is actually an asset of an organization and therefore can be influenced or changed by leadership. Leaders must understand the culture and the maturity of the organization to allow change. They must also be knowledgeable about change concepts and models to steer and guide the change to the organization's culture.

What is the impact of organizational culture to high reliability? High reliability depends on a strong safety culture of anticipation and effective containment of events (Weick and Sutcliffe, 2007). Singer et al. (2009) studied the correlation between organizational cultures and safety cultures. The authors found a strong association between organizational culture and patient safety culture. Furthermore, a higher level of group culture was related to higher levels of safety culture, while the opposite was found with hierarchical cultures. The conclusion made was that a mix of culture with a higher emphasis on group values such as teamwork, collaboration, shared decision-making, and participation leads to a higher safety culture. Implications for practice include the implementation of interventions to improve teamwork and reduce hierarchy, leading to substantial improvements in patient safety. Perhaps not coincidentally, these interventions are highly valued in highly reliable organizations.

Culture can be an ambiguous and elusive term. It can be considered a "soft" concept, particularly in a world of "hard" science. However, culture is often a factor that holds an organization back or moves it forward toward high reliability.

STAGES OF LEARNING

Leaders must possess a basic knowledge of the general processes of organizational change in order to lead a true change effort. Schein and Bennis defined the stages of learning and change in 1965, and these stages still apply today. The stages are as follows:

1. Individuals within an organization must be motivated to change. For this to occur, they must feel a sense of safety and security. Change is disconcerting and provokes anxiety.

2. Individuals in the organization must learn new concepts, understand new meanings for old concepts, and evaluate concepts with a new lens. Experimentation and small trials become relevant.

3. Individuals in the organization must embrace and internalize the "new" or incorporate new concepts into the culture.

JOURNEY TO HIGH RELIABILITY: ASSESSING HRO MATURITY

So how does an organization or integrated delivery network launch the culture change needed to embark on the journey to high reliability? First, leaders within the organization must understand the change model. They must also realize that to lead change, they need additional information and understanding of the organization.

The first step is an assessment of readiness and an understanding of the current state of the culture of safety—in other words, its level of high reliability organization (HRO) maturity. The Agency for Healthcare Research and Quality (AHRQ) Hospital Survey on Patient Safety Culture (Sorra and Nieva, 2004; Sorra and Dyer, 2010) is one tool that can assist with gathering data and assessing the organization's strengths with regard to a culture of safety as well as areas where improvement is needed. This survey provides benchmarks for the various questions as well as the ability to perform comparisons with like organizations. This validated survey tool measures a culture of safety in 12 different dimensions. These dimensions cover communication, teamwork, management support of safety efforts, organizational learning or improvement efforts, and non-punitive response to error, to name a few. Questions support non-punitive error reporting versus the concepts of Just Culture and accountability.

 In some cases, the wording of the questions in the survey may be challenging for staff to decipher.

It is also wise to perform an internal HRO maturity survey that asks members in leadership positions, board members, clinical staff, and non-clinical staff for their views on organizational activities related to reliability. Our organization, Centura Health, conducted one such survey. At the time, there were few tools to measure readiness in this area, so we used the Chassin and Loeb (2013) framework to create our own measurement tool. It included 14 framework components in three domains, as noted in Table 4.1.

TABLE 4.1 DOMAINS AND COMPONENTS REFLECTIVE OF HIGH RELIABILITY

Domains	Components
Leadership commitment	Board of trustees
	CEO and all senior management, including nursing leaders
	Engagement of physicians
	Hospital's quality strategy
	Hospital's use and dissemination of data on measures of quality
	Hospital's use of IT to support quality and safety improvements
Safety culture	Trust
	Accountability
	Identification of unsafe conditions
	Strengthening of systems
	Assessment
Robust process improvement	Lean
	Six Sigma
	Change management

Adapted from Chassin and Loeb (2013)

Our HRO maturity survey consisted of questions that focused on three primary components:

- Leadership engagement and involvement
- Culture
- Application of robust improvement efforts

We evaluated the following:

- Our ability to address quality and safety through our IT solutions
- Involvement by various professionals in process improvement activities
- Our measurement of safety
- Our application of critical event analysis, failure mode effects, and root cause to determine needed improvement

Although not scientifically tested, our internal survey enabled us to assess the activities in these areas that were underway, gain knowledge of the maturity of the entities engaged in quality and safety activities, and build a plan to move forward. We needed a way to "take the temperature" of our current activities as well as discover any areas that were not aligned with our journey to reliability. The survey also provided information on system themes that we could address in our task force.

We performed a limited electronic survey of clinical leadership, board members, and key physicians. Participants were asked to evaluate the questions based on four stages of HRO maturity, with answers of 1 being least mature and 4 being fully mature. Table 4.2 contains an example of a question from each domain.

TABLE 4.2 EXAMPLES OF SURVEY QUESTIONS IN EACH DOMAIN

	1 (Least Mature)	2	3	4 (Fully Mature)
Leadership Commitment				
Select the statement that most closely characterizes board leadership at our hospital.	Board and CEO/management quality focus is nearly exclusively on regulatory compliance.	The full board's involvement in quality is limited to hearing reports from its quality committee.	The full board is engaged in the development of quality goals and the approval of the quality plan and regularly reviews adverse events and progress on quality goals.	The board commits to the goal of high reliability for all clinical services.

Safety Culture				
Select the statement that most closely characterizes our hospital's safety culture related to trust.	There is no assessment of trust or intimidating behavior.	Codes of behavior (behavioral standards) are adopted in some clinical departments.	CEO and physician leaders establish a trusting environment among all staff by modeling appropriate behaviors and championing efforts to eradicate intimidating behaviors.	High levels of measured trust exist in all clinical areas, and self-policing of codes of behavior is in place.

Robust Process Improvement				
Select the statement that most closely characterizes our hospital's performance-improvement methods.	No formal approach to quality management has been adopted by the organization.	Exploration of modern process-improvement tools has begun.	An organizational commitment exists to adopt a full suite of robust performance-improvement tools.	Adoption of robust performance-improvement tools has occurred throughout the organization.

As a large integrated delivery network in Colorado and Kansas, we expected variability in responses across our entities. However, we also hoped this assessment would provide us with more information to formulate system-wide actions that we could use to formulate a road map. The timing of this assessment aligned with our Joint Commission survey cycle. We knew we had many high performers in safety activities and wanted the ability to share best practices and learning across our continuum.

For us to develop and implement our own maturity survey, leadership support and backing were necessary. Our first step was to create the needed platform for HRO. As stated, our ability to move forward was spurred by our Joint Commission survey cycle, which prompted more dialogue and interest in high reliability. We used our own clinical system leadership group as our approval body for this internal survey and brought the results back to this group with a plan for next steps.

CONTINUING THE JOURNEY: HRO TOOLKIT

Our survey results demonstrated that on the maturity survey scale of 1 to 4, with 1 being least mature and 4 being fully mature, we hovered between 2 and 3 in the three main dimensions of leadership commitment, safety culture, and robust process improvement. Analysis of our results revealed that visibility of leadership and the board's commitment to safety were important to our staff. We needed to create more opportunities for this visibility in addition to holding town halls and meetings. It was also clear that we needed a refresh on Just Culture principles and concepts and that we needed our human resources and talent management professionals to partner in this area. We also were able to identify very strong safety work that was already in existence that could be shared across our entities.

We did not want this journey to be a "project of the month" or to minimize the importance of high reliability. We knew we needed to generate interest and enthusiasm. We had experience in putting together chartered and focused evidence-based practice (EBP) teams in the past; this became our platform for putting together a task force dedicated to this effort. Our EBP project teams were designed with Dr. David Sackett's definition of EBP in mind: "Evidence-based medicine is the integration of best research evidence with clinical expertise and patient values" (Sackett, Straus, Richardson, Rosenberg, and Haynes, 2000, p. 1.). We assembled a team of safety and quality experts across our healthcare continuum to put together an intentional plan for our journey to high reliability.

We established a charter and identified our next steps. The charter enabled our team to identify our mission statement and priorities and created guardrails for the project. The charter defined the purpose of the group as providing a toolkit based in the literature that would support the principles of HRO outlined by Weick and Sutcliffe (2007). We further defined the membership as well as their roles and expectations. Finally, we ensured that the charter supported our organizational values and mission. Chartering created the necessary guiding principles that enabled the team to come together, divide the components of our work, and create what we termed our HRO toolkit.

After our charter was approved, we spent several meetings reviewing both the principles of high reliability and the results from our internal survey and an AHRQ Culture of Safety Survey. We then used the five principles of reliability to create a grid of current work and proposed future work for our healthcare system. We also performed a thorough search of the literature to create a bibliography to support the toolkit components devoted to each principle.

We wanted to use the toolkit to provide a platform for sharing leading practices by our entities and for disseminating information on leading practices outside our industry that supported high reliability. We also wanted the toolkit to offer flexibility in the adoption of various tools based on the organization's environment and culture. That is, we wanted each healthcare entity to choose from a menu of items to implement to support each of the five principles. Our goal was to create accountability for implementation but also to offer flexibility to fit both the culture and stage of maturity of each organization. Table 4.3 lists the components we provided in our toolkit.

TABLE 4.3   COMPONENTS IN THE HRO TOOLKIT

HRO Characteristic	Toolkit Contents
HRO overview	Information about HRO core principles and the science of safety education
Preoccupation with failure	Daily safety huddle template
Reluctance to simplify	Information about Good Catch program
	Event debriefing guidelines
	Standardized RCA template
	Five Whys template
	Event investigation training
Sensitivity to operations	Leadership rounding tools
Resilience	Failure mode and effects analysis (FMEA) templates
Deference to expertise	Safety imperatives and accountability policy
	Team training

EXAMPLE: SAFETY HUDDLE

In the area of preoccupation with failure, we provided a template and literature to support the carrying out of patient safety huddles. The intent was that individual hospitals could use the template and related instructions to start doing daily safety huddles right away. The result was that within a year, almost all of the organization's hospitals were doing a daily huddle, which led to a significant difference in the safety culture. Table 4.4 reveals the topics we consistently discuss in our daily huddles.

TABLE 4.4   SAFETY HUDDLE FORMAT

Topic	Content	Example
Celebrations	Acknowledgment of safety successes, good catches, and near misses that provided an opportunity for learning	An OR physician stopped a procedure when there was a question regarding how to prepare a specimen that was to be obtained during the surgery. Incorrect preparation would have invalidated the biopsy results in an irretrievable specimen.
Look back	Significant safety or quality issues found within the last 24 hours	These might include reported medication errors or near misses.

continues

TABLE 4.4 SAFETY HUDDLE FORMAT (CONTINUED)

Topic	Content	Example
Look ahead	Safety or quality issues that could arise within the next 24 hours	These might include infection risks, staffing and coverage issues, and errors that might occur in areas under leadership transition.
Follow up	Status update on issues brought up in previous huddles but not resolved at that time	This might include answers to questions like, "Are the call lights fixed?" or "Did we adjust the upper limits on vancomycin infusions?"
Announcements	Facility-specific messages for the day or week	An example might be, "The AHRQ Safety Survey is available now!"

One aspect of daily huddles is to recognize good catches and encourage near-miss reporting. Our organizations used theme-based materials that they felt fit their culture. These included baseball- and soccer-themed "Good Catch!" certificates to recognize the preemptive reporting of potential patient safety issues. (See Figure 4.1 and Figure 4.2.) One hospital gave away a T-shirt with a "Safety MVP" logo each month. Other hospitals gave away prizes for the "best" catch or allowed all good catch–award recipients to enter a drawing for a giveaway. Either way, because of this good-catch and near-miss reporting and the celebration of these reports during safety huddles, the organizations realized an increase in event or near event reporting.

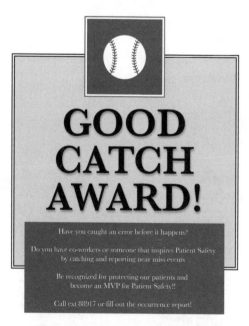

Figure 4.1 Good Catch flyer.

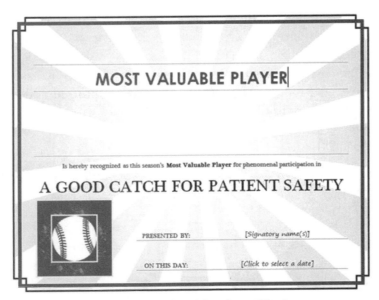

Figure 4.2 Good Catch certificate.

EXAMPLE: RED RULES TO SAFETY IMPERATIVES

Red rules are rules that cannot be broken and must be followed exactly as specified without exception. In our case, the HRO task force also tackled a long-standing history of the use of red rules as a part of our patient safety structure and reevaluated how we would shift our reliance on red rules to our patient safety imperatives. The use of red rules began early in our journey in patient safety. We had identified a need to tighten our accountability around patient identification. What we learned was that rather than leading to more reporting of potential system issues, the policy was used more for corrective action. We wanted our culture to support accountability but to improve patient safety areas to identify system breakdowns and opportunities to prevent errors. To do this, we needed our staff to feel comfortable providing feedback and ideas and reporting near misses.

We retired our red-rules policy in favor of a new policy that focused on shared accountability and empowering staff to act. This policy stressed speaking up (and being supported for doing so) if a violation of a safety imperative such as hand hygiene or wearing personal protective equipment occurred. We wanted to break from the language we had used in the past and to update our policy on associate performance to include a more thorough explanation of the use of a Just Culture algorithm. The task force included members of our human resources department to help us revise these policies and to assist in incorporating training on Just Culture and high reliability principles in our new manager and leader orientation.

The task force recognized that although we had designed programs that were safety oriented in the past, these did not involve safety training for the physicians who worked with us. We worked with a local large malpractice carrier for several providers to design a very thorough training curriculum that supported high reliability for physicians. Physicians who attended the training became eligible for potential malpractice discounts, providing additional motivation. This training was scenario- or situation-based, which helped with the practical translation of the principles of high reliability.

 A future goal of the task force is to provide greater visibility to Just Culture principles within the peer review structure and functions. Although not fully completed, this is a part of our map for next steps.

There is no one-size-fits-all approach to achieving greater reliability. It is a continuous journey that should be aligned with the organization's state of readiness. The culture of readiness and maturity must be assessed.

Leadership engagement and executive support are non-negotiable aspects of this journey and should be the highest priority, or the burning platform, to advance HRO principles. This burning platform must move the organization toward a program to realize the capability and quest to have zero harm. We recognize that given the complexity and reliance on human intervention and science in healthcare, errors will occur. As noted by Weick and Sutcliffe, "The hallmark of an HRO is not that it is error-free but that errors don't disable it" (2007, p. 14). Other industries have proven that with effort and commitment, improvements in prevention and safety can occur. In healthcare, we must embrace this journey. We must commit the necessary efforts and resources to provide our caregivers with the support and training to deploy HRO tactics and principles in their everyday practice.

In this age of value versus volume in healthcare, providing our patients and consumers with a safer healthcare system that has greater reliability, teamwork, and accountability will translate with ease to the value proposition we all want to offer our patients. Today, healthcare organization culture leaders are visibly driving safety through daily safety huddles and rounding. They lead their meetings with good catches and near-miss reporting and include staff in solutions to improve patient safety and reliability. Embracing the lessons of industries outside healthcare will help guide the healthcare environment toward improved safety. Value does not always mean the least expensive; it should mean providing the best care and service to our patients without introducing risk and harm. Accountability and leadership will help us drive toward the goal of zero harm and inspire us to address risky behavior or patterns that set us up for failure. High reliability is a journey that does not end but moves us toward better delivery of value-based care to those we serve!

SUMMARY

Achieving high reliability involves a continuous journey of improvement. An organization must evaluate a sense of readiness for change through an assessment of maturity and some measurement of the aspects of the culture of safety. Leadership must believe and embrace the idea that this is the highest priority, support a learning environment, and support an accountable culture that is foundational to a Just Culture. Each organization's path to reliability will vary. It is important to evaluate the efforts currently underway in the organization and remove barriers to adopt leading practices in safety and reliability. Healthcare is complex. Understanding that high reliability is a journey can help an organization to draft a road map to enable it to deliver more reliable and safer care.

KEY POINTS

- High reliability is a journey. Thoughtful planning and a burning platform are needed to move an organization through that journey.

- High reliability is not a one-size-fits-all process. It's imperative to assess the HRO maturity of an organization before embarking on the journey.

REFERENCES

Bellot, J. (2011). Defining and assessing organizational culture. *Nursing Forum*, *46*(1), pp. 29–37.

Cameron, K. S., and Quinn, R. E. (2006). *Diagnosing and changing organizational culture based on the competing values framework*. San Francisco, CA: Jossey-Bass.

Chassin, M. R. (2013). Improving the quality of health care: What's taking so long? *HealthAffairs*, *32*(10), pp. 1761–1765.

Chassin, M. R., and Loeb, J. M. (2013). High-reliability health care: Getting there from here. *The Milbank Quarterly*, *91*(3), pp. 459–490.

Institute of Medicine. (1999). To err is human: Building a safer health system. Washington, DC: The National Academies Press.

Rousseau, D. (1990). Assessing organizational culture: The case for multiple methods. In L. Goldstein (Ed.), *Frontiers of industrial and organizational psychology*. San Francisco, CA: Jossey-Bass.

Sackett, D. L., Straus, S. E., Richardson, W. S., Rosenberg, W., and Haynes, R. B. (2000). *Evidence-based medicine: How to practice and teach EBM* (2nd Ed.). London: Churchill Livingstone.

Schein, E. H. (2010). *Organizational culture and leadership* (4th Ed.). San Francisco, CA: Jossey-Bass.

Schein, E. H., and Bennis, W. G. (1965). *Personal and organizational change*. New York, NY: John Wiley & Sons.

Singer, S. J., Falwell, A., Gaba, D. M., Meterko, M., Rosen, A., Hartmann, C. W., and Baker, L. (2009). Identifying organizational cultures that promote patient safety. *Health Care Management Review*, *34(4)*, pp. 300–311.

Sorra, J. S., and Dyer, N. (2010). Multilevel psychometric properties of the AHRQ hospital survey on patient safety culture. *BMC Health Services Research*, 10, pp. 199–212.

Sorra, J., and Nieva, V. (2004). Hospital survey on patient safety culture. Agency for Healthcare Research and Quality. Retrieved from http://www.ahrq.gov/sites/default/files/wysiwyg/professionals/quality-patient-safety/patientsafetyculture/hospital/resources/hospcult.pdf

Weick, K. E., and Sutcliffe, K. M. (2007). *Managing the unexpected: Resilient performance in an age of uncertainty*. San Francisco, CA: Jossey Bass.

PART 2

HRO CONCEPTS AND APPLICATION TO PRACTICE: PREOCCUPATION WITH FAILURE

CHAPTER 5

USING FAILURE MODE AND EFFECTS ANALYSIS TO PREDICT FAILURE

Katherine Bilys, MBA, CPHQ

James Reason, noted human factors expert, has helped healthcare institutions and other high-risk industries understand that the human species is largely optimistic and has difficulty anticipating failures, particularly in complex environments such as operating rooms and intensive care units (Reason, 1990). A useful antidote to our optimism is the failure mode and effects analysis (FMEA) tool, which has been used in process engineering since the late 1950s to design and refine critical processes.

FMEA is a favorite tool of people who work in high reliability organizations (HROs). Their preoccupation with failure compels them to look for potential hazards before they occur. HROs work vigilantly to deeply understand a process' potential failures (failure modes) and to identify the consequences of the failure (effects analysis) to develop and implement solutions *before* the failure occurs and affects the patient (Weick and Sutcliffe, 2007). In this chapter, you will learn when and how to conduct an FMEA.

FMEA has endured as a process tool because it is adaptable and flexible. An evidence-based tool, FMEA is endorsed by such organizations as The Joint Commission (TJC), the

> Accidents do not occur because people gamble and lose, they occur because people do not believe that the accident that is about to occur is at all possible.
>
> —James Reason

Institute of Healthcare Improvement, and the Agency for Healthcare Research and Quality (AHRQ) because of its effectiveness in identifying and prioritizing hazards. FMEA has been used to identify latent risks in various clinical areas, including the following:

- Emergency department care (Thornton et al., 2014)

- Blood transfusions (Lu, Teng, Zhou, Wen, and Bi, 2013)

- Medication administration (Lago et al., 2012)

- Handoff communication (Steinberger, Douglas, and Kirschbaum, 2009)

- Smart pump implementation (Wetterneck et al., 2006)

- Radiology procedures (Thornton, Brook, Mendiratta-Lala, Hallett, and Kruskal, 2011)

In addition, there are many other applications for FMEA in healthcare. Following are yet more examples of how FMEA can be used in healthcare:

- **To map processes for a new telemetry system with expanded remote monitoring capabilities:** You likely already have a telemetry system and are aware of some process and technological issues. You can use FMEA as part of the implementation plan to take advantage of its new capabilities and to troubleshoot current issues for a stronger (that is, less problem-prone) transition.

- **To evaluate infant security systems from banding babies with sensors to discharge:** Maternity units perform regular drills and vulnerability assessments. You can use FMEA to truly evaluate how your infant security technology and processes interact with the human processes.

- **To define post-operative management of a new surgical population:** Suppose your hospital has recruited a surgeon to perform liver transplants, a new procedure for your hospital. You must plan for post-operative care and meet the transplant regulations of the Centers for Medicare and Medicaid Services (CMS) and the Organ Procurement and Transplantation Network (OPTN). FMEA can assist in this.

- **To implement barcode scanning in the administration of blood products:** Using FMEA can assist if you are adding barcode scanning for blood administration and need to define the process and procedures to integrate the technology into nursing practice.

Notice that these examples are not in response to any event. FMEA is a proactive tool that enables healthcare organizations to look at processes more holistically, hunting for potential failures. Reactive reviews—for example, after an event—use root cause analysis to find contributing factors to a specific outcome. Hospitals accredited by TJC are required to proactively assess a high-risk process every 18 months (TJC, 2014). The FMEA tool is a perfect tool for meeting this requirement.

QUALITY-IMPROVEMENT TOOLS

FMEA uses a number of common quality-improvement tools:

- **Multidisciplinary improvement team:** The FMEA team should be multidisciplinary and represent *all* stakeholders. For example, in the aforementioned barcode project for blood administration, you would want representatives from your IT, biomed, blood bank, and nursing departments at the table.

- **Process mapping:** FMEA uses a visual process map to focus the team on a sequence of events.

- **PDCA:** The Plan, Do, Check, Act (PDCA) approach offers an important structure for the solution-building and implementation phases. Your organization may use Six Sigma's Define, Measure, Analyze, Improve, Control (DMAIC) or FOCUS-PDCA methodology. Any quality-improvement framework will do—the important point is that you use one.

- **Brainstorming:** This tool is particularly useful in the solution-building phase.

- **Five Whys:** This tool is used to develop solutions.

This chapter does not go into any technical depth on these tools. There are many other resources to help you learn how to use them.

PERFORMING AN FMEA

These are the basic steps to performing an FMEA:

1. Identifying a process

2. Forming the FMEA team

3. Mapping the process

4. Analyzing each process step for potential failures, the consequences of said failures, and the probability the failures will occur, and calculating each failure's hazard score to prioritize attention and resources

5. Using an improvement framework such as PDCA to mitigate or eliminate failures with high-value hazard scores

Read on for instructions on conducting each step.

STEP 1: IDENTIFYING A PROCESS

Although you can use FMEA to evaluate any process, you should use your time and resources strategically. Your selected process should have the following characteristics:

- It should have a high degree of risk.

- It should not be in response to an event.

- It should be viewed by senior leaders and medical staff leadership as a priority for resources and focus.

 In this example, a process that involves scanning barcodes of blood products before transfusion will be used to illustrate an FMEA.

STEP 2: FORMING THE FMEA TEAM

The ideal size for an FMEA team is 8 to 10 people. Fewer than 8 may limit diversity, and more than 10 may make it too cumbersome and time-consuming to move through the process. To ensure continuity, it is advisable to have the same team members attend each meeting (Ashley, Armitage, Neary, and Hollingsworth, 2010).

Select team members who represent the stakeholders in the process. These individuals will have an expertise in some or all aspects of the process. Make it a priority to identify front-line staff and minimize management. You want to provide a non-threatening atmosphere for the people who do the work to speak freely. For large stakeholder groups, such as nurses, consider including representatives from different shifts (for example, days, nights, and weekends) and different units (for example, ICU, medical/surgical, and the operating room) to minimize focus on nuances unique to a unit or shift.

For the project in this example—scanning barcodes before administering blood products—we recruited the following members:

- One nurse from the intensive care unit (day shift)

- One nurse from the medical/surgical unit (night shift)

- One nurse from the emergency department (day shift)

- One nurse from the operating room (weekend)

- One representative from the IT/biomedical engineering department (which supports the scanners)

- One representative from the blood blank (which issues the blood armbands)

- One nurse informaticist (they support the EMR and scanning interface)

- One representative from the quality department to facilitate the FMEA and improvement work

 When recruiting members, establish a commitment to attend all meetings. Schedule 3 to 5 meetings several days apart or over 2 to 3 weeks so members and managers can plan accordingly. The longer it takes to complete the analysis, the more difficult it will be to keep the team's attention and interest.

STEP 3: MAPPING THE PROCESS

A *process map* is a visual description of a process. Each step in the map is composed of a verb and a noun, like "map process." Many processes are complex and have multiple subprocesses. You will want to be sensitive to the scope and complexity of the process, knowing that a bigger or more complex process will take more time to map than a smaller, less complex process.

With respect to the mapping process, there are two central questions:

- **What are the start and end points?** The start and end points will be determined by two factors: the aspects of the process you believe to be the riskiest and where a logical separation from other processes exists. If you select too large a process, the FMEA will take too long and your team will lose enthusiasm. If you select too small a process, you will likely not have any real impact on patient safety. As the first order of business, the facilitator should recommend a scope but obtain input from the team.

- **How detailed should the process be?** As with the project scope, you want to find a middle ground in the level of detail. If the process detail is too high level, there will be dozens of things that can go wrong in one process step. If it is too detailed, the team will get bogged down. If your team starts getting into too much detail, defining decision points and alternate paths, remind them of the intent of the process map. It is not to document a procedure for training and education purposes but to analyze the major functions that are performed.

Gathering Materials

You will need the following materials to map the selected process:

- Large sticky notes (4×6 inches is ideal)

- Markers (medium point permanent markers work well)

- Flip-chart paper or, ideally, a 10-foot roll of white butcher paper

Setting Up the Room

You will map the process as a group, during the meeting. Set up the meeting room as follows:

1. Tape the paper on the wall. If it's flip-chart paper, tape up multiple pieces side by side. If it's butcher paper, tape a good-sized length of it on the wall. You will place the sticky notes on this paper, and you will want to be able to take the paper down without disturbing the sticky notes.

2. Organize the tables and chairs in a U-shape facing the flip-chart or butcher paper.

Completing Step 3

As mentioned, each process step should consist of a brief verb-noun combination. To map the process, follow these steps:

1. Place the sticky note containing the first process step on the far left side of the paper.

2. Place the sticky note with the last process step on the far right side of the paper.

3. Fill in the process steps in between, allocating one sticky note per process step.

Discuss the level of detail as you are going and adjust accordingly. The sticky notes make it easy to add or subtract steps or to move steps around.

4. When you believe you are finished, walk through the map one final time.

5. Number each process step.

Depending on the scope of your process, this may require all the time and energy your team has. If so, this is a good time to break. You can always resume later. If your break is long enough, you can transcribe your process into electronic format using word-processing software or a more sophisticated process-mapping program. For our example, Figure 5.1 shows the steps of the blood-scanning process:

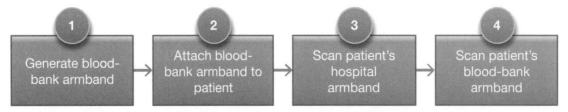

Figure 5.1   Steps for the blood-scanning process.

Notice the scope and level of detail in Figure 5.1. Specifically, note that it does not start with entering the order for blood, nor does it include steps after scanning the patient's blood-bank armband, such as transfusing or vital sign monitoring. It also does not describe the individual steps involved in generating the blood-bank armband. It may be that as we get into the details, we find we need to expand on a process step, but this is where we are starting.

Engage all participants to minimize the impact of what can be tedious work. Give each participant sticky notes and markers and have them place them on the paper.

STEP 4: ANALYZING EACH PROCESS STEP AND CALCULATING A HAZARD SCORE

We now get into the heart of the FMEA. For each step, you will identify all possible failures. In addition, for each failure, you will determine the following:

- How the failure will affect a patient, staff member, visitor, etc. (effects analysis)
- The probability that the failure will occur (occurrence)
- How likely it is that anyone will know the failure occurred (detection)

Gathering Materials

You will need the following materials to analyze each process step:

- **The process map:** You generated this in the previous step.
- **An FMEA grid:** You can create your own FMEA grid (see Table 5.1) using word-processing or spreadsheet software. Calculating the hazard score involves very simple math. Spreadsheet software is not required to calculate these formulas.
- **Severity, occurrence, and detection (SOD) scales:** You can create your SOD scales (see Table 5.2). You will then provide them to participants so they can make notes and follow along. Table 5.2 relates a score for severity, occurrence, and detection to more objective data (Tennessee Center for Patient Safety, 2013).

You may have team members who want to gather more data before committing themselves to a score. If this happens, reassure the group that estimates are acceptable and that the payoff for more concrete data is rarely worthwhile.

TABLE 5.1   FMEA GRID

Process Step	Failure Modes (What might happen?)	Causes (Why?)	Effects (What will the impact on the patient be?)	S (Severity)	O (Occurrence)	D Detection)	S×O×D (Hazard score)
1							
2							
3							
…							

TABLE 5.2   SOD SCALE

Category Score	Severity (What impact will failure have on the patient?)	Occurrence (What is the likelihood the failure will occur?)	Detection (If the failure occurs, how likely is it that we will know it occurred?)
1	Did not reach patient; near miss	≥ 1 in 150,000	Almost certain
2	Reached patient, no harm	1 in 150,000	Very high
3	Reached patient, caused emotional distress or inconvenience	1 in 15,000	High
4	Patient required mild treatment (for example, a few sutures) as a result of the event	1 in 2,000	Moderately high
5	Patient required more significant treatment (for example, surgery) as a result of the event	1 in 400	Moderate
6	Event resulted in temporary harm (bodily or psychological)	1 in 80	Low
7	Event resulted in mild permanent harm	1 in 20	Very low

8	Event resulted in moderate permanent harm	1 in 8	Remote
9	Event resulted in severe permanent harm	1 in 3	Very remote
10	Event resulted in death	≤ 1 in 2	Absolute uncertainty

Completing Step 4

This section demonstrates how to use the FMEA grid and SOD scale using the example of the blood-scanning process. We'll start with step 1, "generate blood-bank armband." Analyze the process step by asking the following questions:

- How can this step fail?

- Why can that failure occur?

> Although it may seem like it, you are not using the Five Whys here. However, the Five Whys will become an important tool during the solution-building phase.

- What impact will failure have on the patient?

- What is the severity score of that effect? Use the severity guidelines in the SOD scale to identify this. (You may identify a variety of effects, from least severe to most severe. To keep things simple, enter the highest severity in this example.)

- How often does this failure occur? Use the occurrence guidelines in the SOD scale and have the group estimate the frequency of occurrence. If there is a range, enter the higher score.

- If this step fails, how likely are you to know it failed? Use the detection guidelines in the SOD scale to select a score.

> Each element of the SOD scale is evaluated independently. They are presented here as a single table simply for ease of reference. If you determine the severity score is 6, this does not mean that the occurrence and detection scores are also 6.

Transcribe your answers into the FMEA grid (see Table 5.3).

TABLE 5.3 FMEA GRID EXAMPLE

Process Step	Failure Modes (What might happen?)	Causes (Why?)	Effects (What will the impact on the patient be?)	S (Severity)	O (Occur- rence)	D (Detection)	S×O×D (Hazard score)
1 Generate blood-bank armband.	The armband can't be printed.	The patient is not registered. The printer is not working. We are out of armbands.	We are unable to use scanning for the admin-istration of blood and will have to perform re-cord keeping manually. Without scanning, the blood could be administered to the wrong patient. Giving blood to the wrong person could be life-threat-ening.	10	6	1	10×6×1 = 60

As shown in Table 5.3, step 1, "generate blood-bank armband," noted one failure: The armband cannot be printed. The team brainstormed possible reasons why this could happen and iden-tified three. (In this phase, we do not concern ourselves with why the *causes* occur; we will get into contributing factors during the solution-building phase.) As the team discussed the impact the failure could have on the patient, we identified the effects from the mundane (manual documentation) to the catastrophic (death). As mentioned, you should always score based on the most severe potential outcome. The team moved on to discuss how frequently staff are unable to generate an armband. In this case, we asked the team member who worked at the blood bank how many times in the last month that has occurred and roughly how many blood-bank armbands they generate on a monthly basis. You are looking for rough estimates here. In this example, the blood-bank representative guessed that 1 out of 80 blood-bank armbands could not be printed with a barcode and had to be handwritten, so we gave occurrence a score of 6.

Our last step in the analysis was to discuss detection—that is, how likely we were to know the failure occurred. In our example, it would be very obvious if the error occurred, so we scored it 1. We then multiplied each score—10×6×1—to calculate a hazard score of 60.

 Technically, the most critical hazard score would be 1,000 (10×10×10). However, the actual score means less by itself than it does in the context of other process-step hazard scores.

Suppose that at this point, the team suggested another process step should be added: "Identify patient." This is a completely legitimate suggestion, and you can easily accommodate it by labeling a sticky note "Identify patient" and inserting it between steps 1 and 2 on the paper. In this case, the last two items under "Effects" in Table 5.3 would be moved to step 1.1. (Technically, this should be step 2.1, but we'll keep things simple here.) Figure 5.2 shows our modified process.

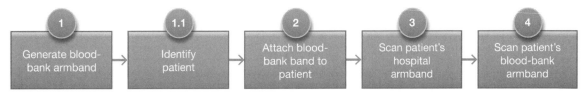

Figure 5.2   Revised process.

Adding step 1.1 changes the scoring for step 1 as shown in Table 5.4. The severity of manual record keeping is benign in that it does not impact the patient. As a result, we change the score for severity to 1, resulting in a hazard score of 6.

TABLE 5.4   REVISED FMEA SCORING

Process Step	Failure Modes (What might happen?)	Causes (Why?)	Effects (What will the impact on the patient be?)	S (Severity)	O (Occurrence)	D (Detection)	S×O×D (Hazard score)
1 Generate blood-bank armband.	The armband can't be printed.	The patient is not registered. The printer is not working. We are out of armbands.	We are unable to use scanning for the administration of blood and will have to perform record keeping manually.	1	6	1	1×6×1 = 6

Your team will then move on to step 1.1, "identify patient," and analyze that step. Then you will analyze each remaining step, including performing hazard scoring, through step 4. Table 5.5 illustrates the findings and analysis.

TABLE 5.5 FMEA FINDINGS AND ANALYSIS

Process Step	Failure Modes (What might happen?)	Causes (Why?)	Effects (What will the impact on the patient be?)	S (Severity)	O (Occurrence)	D (Detection)	S×O×D (Hazard score)
1 Generate blood-bank armband.	The armband can't be printed.	The patient is not registered. The printer is not working. We are out of armbands.	We are unable to use scanning for the administration of blood and will have to perform record keeping manually.	1	6	1	6
1.1 Identify patient.	The patient is not properly identified.	The nurse chooses not to follow the patient-identification process (reckless behavior).	The band is attached to the wrong patient.	2	5	8	80
2 Attach blood-bank armband to patient.	The blood-bank armband cannot be attached.	The patient is edematous. The armband extender is out of stock. The peds/NICU patient is too tiny for the band to stay on.	Staff must find an alternative way to attach the armband to the patient. Transfusion is delayed.	6	5	1	30

3 Scan the patient's hospital armband.	The hospital armband is not scanned.	The arm is under a sterile drape, so blood must be administered without scanning. It is an emergent administration.	The blood-bank armband cannot be scanned.	1	4	1	4
4 Scan the patient's blood-bank armband.	The blood-bank armband is not scanned.	The arm is under a sterile drape, so blood must be administered without scanning. It is an emergent administration.	The blood could be administered to the wrong patient. The wrong blood product or type could be administered.	10	4	10	400

Let's discuss step 1.1 in Table 5.5, "identify patient." Here, the scoring can get tricky. Our minds want to go to the worst-case scenario of administering blood to the wrong patient. However, in this process, there are two additional steps that serve as a safety net:

- **Scanning the patient's hospital armband:** This informs the electronic charting system which patient we are working with.

- **Scanning the patient's blood-bank armband:** This causes the system to check for an order and match the units of blood to what is in the system. If the system does not find issued blood products, the nurse is alerted.

So in this example, identifying the wrong patient does not necessarily result in catastrophe. Not scanning the patient's hospital armband might not cause harm. In this system, if you do not scan the hospital armband, then scanning the blood-bank barcode will not work. As you complete your FMEAs, it is important to make these types of distinctions because accurate hazard scores prioritize energy and focus.

As shown in Table 5.5, failing to scan the blood-bank armband may have the most hazardous outcome. In fact, step 4 has a hazard score of 400, compared to scores of between 4 and 80 for the preceding steps. At this point, FMEA does not provide answers on specific risk-mitigation tactics. It simply tells you where to place your energy and attention for improvements to reduce risk.

This ends the analysis phase, which may take between 3 and 10 hours depending on the scope and complexity of your process. This example is very simple, but it should give you an idea of the FMEA flow and how to use it to understand your specific process.

> You should facilitate the session to keep the analysis moving forward, but do allow for discussion. Some team members may need to think out loud to articulate their thoughts, whereas others may simply like to hear themselves talk. You should feel comfortable moving things along! Note, too, that the analysis phase should not be used for problem-solving. If the team starts identifying solutions, use a flip chart marked "Parking Lot" to capture those thoughts, but process them later.

STEP 5: USING AN IMPROVEMENT FRAMEWORK TO MITIGATE FAILURES

Your work to this point helps you identify the flaws in your current process. The hazard scores help you prioritize your improvement efforts. Failing to act on this analysis leaves your organization with known patient safety vulnerabilities (not to mention many wasted man hours in conducting the FMEA). In quality improvement parlance, the FMEA is a strategic method to identify *what* to improve.

As your team begins the improvement phase, agree on meeting norms. While it may be challenging to free up staff to work on the improvement phase, resist drawing the project out by meeting only monthly. With this approach, teams rarely find the traction they need to test and refine improvement ideas. Meeting weekly or every few days to quickly discuss and refine "tests of change" creates momentum and compresses the improvement cycle.

> During the improvement phase, it is critical to engage leadership. It is at this point where staff need leadership to support culture change and general change management.

Gathering Materials

You will need the following materials to use an improvement framework to mitigate failures:

- A completed FMEA
- An improvement framework (for example, PDCA)
- The Five Whys

Completing Step 5

Your team may choose to address all hazards, all hazards whose scores are above a certain threshold, or the hazard with the highest score. Regardless, you will want to have a conversation about what your team learned about the potential hazards and, with your executive sponsor, make a determination on the scope of the improvement project. For purposes of this example, we will focus on the hazard with the highest score: bypassing scanning the blood-bank armband.

You will use your organization's designated improvement framework, such as PDCA, to organize and drive the improvement phase. In this phase, you will dig deep to uncover *why* staff bypass scanning the blood-bank armband. The Five Whys technique is very effective, and might go something like this:

- **Why do staff bypass scanning the blood bank armband?** Because the arm is under a sterile drape.

- **Why was the band left on and inaccessible?** Because staff felt the patient had been identified on entry into the OR.

- **Why did staff not feel they needed to scan to ensure the blood product was intended for that patient?** Because they manually checked the product against what was ordered.

- **Why do staff find that process more efficient than scanning?** Because they aren't performing the full manual process.

- **Why aren't they performing the full manual process?** Because that expectation has not been reinforced.

Through the Five Whys, we get to the heart of both process and culture issues. If the team fails to identify these contributing factors, they may develop solutions that ultimately do not address the real problem. In this example, it was revealed that the staff did not have an alternative process to make the armband accessible during the procedure, did not recognize the value of scanning, and has been permitted to bypass scanning and yet not complete the full manual process. These cultural issues have likely evolved over time and may fit the definition of "normalization of deviance," where people knowingly disregard a rule because *no one* is following the rule.

The solution to mitigating this hazard score may be very simple:

- Define an alternative location for OR blood-bank armbands.

- Include the location of the blood-bank armband in the procedure briefing/timeout.

- Provide the "why" of the safety procedure.

- Establish the expectation for this behavior.

- Establish how staff will hold each other accountable.

- Determine how you will assess whether these changes resulted in an improvement (that is, monitor and measure).

Measurement is critical. It tells the team whether the changes were effective. In our project, we measure scanning compliance as one indication of success. There may be other intermediate measures such as an intraoperative checklist of armbands relocated during surgery.

To start, use small tests to gauge the effectiveness of the change. Try using the alternate armband site with one OR team for 1 day or 1 week (depending on the volume of patients who may receive blood products during an OR procedure). Get their feedback on what worked well and what didn't. Then adjust the process and try again, either with that OR team or another one. Repeat until the team feels that the process has been thoroughly tested and any kinks have been worked out. A sound change-management strategy will support the culture changes necessary to get the team on board.

 You will perform the Five Whys for every root cause for staff bypassing scanning—not just one, as was discussed here. You can then use the improvement framework for each identified hazard to keep the team on task.

CHALLENGES

FMEA is a time-consuming process filled with challenges. These include the following:

- The need for an experienced leader

- The commitment of human resources

- Identifying failure modes without data

- Evaluating the complexity and volume of steps in current healthcare processes (Wetterneck, Skibinski, Schroeder, Roberts, and Carayon, 2004)

In addition to these, FMEA can be overwhelming. For best results, see the following suggestions:

- **Expect fatigue:** When done well, FMEA is rigorous. It requires getting in deep just to identify where to focus improvement efforts. Combat the fatigue by setting appropriate expectations. Warn team members that there will be moments when it feels tedious, offer frequent breaks, and offer interactivity where possible (for example, let team members fill out sticky notes, place them on the wall, and so on).

■ **Resist scope creep:** It takes discipline and control to establish and maintain focus on a manageable aspect of a process. It can be so challenging to assemble a team of representative stakeholders without trying to expand the scope because they have "everyone in the room together."

■ **Be aware that there is a time commitment:** FMEA and improvement work cannot be completed in one meeting. The number of meetings needed depends on the scope and complexity of the process as well as what failures you elect to address. This can also be a challenge with team members who work shifts and can only attend when they are off. Consider working with their managers to coordinate work schedules so the FMEA team can have consistent attendance.

■ **Meet often:** The team needs traction, particularly in the improvement phase as risk-mitigation ideas are tested and refined. Meeting only once a month makes it difficult, if not impossible, to achieve and sustain momentum. Meet weekly or even daily, get focused, and "git 'er done"!

SUMMARY

FMEA takes a systems approach to evaluating the vulnerabilities in human-built processes and provides the opportunity to identify what measures are needed to keep your patients safe. It helps staff to think about what is possible and helps push them from their tendency to think about how effectively their processes *usually* work.

KEY POINTS

■ Use FMEA to evaluate a process.

■ Do not use FMEA to understand why an event occurred.

■ Do not use FMEA to understand why a particular outcome is occurring (for example, a higher-than-usual rate of DVTs).

■ Select a process that administration, medical staff leaders, and staff feel is high risk and may potentially harm patients.

■ Engage representation from key stakeholders.

■ Allow adequate time to conduct the analysis.

■ At a minimum, address high-value hazard scores using an improvement framework such as PDCA.

■ Compress your analysis and improvement work into weeks, not months.

REFERENCES

Ashley, L., Armitage, G., Neary, M., and Hollingsworth, G. (2010). A practical guide to failure mode and effects analysis in health care: Making the most of the team and its meetings. *Joint Commission Journal on Quality and Patient Safety*, *36*(8), pp. 351–358.

The Joint Commission. (2014). *Comprehensive accreditation manual: Hospitals*. Oakbrook, IL: Joint Commission Resources.

Lago, P., Bizzarri, G., Scalzotto, F., Parpaiola, A., Amigoni, A., Putoto, G., and Perilongo, G. (2012). Use of FMEA analysis to reduce risk of errors in prescribing and administering drugs in paediatric wards: A quality improvement report. *BMJ Open 2*(6), e001249.

Lu, Y., Teng, F., Zhou, J., Wen, A., and Bi, Y. (2013) Failure mode and effect analysis in blood transfusion: A proactive tool to reduce risks. *Transfusion*, *53*(12), pp. 3080–3087.

Reason, J. (1990). *Human error*. Cambridge, England: Cambridge University Press.

Steinberger, D. M., Douglas, S. V., and Kirschbaum, M. S. (2009). Use of failure mode and effects analysis for proactive identification of communication and handoff failures from organ procurement to transplantation. *Progress in Transplantation*, *19(3)*, pp. 208–214.

Tennessee Center for Patient Safety. (2013). FMEA failure risk scoring schemes. Retrieved from http://www.tnpatientsafety.com/PSO/FMEAWebinarSeries2013/tabid/285/Default.aspx

Thornton, E., Brook, O. R., Mendiratta-Lala, M., Hallett, D. T., and Kruskal, J. B. (2011). Application of failure mode and effect analysis in a radiology department. *Radiographics*, *31*(1), pp. 281–293.

Thornton, V. L., Holl, J. L., Cline, D. M., Freiermuth, C. E., Sullivan, D. T., and Tanabe, P. (2014). Application of a proactive risk analysis to emergency department sickle cell care. *The Western Journal of Emergency Medicine*, *15*(4), pp. 446–458. doi: 10.5811/westjem.2014.4.20489

Weick, K. E., and Sutcliffe, K. M. (2007). *Managing the unexpected: Resilient performance in an age of uncertainty*. San Francisco, CA: Jossey-Bass.

Wetterneck, T., Skibinski, K., Roberts, T. L., Klepping, S. M., Schroeder, M. E., Enloe, M., … Carayon, P. (2006). Using failure mode and effects analysis to plan implementation of smart IV pump technology. *American Journal of Health System Pharmacy*, *63*(16), pp. 1528–1538.

Wetterneck, T., Skibinski, K., Schroeder, M., Roberts, T., and Carayon, P. (2004). Challenges with the performance of failure mode and effects analysis in healthcare organizations: An IV medication administration HFMEA. Proceedings of the Human Factors and Ergonomics Society Annual Meeting, September 2004, vol. 48 no. 15, pp. 1708–1712.

CHAPTER 6

CLOSE CALLS AND NEAR MISSES: WHAT'S THE BIG DEAL?

Sherilyn Deakins, MS, RN, CPPS

Imagine it's just another day in the emergency department. A nurse, Brooke, is at the medication station. She expects to pull a Tranxene 7.5 mg tablet from the bin but notices that it looks different. Brooke asks the clinical pharmacist about it, and they look up the medication online. They discover that the medication is not a 7.5 mg tablet but a 15 mg tablet. Brooke is relieved she caught this potential mistake. Otherwise, she would have given the patient a double dose of Tranxene by mistake.

This type of error happens every day in healthcare settings of all types (Institute of Medicine [IOM], 1999). These errors can reach the point of care and cause injury, harm, and even death to patients (James, 2013). Healthcare organizations waste millions of dollars on preventable adverse events (Eber, Laxminarayan, Perencevich, and Malani, 2010). However, many events are caught and do not reach a patient, even though they are recognized as a potential for actual error (Clark, 2012). These types of mistakes are called *near misses* or *close calls* (IOM, 2003). Near misses hit your gut. You say to yourself, "Wow, that was a close call! I'm glad I was paying attention!"

> To make no mistakes is not in the power of man; but from their errors and mistakes the wise and good learn wisdom for the future.
>
> *—Plutarch*

This chapter answers the following questions about near misses and close calls:

- What are they and how do they occur?

- What's the big deal?

- Why should I report a close call if it doesn't reach the patient?

- What should I do when I experience a close call?

- How do I get more reports about near misses or close calls?

WHAT ARE CLOSE CALLS AND HOW DO THEY OCCUR?

A *patient safety event* is an event that reaches the patient, causing harm up to and including severe harm and/or death (The Joint Commission, 2014). Patient safety events also include events that occur but do not reach the patient. These types of events are known as near misses or close calls (IOM, 2003).

The Institute for Safe Medication Practices defines a near miss as an event, situation, or error that occurs but is caught before it reaches the patient (South, Skelley, Dang, and Woolley, 2015). Another common description of a near miss is a recovery process that involves detecting potential errors or deviations in practice and enacting countermeasures to prevent harm (Jeffs, MacMillan, and Maione, 2008).

Near misses can come in all shapes and sizes. Examples of near misses include the following:

- Wrong medications stocked in the medication dispensing bin, which are caught by a nurse prior to administration

- Medication transcription errors, which are caught by a pharmacist prior to entry into the medication record

- A patient misidentified as a do not resuscitate, which is caught due to family interaction prior to any untoward event (Marella, 2007)

- A patient with a high risk for pressure ulcers who is not on the correct prevention measures but who fortunately does not develop a pressure ulcer during his or her hospitalization (Jeffs et al., 2008)

Many terms may be used to describe near misses. These include *near hits, potential adverse events*, and *close calls* (IOM, 2003). A near miss may be considered a misnomer because it implies a near hit or error. Close call seems to better describe an event that almost reaches the patient but is averted. This chapter refers to these events as close calls.

Following are a few others terms and definitions that relate to close calls.

The Agency for Healthcare Research and Quality (AHRQ) defines a medical error as follows (2015):

> Medical errors happen when something that was planned as part of medical care does not work out or when the wrong plan was used in the first place. Medical errors can occur anywhere in the health care system: hospitals, clinics, outpatient surgery centers, doctors' offices, and pharmacies. Errors can involve medicines, surgery, diagnosis, equipment, and lab reports. They can happen during even the most routine tasks, such as when a hospital patient on a salt-free diet is given a high-salt meal. Most errors result from problems created by today's complex health care system, but errors also happen when doctors and their patients have problems communicating.

Finally, the AHRQ defines an adverse event as follows (AHRQ, 2015):

> Any injury caused by medical care. Examples include pneumothorax from central venous catheter placement, anaphylaxis to penicillin, postoperative wound infection, and hospital-acquired delirium (or "sun downing") in elderly patients. Identifying something as an adverse event does not imply "error," "negligence," or poor quality care. It simply indicates that an undesirable clinical outcome resulted from some aspect of diagnosis or therapy, not an underlying disease process. Similarly, postoperative wound infections count as adverse events even if the operation proceeded with optimal adherence to sterile procedures, the patient received appropriate antibiotic prophylaxis in the perioperative setting, and so on.

How do close calls occur? To answer that, one must understand that healthcare is a complex dynamic environment (South et al., 2015). In this environment, patient safety events and medical errors occur. Multiple factors influence the cause for medical errors.

In 1990, James Reason introduced the model of human error theory, which helps identify the various causes for medical errors (Clark, 2012). This model is commonly known as the Swiss cheese model of accident causation (Reason, 2000). The system side of the theory focuses on creating policies, procedures, and work environments to prevent errors. The people side of the theory focuses on creating safe work habits.

It is critical for those in healthcare not only to admit that errors occur but also to plan for those errors. Human error theory has a proactive focus by emphasizing appropriate and effective layers of defenses to prevent errors. Planning for errors helps put those in healthcare in a proactive mode to stop errors. The defense model layers safety measures such as policy, procedures, checklists, double-checks, and technology on top of human action to prevent errors from getting through the system. The more an organization and the individuals within it are aware of safety technology and behaviors, the more a system can improve, and the less likely it is that errors will reach the patient (Jeffs et al., 2008).

WHAT'S THE BIG DEAL?

Patient safety is an essential element of patient care. When patient safety is compromised due to medical errors, injury and death can occur (IOM, 1999). These medical errors can also lead to increased lengths of stay and other unnecessary costs (Pronovost, 2014). New evidence estimates there are between 210,000 and 400,000 premature deaths per year associated with preventable harm (James, 2013). In addition, James indicates there is a 10- to 20-fold increase in serious harm compared to lethal harm, meaning many individuals are affected by preventable harm. Millions of dollars are wasted on preventable adverse events (Eber et al., 2010).

In 1999, the Institute of Medicine (IOM), an agency of the U.S. government, released a report called "To Err Is Human." This report revealed that between 44,000 and 98,000 Americans die each year due to medical errors (IOM, 1999). Healthgrades, a healthcare quality company, estimated that between the years of 2000 and 2002, the number of deaths related to medical errors was 195,000 (Health Risk Management, 2004). The IOM landmark report described several recommendations critical to the improvement of safety in America's healthcare environment. A key theme in the IOM report was the acknowledgment that humans are prone to error and that those errors most often can be traced back to system failures (IOM, 1999). Effective allocation of human and fiscal resources is necessary to mitigate these adverse events (Pronovost et al., 2008). Positive patient outcomes depend on efficient and cost-effective patient safety measures (Pronovost et al., 2008).

WHY SHOULD I REPORT A CLOSE CALL IF IT DOESN'T REACH THE PATIENT?

When it comes to close calls, a common attitude is "No harm, no foul" (Jeffs, Berta, Lingard, and Baker, 2012). In other words, if it doesn't reach the patient, why does it really matter? This is a variation of outcome bias. *Outcome bias* occurs when one judges an event more severely based on the outcome (Dekker, 2011). For instance, if an event in a hospital reaches a patient and causes harm or distress, the event is judged by staff to be something worthy of reporting. On the other hand, if the event was caught prior to reaching the patient, many think there is no need to pursue the event further.

Consider an example. Suppose Thomas is an RN working on a busy medical/cardiac critical care unit. Every day, the unit is filled with critically ill patients, many on ventilators and receiving vasoactive infusions. Each patient is monitored on cardiac telemetry. Hearing the high-alert alarms is critical to attending promptly to clinical changes. Last month, a small fire in the cafeteria caused the fire alarms to go off throughout the whole house. The alarm was extraordinarily loud—so much so that several people said that they could not hear clinical alarms over the fire alarm. The fire department responded, but the alarm continued for 15 minutes.

Fortunately, the patients in the unit experienced no events during the period when the fire alarm went off. The staff were just happy nothing bad happened. Although they noted the *potential* for something bad to happen, they did not follow up by articulating how the alarm could affect patient safety. How would they feel if the same thing happened again and a critical alarm was missed? Many events that affect patients come with warnings that may have occurred days, weeks, or months prior. Had these warnings been noticed and the associated problem fixed beforehand, these events could have been prevented.

 High reliability organizations (HROs) rely on staff noticing and addressing near misses prior to a bad outcome (Kemper and Boyle, 2009).

In the world of patient safety, close calls occur with higher frequency than adverse events. However, many systems either do not catch close calls or offer no way to report close calls (Chang, Schyve, Croteau, O'Leary, and Loeb, 2005). It is estimated that for every adverse event, there are anywhere from 3 to 300 more close calls (Jeffs et al., 2012; Williamsen, 2013). Because close calls occur more frequently, it makes sense to promote reporting. This would allow for a greater opportunity for learning than that which currently exists in most event reporting systems (Jeffs et al., 2012).

How will we learn if we don't report? Because this book is about high reliability, I want to take the opportunity to link this issue to the characteristic of preoccupation with failure. Preoccupation with failure is not a bad thing. In fact, from the patient's perspective, it is a great characteristic of a caregiver. I would much rather have a caregiver who thinks about what could go wrong ahead of time rather than reacting to something that does go wrong after the fact. Which kind of caregiver would you rather have? Which kind of caregiver would you rather *be*?

Some people think it takes too much time to report or even to pay attention to possible close calls (Clark, 2012). If you have been involved in an event that causes harm to a patient or, worse, contributed to a patient's death, you will soon realize that the few minutes it takes to report a close call is far easier to deal with than the amount of time required to review, analyze, and make improvements after a harmful event. Besides, in addition to the patient impact, the toll of an adverse event on the family and caregivers involved is far greater than any inconvenience associated with reporting a close call (Clark, 2012).

Other common barriers or attitudes with regard to reporting close calls include the following:

- **Quick fixes:** Clinicians know there is an error but are so used to doing the "quick fix" that they fail to think of the event as a close call or error at all.
- **The black hole:** Often, even if a close call is reported, the clinician does not hear of a fix or whether the reporting made a difference. As a result, the clinician stops reporting these types of events. Clinicians may also be uncertain whether the data they report is used or whether the organization values this type of reporting.

■ **Stigmas:** Some clinicians fear being stigmatized if they report a problem they made themselves or if they report on a colleague.

■ **Competing priorities:** Clinicians who are very busy may forget to report due to other competing tasks (Jeffs et al., 2012).

Williamsen (2013) lists five reasons why close calls are not reported:

■ Fear of punishment and retaliation

■ Lack of recognition/feedback

■ Peer pressure

■ Concerns about one's record and reputation

■ A desire to avoid work interruption

 These characteristics are not demonstrated only with nursing. The literature indicates that these barriers and attitudes also exist among physicians and pharmacists (Patterson and Pace, 2014; Smith et al., 2014).

Close calls are an important way to learn where an organization's safety systems are vulnerable or non-existent (Speroni, Fisher, Dennis, and Daniel, 2014). Healthcare has much work to do in the field of reporting and analyzing near miss events. As stated, the ratio of actual events to close calls can be as much as 1 actual event to 300 close calls. However, if you look at most healthcare facilities, there is a good chance that the ratio is flipped: More events are reported that cause harm than close calls. Imagine if healthcare righted that ratio. How much more would we learn? How many more events would we avert? Would our harm rates decrease? Could we get to a point of zero harm for all patients? Understanding what behavior and/or process prevented the event from reaching the patient is important for patient safety and the organization's journey toward high reliability (Kemper and Boyle, 2009). It is much easier to be thankful the patient was *not* harmed than to explain to the patient and family why the patient *was* harmed. Ultimately, this is why you should report. It matters to your patients.

WHAT SHOULD I DO WHEN I EXPERIENCE A CLOSE CALL?

The sequence of events that led to a close call is likely the same series of events that could harm a patient (South et al., 2005). Analyzing near miss events against Reason's defense theory will enable you to determine where the system or individual was vulnerable or failed. When you know where the failure lies, you can identify a fix (Clark, 2012).

A close call represents an opportunity for the organization to understand the vulnerabilities in its culture and to be proactive on event avoidance (Clark, 2012). Another important reason to report is to be transparent. This gives you a chance to share your story with others. When stories are shared, it leads to others learning without having to experience the actual event. This may lead to increased safety for patients. It also increases organizational wisdom, which leads to the organization becoming more reliable in the delivery of quality healthcare (Kemper and Boyle, 2009).

One attribute of an HRO is a state of mindfulness (Kemper and Boyle, 2009). This is an increased awareness of the environment in which you work and of the people with whom you work. Analyzing close call events may enable you to glean understanding of events that reach the patient (South et al., 2005). Another reason to analyze close calls is that it serves as an indirect measurement of a safety culture (Williamsen, 2013). The impact of medical errors on patients' lives is devastating (Eber et al., 2010). Understanding how close calls occur brings you one step closer to preventing future events and harm.

HOW DO I GET MORE REPORTS ABOUT CLOSE CALLS?

A robust safety program has been shown to reduce harm and to improve safety and quality of care (Richman, Mason, Mason-Whitehead, McIntosh, and Mercer, 2009). A robust reporting system is an important part of any safety program. Such a reporting system consists of many factors, including the following:

- A clear definition of events to report

- An understanding by end users as to how to report

- A willingness to report

- An ability to aggregate and analyze data

- An ability to interpret data for the implementation of improvements

- An ability to share data for learning opportunities

- Continuous evaluation of all aspects of the reporting system for further improvements (IOM, 2003)

After an organization has been educated with regard to the reporting process (including what and how to report) and has addressed barriers that may prevent reporting, the next step is to increase reporting. The literature suggests various strategies for increasing close call reporting. These include the following (Aston and Young, 2009; Jeffs et al., 2008; Sanghera, Franklin, and Dhillon, 2007):

- Developing award and recognition programs

- Proper awareness and education of safety events

- Ensuring timely feedback to clinicians reporting into the system

At my organization, we tried for years to educate staff about the importance of reporting close calls. We rounded with flyers. We discussed the issue in committees and unit-based meetings. It was all to no avail. Finally, we introduced a daily hospital-wide safety huddle. This was an informal forum for all non-clinicians, clinicians, management, and executive leaders. In the safety huddle, participants are encouraged to share safety issues with no restrictions and no threat of recriminations. Through this 15-minute venue, we increased close-call reporting per 1,000 patient days by 93%—over 300 more close call events reported than before. Our hospital also saw an improvement in the "non-punitive response to error" category on the AHRQ safety culture survey just 6 months after we initiated the daily safety huddle. The safety huddle offers an effective means of learning and sharing events throughout the organization. We also encourage transparency by recognizing those units with the most reports of unsafe or close call events (see Figure 6.1). The numbers don't lie. According to the literature, driving awareness and transparency and sharing our learning via a safety huddle offers hope when it comes to reducing medical error (Goldenhar, Brady, Sutcliffe, and Muething, 2013).

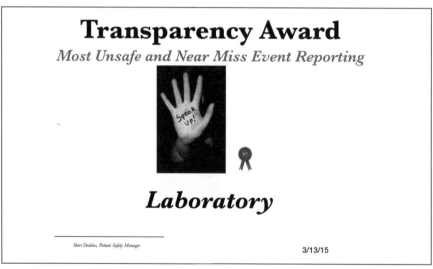

Transparency Award

Most Unsafe and Near Miss Event Reporting

Laboratory

Sheri Deakins, Patient Safety Manager

3/13/15

Figure 6.1. A "Transparency" award for the most reported close calls.

Remember Brooke from the beginning of this chapter? She found what she thought was the wrong dose of Tranxene. Further investigation revealed, however, that the medication she found *wasn't* the wrong dose. In reality, the pharmacy had switched suppliers of the medication, and the new manufacturer's tablet came in a different form and color from what she was used to. Brooke felt bad for what she thought was "wasting people's time." However, she was informed that her preoccupation with failure was more important than whether her report was accurate. Brooke was acknowledged for a great catch and for demonstrating the highly reliable characteristic of preoccupation with failure (see Figure 6.2). These behaviors lead to a state of mindfulness—that is, of being in the present with all attention focused (Howland and Bauer-Wu, 2015). Being mindful during your clinical practice can enhance your awareness of clinical situations and relationships with colleagues. This behavior saves lives and prevents harm (Howland and Bauer-Wu, 2015).

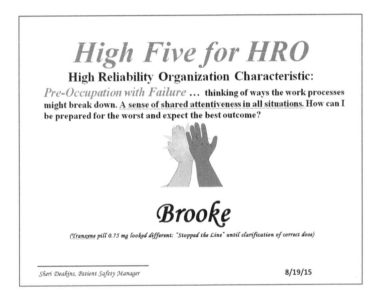

Figure 6.2.   A "High Five" award for the demonstration of a high reliability characteristic (preoccupation with failure).

SAFETY IMAGINATION

Psychologist Nick Pidgeon (2010) described the term *safety imagination*, meaning an exercise or thought process practiced by a mindful organization. He references the Challenger space shuttle disaster, noting that the culture at NASA was to see what people chose to see and to ignore what they did not want to address. This furthers the argument that organizations are defined by what they tolerate. Using a practice of safety imagination in meetings and when discussing high reliability is a way to increase the importance of close call reporting. Safety imagination is defined as engaging in the following practices:

- Attempting to fear the worst
- Using good meeting management techniques to elicit varied viewpoints
- Playing the "what if" game with potential hazards
- Allowing no worst-case situation to go unmentioned
- Suspending assumptions about how the safety task was completed in the past
- Tolerating ambiguity (because newly emerging safety issues will never be clear)
- Visualizing the development of near-miss into accidents (Pidgeon, 2010, p. 215)

SUMMARY

Preventable medical errors are devastating to both the patient and the care provider (Eber et al., 2010). Organizations must continually evaluate the use of current resources to ensure positive patient outcomes while maintaining financial integrity (Pronovost, Weast, and Rosenstein, 2005). Assessing the existing structure and processes and comparing them to new evidence-based strategies is imperative to ensuring the effectiveness of an organization's patient safety program (Speroni et al., 2014). Healthcare organizations must realize that conditions in healthcare environments are very fluid and dynamic. Many interruptions and distractions occur throughout the day, which may lead to close calls or medical errors. Healthcare workers must create safe, protective habits and practice patterns that instill proper defenses to avert errors. Policies and procedures must be scrutinized for conditions that could lead to error-producing conditions. Research focusing on effective error management, including close calls, can be valuable to patient safety.

KEY POINTS

- Close calls are safety events that do not reach the patient.
- Close calls matter in part because they may serve as warning signs for the next potential medical error.
- Close calls should be reported even though they do not cause harm because they may help to reveal individual and/or system fixes prior to patient harm.

- Recovering from an error involves more time than reporting a close call. It is important to speak up in the event of a close call. If you made the mistake, someone else can, too. Your transparency in reporting may save a colleague from making the same mistake, which may end up hurting a patient.

- Literature supports many causes for close calls. These include both individual and system factors. Organizations can improve the safety culture with more close call reporting.

- Close calls allow an organization the opportunity for individual and system learning.

REFERENCES

Agency for Healthcare Research and Quality. (2015). Patient safety glossary. Retrieved from psnet.ahrq.gov/glossary.aspx

Aston, E., and Young, T. (2009). Enhancing the reporting of "near miss" events in a children's emergency department. *Journal of Emergency Nursing, 35*(5), pp. 451–452.

Chang, A., Schyve, P. M., Croteau, R. J., O'Leary, D. S., and Loeb, J. M. (2005). The JCAHO patient safety event taxonomy: A standardized terminology and classification schema for near misses and adverse events. *International Journal for Quality in Health Care, 17*(2), pp. 95–105.

Clark, C. (2012). The near miss: Healthcare leaders are looking at ways to catch adverse events before they happen. *HealthLeaders*, Dec., pp. 58–62.

Dekker, S. (2011). *Patient safety: A human factors approach.* Boca Raton, FL: CRC Press, Taylor and Francis Group.

Eber, M. R., Laxminarayan, R., Perencevich, E. N., and Malani, A. (2010). Clinical and economic outcomes attributable to health care–associated sepsis and pneumonia. *Archives of Internal Medicine, 170*(4), pp. 347–353.

Goldenhar, L. M., Brady, P. W., Sutcliffe, K. M., and Muething, S. E. (2013). Huddling for high reliability and situation awareness. *BMJ Quality & Safety, 22*(11), pp. 899–906. doi: 10.1136/bmjqs-2012-001467

Health Risk Management. Medical error rate may be higher than IOM estimate. *Health Risk Management, 26*(9), p. 106.

Howland, L. C., and Bauer-Wu, S. (2015). The mindful nurse. *American Nurse Today, 10*(9), pp. 12–13.

Institute for Safe Medication Practices. (2009). Acute care ISMP medication safety alert. Retrieved from https://www.ismp.org/Newsletters/acutecare/articles/20090924.asp

Institute of Medicine. (1999). To err is human: Building a safer health system. Washington, DC: The National Academies Press.

Institute of Medicine. (2003). Patient safety: Achieving a new standard for care. Washington, DC: The National Academies Press.

James, J. T. (2013). A new, evidence-based estimate of patient harms associated with hospital care. *Journal of Patient Safety, 9*(3), pp. 122–128.

Jeffs, L., Berta, W., Lingard, L., and Baker, G. R. (2012). Learning from near misses: From quick fixes to closing off the Swiss-cheese holes. *BMJ Quality & Safety, 21*(4), pp. 287–294.

Jeffs, L., MacMillan, K., and Maione, M. (2008). Leveraging safer nursing care by conceptualizing near misses as recovery processes. *Journal of Nursing Care Quality, 24*(2), pp. 166–171.

Jeffs, L., Rose, D., Macrae, C., Maione, M., and MacMillan, K. M. (2012). What near misses tell us about risk and safety in mental health care. *Journal of Psychiatric and Mental Health Nursing, 19*(5), pp. 430–437.

The Joint Commission. (2014). Social aspects of clinical errors. *The Source, 12*(9), pp. 1–10.

Kemper, C., and Boyle, D. K. (2009). Leading your organization to high reliability. *Nursing Management, 40*(4), pp. 14–18.

Marella, W. M. (2007). Why worry about near misses? *Patient Safety and Quality Health Care*, Sept/Oct(4), pp. 22–26.

Patterson, M. E., and Pace, H. A. (2014). A cross-sectional analysis investigating organizational factors that influence near-miss reporting among hospital pharmacist. *Journal of Patient Safety, Aug.*

Pidgeon, N. (2010). Systems thinking, culture of reliability and safety. *Civil Engineering and Environmental Systems, 27*(3), pp. 211–217.

Pronovost, P. (2014). Unit-based safety program improves safety culture, reduces medication errors and length of stay. Retrieved from https://innovations.ahrq.gov/profiles/unit-based-safety-program-improves-safety-culture-reduces-medication-errors-and-length-stay#contactInnovator

Pronovost, P., Rosenstein, B. J., Paine, L., Miller, M. R., Haller, K., Davis, R., ... Garrett, M. R. (2008). Paying the piper: Investing in infrastructure for patient safety. *Joint Commission Journal on Quality and Patient Safety, 34*(6), pp. 342–348.

Pronovost, P., Weast, B., and Rosenstein, B. J. (2005). Implementing and validating a comprehensive unit-based safety program. *Journal of Patient Safety, 1*(1), pp. 33–40.

Reason, J. (2000). Human error: Models and management. *British Medical Journal, 320*(7237), pp. 768–770.

Richman, J., Mason, T., Mason-Whitehead, E., McIntosh, A., and Mercer, D. (2009). Social aspects of clinical errors. *International Journal of Nursing Studies, 46*(8), pp. 1148–1155.

Sanghera, I. S., Franklin, B. D., and Dhillon, S. (2007). The attitudes and beliefs of healthcare professionals on the causes and reporting of medication errors in a UK intensive care unit. *Anaesthesia, 62*(1), pp. 53–61.

Smith, K. S., Harris, K. M., Potters, L., Sharma, R., Mutic, S., Gay, H. A., ... Terezakis, S. (2014). Physician attitudes and practices related to voluntary error and near-miss reporting. *Journal of Oncology Practice, 10*(5), pp. 350–357.

South, D. A., Skelley, J. W., Dang, M., and Woolley, T. (2015). Near-miss transcription errors: A comparison of reporting rates between a novel error-reporting mechanism and a current formal reporting system. *Hospital Pharmacy, 50*(2), pp. 118–124.

Speroni, K. G., Fisher, J., Dennis, M., and Daniel, M. (2014). What causes near-misses and how are they mitigated? *Plastic Surgery Nursing, 34*(3), pp. 114–118.

Williamsen, M. (2013). Near-miss reporting: A missing link in safety culture. *Professional Safety*, May, 46–50.

PART 3

HRO CONCEPTS AND APPLICATION TO PRACTICE: RELUCTANCE TO SIMPLIFY

ROOT CAUSE ANALYSIS: A TOOL FOR HIGH RELIABILITY IN A COMPLEX ENVIRONMENT

Jane S. Braaten, PhD, APRN, CNS, ANP, CPPS

Healthcare today creates a "perfect storm" for error to occur by blending an extremely complex system with human beings to meet the needs of those seeking care. Complexity creates the conditions, whereas humans are put in a position of making errors, causing the storm (Woods, Dekker, Cook, Johannesen, and Sarter, 2012). Human nature leads us to seek easy solutions. As a result, when human beings are caught in this storm, they are often quick to blame the event on human error. But as suggested in the opening quote, safety advances when human error is recognized as merely an attribute of the system rather than the cause of an adverse event (Woods et al., 2012).

High reliability organizations (HROs) rely on finding system and process solutions to prevent human error in a proactive rather than reactive manner (Weick and Sutcliffe, 2007). In contrast, root cause analysis (RCA) has typically been used in a reactive manner—looking backward at an error that has occurred instead of looking forward to anticipate problems that have not yet transpired. The problem with RCA is that in a complex system, conditions

> Progress on safety comes from going behind the label 'human error' where you discover how workers and managers create safety, and where you find opportunities for them to do it even better.
>
> —David Woods, Sidney Dekker, Richard Cook, Leila Johannesen, and Nadine Sarter

are rarely static, so solving problems of the past may not translate to a stable solution for the future (Dekker, 2011). Proactivity in RCA is now imperative to achieve sustainable change. This chapter explains the background, process, and challenges of using RCA as a tool to advance safety in an HRO.

HUMANS AND COMPLEXITY: A PERFECT STORM FOR ERROR

Hospitals are complex systems. In addition to supporting many providers, hospitals face emergent conditions and high-risk situations each day. Furthermore, patient conditions change rapidly. A hospital day that starts casually can shift into high gear without warning. These factors lead to a system with many interrelatable parts that continually change and move.

Woods (1988) described complex environments as having four key characteristics. The characteristics are listed below with their application to the hospital environment:

- **High risk:** Hospitals are known for conducting technologically intense procedures and surgeries.

- **Dynamic and emergent:** Patients may experience quick deterioration of clinical conditions. In addition, resource availability, such as staffing levels, varies.

- **Interdependent parts:** Hospitals support numerous people and disciplines involved in the delivery of care.

- **Uncertain:** Conditions in the hospital can change quickly. For example, an accident that brings many trauma victims to the emergency department is not predictable.

Another important characteristic of complexity is that a complex system cannot be reduced to its parts. A complex system is interdependent. It can be explained only by the interaction between the parts and the whole, not by reducing the parts individually (Dekker, Cilliers, and Hofmyer, 2011). This makes it extremely difficult to consider error-causing events. A simple cause and effect investigation is impossible.

Consider the following example of complexity and interdependence leading to error:

> *A nurse was concerned because her patient was complaining of itching and hives on his face. She assessed the situation and found that the hives were spreading. She associated it with the antibiotic that was infusing. She stopped the infusion, informed a physician, and administered an antihistamine. The reaction cleared. When evaluating the data from the infusion pump (Smart Pump), it was found that the dose of antibiotic went in over 45*

minutes when it should have infused over 2 hours. The nurse had used the drug library provided on the pump and overridden a soft limit in the rate setting. When investigating the event, the first response from the investigating body was that she shouldn't have over-ridden the soft limit. It asked, "Didn't she know that the infusion should go over 2 hours?" The investigating body then took action by educating the nurse. After the investigation, however, it was revealed that the label on the antibiotic contained instructions to infuse the drug over 45 minutes. The nurse followed the instructions on the label. The mistake had originated in the pharmacy. The pharmacy discovered a system error that led to the error in the printing of labels.

Here's another example of complexity and interdependence leading to error:

A nurse and physician working in a very busy emergency department (ED) admitted two patients during the same time period over a shift change. One patient was a young man with changes in mental status. The other was an elderly woman with knee pain. The physician saw both patients and then placed orders for both. (The ED was working on an improvement priority to reduce wait times for patients, so physicians often placed orders after seeing multiple patients.) The physician mistakenly ordered a CT scan of the head for the knee patient and a knee X-ray for the patient with changes in mental status. The CT technician, attempting to quickly complete ED tests (another improvement priority), immediately administered the CT scan of the elderly patient's head. Similarly, the X-ray technician quickly captured an X-ray of the young man's knee. Neither patient questioned these tests. It was not until the results of these tests were returned that the nurse and physician realized the error. This occurred within a span of 30 minutes.

The key concept illustrated in these examples—and in many other adverse events that occur in healthcare—is that simply reducing a problem to a simple cause, such as human error, fails to recognize the complex factors that exist in healthcare. Our natural inclination is still to look at the individual rather than the system because it gives us an illusion of control (Dekker, 2012). However, the situation behind the error was most likely present and evolving long before the unfortunate individual experienced the error. Think about your first reaction to these cases. Was it difficult to abstain from passing judgment on the providers or staff members in question? Thus the need for RCA to dig deeper to discover the system and relationships that led to the errors. Perhaps Henriksen, Dayton, Keyes, Carayon, and Hughes (2008, p. 4) said it best:

…the error is just the tip of the iceberg; it's what lies underneath that we need to worry about. When serious investigations of preventable adverse events are undertaken, the error serves as simply the starting point for a more careful examination of the contributing system defects that led to the error. However, a very common but misdirected response to managing error is to "put out the fire," identify the individuals involved, determine their culpability, schedule them for retraining or disciplinary action, introduce new procedures or retrofixes, and issue proclamations for greater vigilance.

ROOT CAUSE ANALYSIS: DISCOVERING THE SYSTEM ISSUES (ROOTS) OF THE PROBLEM

An RCA is a systematic team event to thoroughly analyze a problem using standardized tools and techniques to find the system issues that led to an adverse event (Andersen and Fagerhaug, 2006). An RCA involves asking the following questions:

- What happened?
- How did it happen?
- Why did it happen?

RCA investigations can be traced back to the 1950s. They started with Toyota and spread to the engineering, production, and aviation industries (Fatima, 2015). Healthcare adopted the process in part due to the Institute of Medicine's (IOM's) report "To Err Is Human" (1999). It stated that errors are not the result of bad people but poor oversight and poor systems. The seminal "Swiss cheese model" developed by John Reason (1990) helped define the approach for healthcare. This model illustrates how errors begin higher up in the system, presenting themselves when all the system issues and human issues, or holes, line up to allow them to become visible, often through an adverse event.

Reason (1990) describes two types of errors:

- **Active errors:** Active errors are those errors that involve practitioners close to the bedside. These practitioners are often the most closely involved or the most proximate factor to the error.
- **Latent errors:** Latent errors occur higher up in the system. They involve factors such as structural components of the organization, the work environment, the workload, and the culture. Latent errors may exist in the system for days, weeks, months, or years before the error surfaces in an active event that affects a patient.

Active and latent errors are also categorized as sharp-end failures (active failures) and blunt-end failures (latent failures) (Cook and Woods, 1994). This depiction is actually more telling of the type of emotional response that occurs as a result of an error. The person at the sharp end is often the victim of system issues and experiences anger, fear of blame, and helplessness.

More often than not, nurses are sharp-end inheritors of a problem that started at the blunt end (Hughes, 2008). For example, consider the following scenario:

> *An RN in a busy ICU was caring for two busy patients. One required multiple antibiotics. The other needed insulin. These infusions were delivered and stored together in the medication area. When the nurse picked up one of the antibiotics, her phone rang. It was a call she needed to answer, so she set the antibiotic down to take the call. After the call was over, a nurse's aide asked the nurse a question, which she answered. After these interruptions, the nurse returned to the task of administering the antibiotic. But instead of picking up the antibiotic she had set down, she accidentally picked up the insulin drip. She hung the insulin drip and programmed it at the antibiotic rate. She caught the error only when she went to find the insulin drip for the other patient. The first patient, who had been given insulin by mistake, experienced an immediate drop in his blood sugar and required hours of extra treatment and monitoring.*

Blunt-end factors that affected the bedside nurse in this situation included the workload, a work environment that tolerated frequent interruptions, and high-risk medications that were not easily differentiated from antibiotics. The nurse in this situation felt horrible afterward and received training to "be more careful next time." After the event occurred another time, insulin drips were marked with a bright pink label.

Focusing on the sharp end and not the blunt end is an inadequate approach to dealing with failure. Reason (2000) likens blaming individuals for these types of events to swatting mosquitoes. You can continue to swat mosquitoes, but the root cause of the mosquitoes lies ignored: the swamp.

RCA: A BRIDGE TO THE "NEW VIEW" OF SAFETY

The importance of RCA is made evident in Sidney Dekker's work contrasting two views of safety (2002). The old view sees errors as competency problems. It holds to believing our systems are safe and that incompetent people are to blame for errors. This view protects the system from unreliable individuals. In contrast, the new view sees human error as an organizational problem. This view holds that our systems are not inherently safe and that human error derives from the relationship between humans and the system. In the new view, human error is indicative of trouble higher up in the system and should be investigated as such.

With respect to high reliability, RCA should be designed to investigate events through this new lens. RCA can be used as a bridge to advance safety toward Dekker's new view, with an emphasis on fixing systems and investigating their effects on the individual (see Figure 7.1).

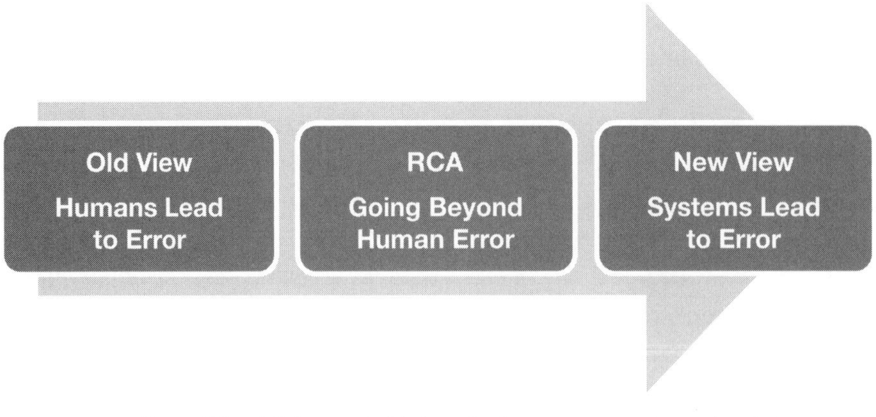

Figure 7.1 RCA as a bridging factor to a new view of safety.

ARE HOSPITALS WITH MORE RCAS SAFER?

The ability of the RCA process to affect safety outcomes in hospitals is not fully understood. This is due to a lack of studies to evaluate its effectiveness (Percarpio and Watts, 2013; Percarpio, Watts, and Weeks, 2008; Wu, Lipshutz, and Pronovost, 2008). In addition, RCA may be implemented ineffectively due to constraints such as lack of resources and training, incomplete results, and incomplete solutions (National Patient Safety Foundation [NPSF], 2015; Wu et al., 2008). RCA may also be ineffective if it does not consider multiple causes and the complexity of systems (Dekker et al., 2011).

One of the first large-scale attempts to correlate RCA frequency with patient safety indicators was performed by the Department of Veterans Affairs Medical Centers (VAMCs) (Percarpio and Watts, 2013). It found that larger VAMCs conducted more RCAs with stronger interventions than smaller VAMCs. At these larger VAMCs, three patient safety indicators (postoperative sepsis, postoperative physiologic or metabolic derangement, and postoperative hemorrhage) were lower than at the smaller facilities. VAMCs with the highest frequency of RCAs did not have significant differences in outcomes from those with a moderate number. Researchers concluded that there did appear to be an association between patient safety and fewer (less than three per year) RCAs performed. However, the low numbers were in the smaller VAMCs. These may also have had fewer resources for patient safety, which may have affected safety more than the number of RCAs.

There is a need to correlate RCAs with improved safety in hospitals as well as a need to find an adequate measure of RCA's effectiveness. The actual impact of RCA and how to measure it is elusive. Percarpio and Watts (2013) state that perhaps RCAs should be studied as affecting a broader range of patient safety indicators. They also suggest comparing RCA effectiveness against other methods of improvement. Because RCA has become the acceptable and mandated (see the next section) method for investigating events, study on its effectiveness and best practice in implementation is imperative.

THE JOINT COMMISSION AND THE RCA

The Joint Commission (TJC) has a policy to address sentinel events for accredited organizations. *Sentinel events* are defined as events that are not related to the normal course of the patient's illness that result in death, severe harm, or temporary harm (TJC, 2015). When a sentinel event is identified, the accredited organization must perform a systematic review. The review does not have to be an RCA, but RCA is the most common method used. RCAs are then voluntarily submitted to TJC for review. The RCA is reviewed by TJC, which documents root causes in a database. Reporting of these events is voluntary and does not represent a comprehensive data set. However, the trends may reflect the tip of the iceberg.

Top root causes of sentinel events from 2012 to 2014 identified by TJC include the following:

- Human factors
- Leadership
- Communication
- Assessment and information management
- Physical environment
- Care planning
- Continuum of care
- Operative care
- Medication use
- Information technology (TJC, 2015)

When an RCA or other systematic analysis is submitted to TJC, it is reviewed for thoroughness, credibility, and acceptability. Key points for this review are as follows:

- **Thoroughness:** Does the analysis
  - Ask a series of "why" questions until system causes are revealed?
  - Focus on system and processes, not just on individuals?
  - Determine human and other factors (systems and processes) most proximate to the event?
- **Credibility:** The RCA must
  - Include participation by a senior leader or someone outside of the team.
  - Include those most closely involved in the process involved.

- **Acceptability:** The RCA must

  - Identify changes that reduce risk or provide appropriate rationale for not undertaking changes.

  - Identify who is responsible for implementation, timeline, effective measurement of actions, and how sustainability will occur (TJC, 2015).

These recommendations provide structure and standardization for an effective RCA. Most recently, the National Patient Safety Foundation (NPSF) (2015) published comprehensive guidelines titled "Root Cause Analysis and ACTION (RCA²)." These guidelines highlight a standardized approach based on risk rather than immediate severity, with strong actions and follow-up to produce sustainable results. This report suggests that the effectiveness of the RCA is found in the process of the RCA, with a focus on identifying system issues as causes of human error with strong causal statements. Furthermore, effectiveness relies on the last steps of the process: the action, how well the action addresses the problem, and how the action is achieved, supported, and measured for sustainability. The next section explains the steps to an effective RCA to meet these criteria.

THE STEPS TO AN EFFECTIVE RCA

The steps to an effective RCA are published in many accounts in the literature. Broadly, the RCA process can be broken down into the steps outlined in Figure 7.2.

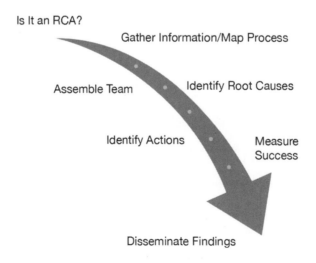

Figure 7.2   Steps to an RCA.

STEP 1: IS IT AN RCA?

The first step in the process is to decide whether RCA is the appropriate method of evaluation for the problem. As noted, TJC requires a systematic review such as an RCA for sentinel events. However, not all events require an RCA. The NPSF (2015) recommends that organizations define for themselves what events are deemed to be "blameworthy." It further recommends that organizations handle these events in a human resources or disciplinary forum rather than with an RCA.

Events discovered through a Just Culture process that are found to be clearly due to reckless behavior with no system or process implications should not be subject to an RCA-type review. These include the following:

- Criminal acts such as theft or abuse

- Acts due to impairment or substance abuse

- Unsafe acts in which providers intended to cause harm or were fully aware of the harm that could occur but purposely chose the action anyway (Department of Veterans Affairs, 2011)

This line can be tricky, however. For example, acts due to substance abuse or instances of drug diversion seem fairly clear-cut in terms of individual accountability and lack of system responsibility. But suppose someone is hired and is permitted to work while impaired or is able to divert drugs until he or she makes a mistake that harms a patient. How do you know your system of oversight or detection is not at fault? Even when reckless behavior is the cause of an error, there may still be room to examine your system for issues regarding early detection and mitigation of said behavior.

RCA is resource-intensive and can't be used for every event. Most often, we use RCA when the resulting harm is judged to be severe, as required by TJC. However, the NPSF has recommended a prioritization system based on risk, thereby including close calls or near misses that could have led to severe harm. You can find further information and an example of a risk matrix at www.npsf.org.

The rationale for using a risk matrix to decide whether to perform RCA rather than choosing to perform RCA based on the severity of injury is sound. Completing an RCA for near misses and close calls is important for high reliability and proactivity. HROs focus on preventing and identifying events *before* they reach a patient (Chassin and Loeb, 2013). Using RCA for only those events that reach patients likely ignores many events that will reach patients in the future. How would you feel if you were told by your surgeon, "We have never had anything bad happen to a patient with this procedure. If something does go wrong, you can rest assured that we haven't planned for it, won't know what caused it, and won't know what to do!" RCA can be proactive and preventative if used to investigate close calls and near misses.

STEP 2: GATHERING INFORMATION

The goal for this phase of RCA is to obtain as much information as possible. To ensure that all versions of the event are investigated, Dekker et al. (2011) state that an investigation should seek multiple sources and multiple points of view without attempting to ascertain who is right or who is wrong. Limiting the information gathered will lead to bias and an RCA with limited effectiveness.

Gathering information may include obtaining policies, procedures, and meeting minutes. It may also involve taking pictures of faulty equipment, obtaining logs from technical devices such as IV pumps, examining electronic medical records, and interviewing staff involved in the event. Interviewing those involved is the most crucial and technical item on this list. As soon as the investigation begins, investigators should interview those with the most knowledge of the event. Interviews should be set up promptly and conducted one on one, preferably face to face in a private setting that is comfortable for the interviewee. Potential candidates for interviews include the following:

- The person most closely involved or who experienced the event

- Witnesses to the event or those in the area when the event occurred

- Family or patients who have knowledge of the event

- Those involved in creation, education, or implementation of the system or process that led to the event

 The ability to interview staff about a safety event is not an inherent skill. Experience and practice with a mentor can help improve skills.

When interviewing staff, ensure that the purpose of the interview is not to assign blame but to find system causes that led to the event. Also, do not ask why the individual made the error. Instead, ask why the action taken made sense to the individual at the time (Dekker, 2011). This helps to reveal system issues. Questions should be designed not only to obtain the facts in the case but also to dig deeper to reveal information about resources available, the physical environment, information accessibility, time pressures, and the culture of safety.

Before interviewing, it is important to prepare the interview questions. Start the interview by asking the participant to describe what happened. Then ask more probing questions to allow system issues to emerge. For example:

- How many other patients were you taking care of?

- What were your other duties on that day?

- What kind of training were you given to perform that procedure?

- Who do you go to for assistance and expertise when you need help?

- Were the orders clear?

- Where do you find that policy and how easy is it to understand?

- Was information in the electronic record easily found?

- What equipment was needed? Was it available?

- Do you feel it is easy to speak up when you are uncomfortable with a situation?

Creating a document to record the interviews, data gained, and data needed is an important step of RCA. Table 7.1 shows an example from a patient who experienced a failure to rescue event due to a severe gastrointestinal bleed. The nurse did not make a rapid response team (RRT) call prior to the patient becoming unresponsive. After noting a heart rate and breathing change, she consulted her charge RN. Both agreed that this was not a significant enough change to call for help because "we don't usually call the team unless we really have to."

TABLE 7.1   SAMPLE INTERVIEW NOTES

Type of Information	Name	Relevance to Event	Significant Points	Further Data Needed
Interview	J. B.	Staff member who found patient and eventually called RRT and then Code Blue	Subject did not feel the patient met RRT criteria.	Interview other staff members involved in care and RRT team members who responded.
			Subject had the charge nurse look at patient; he agreed.	Check for acceptance of calling for help and calling the RRT team.
				Check charting for RRT criteria.
				Check assessments/labs.
Policy	Rapid Response Team (RRT) Policy	Describes protocol for calling RRT	Policy contains calling criteria.	Check availability of protocol to staff.
				Ask staff how they interpret the criteria.

continues

TABLE 7.1   SAMPLE INTERVIEW NOTES   (CONTINUED)

Type of Information	Name	Relevance to Event	Significant Points	Further Data Needed
Chart documen-tation	Vital signs Labs Assessments	Looking for trends in blood-pressure rate, heart rate, and labs values before event and indicators of deterioration	BP was trending lower and heart rate was trending toward intermittent tachycar-dia with activity. Hematocrit was ordered but not completed.	Check with staff on use of trending functions. Why wasn't hematocrit completed?

STEP 3: MAPPING THE PROCESS

One of the most important steps in RCA is mapping the event. This can be done with a simple timeline or flow chart. The keys to this process are accuracy, transparency, and diversity of information. The map should have enough detail to allow team members to place themselves in the shoes of the individual involved in the situation. The review team should feel the same physical stressors, barriers, limits, and lack of resources that the individual felt at the time of the event. This will help them to understand the "local rationality" affecting actions—that is, how situational factors lead to an interpretation of events that ultimately prompts actions (Dekker, 2011). Dekker states that the challenge lies in understanding how decisions made sense at the time. This understanding arises only through details obtained during interviews, verbatim narrative accounts, pictures, documentation cited, and a review of pertinent processes or policies.

Consider the following scenario (see Table 7.2):

> *Mr. R. was a 60-year-old gentleman awaiting discharge from a cardiac stepdown unit. He was to remain on telemetry monitoring until discharge. His family had been visiting but left to get lunch. The nurse taking care of him had two other patients who were keeping her very busy and was in another room. The telemetry technician noted that Mr. R. was off the monitor but had seen the patient's family in the room earlier, knew the patient was going home, and didn't see the patient's nurse, so he did not alert anyone. The technician then went to lunch after giving report to a covering technician. The covering technician also noted that the patient was off monitor but saw the discharge note and thought he was gone. Twenty minutes later, the nurse walked by the room and saw the patient on the floor, unresponsive.*

TABLE 7.2: SAMPLE TIMELINE

	1200	1205	1210	1220	1230	1240
Patient	Awaiting discharge. Family in room.	Family left room. Did not tell anyone at desk that they were leaving.	On telemetry monitor.	"Leads off" reading on telemetry.	"Leads off" reading on telemetry.	Found unresponsive.
Nurse	This patient was stable. Had two other higher-acuity patients.	Taking care of other patient.	Taking care of other patient.	Did not see this because she was in another room and counted on someone to notify her if something was needed.		Walked by room on way to desk and saw patient on floor.
Telemetry technician 1	Watching telemetry but also answering phone and entering orders per job description.		Needing lunch.	Thought this patient was going home so assumed nurse was in room to discharge.	Gave report to oncoming telemetry technician. Mentioned that the patient was being discharged.	
Telemetry technician 2	Watching telemetry on other side of unit.				Watching telemetry but also answering phone, entering orders as per job description. Thought patient was being discharged.	Called Code Blue when nurse called out of the room to do so.

STEP 4: ASSEMBLING THE TEAM

With respect to assembling teams, there are two current practices:

- Assembling a team that includes those involved in the event
- Assembling a team that includes experts on the subject matter who were not involved

Current NPSF guidelines prefer the latter. In this model, the review team should be made up of no more than four to six people. This both increases efficiency and minimizes resources used. Team members should consist of the following:

- A team lead with training and expertise in the RCA process

- An expert in the subject matter at hand

- An individual in the organization who has little knowledge of and is not a stakeholder in the process at hand

- Front-line staff familiar with the process at hand

- A patient representative who represents the interests of the patient and family affected

This model does not include staff directly involved in the event to avoid possible conflicts of interest or the introduction of bias.

The benefits of this model are that it reduces bias and ensures an objective review. When staff who were involved in the event are present, it may introduce bias. For example, the review team might sidestep delicate questions or skirt around controversial issues to avoid making the individual feel uncomfortable. Many RCAs uncover intense emotions as individuals place themselves back into the scene or experience grief or remorse. This can lead to the individual claiming ownership of the situation and denying system issues. On the other hand, the individual could become defensive, causing the team to dismiss issues that need to be addressed to ensure harmony.

 An outside review (that is, a review by a team not involved in the event) may be subject to a different type of bias: hindsight bias—in other words, a tendency to pass judgment when looking at a situation with information that was not available at the time.

This model demands a great deal of work, both up front and during meetings. The RCA facilitator must be skilled in interviewing and mapping events. All information must be available for the team to evaluate because those people who were involved are not there to refute or dispute facts. This involves a meticulous mapping of the event and evidence prior to the meeting. A review with those involved to ensure the integrity of presented material before the meeting is also necessary.

 Staff involved in an adverse event deserve a debriefing where they can grieve if necessary. Debriefing is not the intent of the RCA. Debriefing sessions should be scheduled and facilitated with appropriate staff leads to allow staff to grieve without allowing that grief to compromise the RCA.

Organizational support of the RCA team is critical. This ensures team members are willing to participate. When an event touches an individual, that individual will likely be willing or even required to participate in the analysis. However, when team members are *not* involved in the event, they must understand that their involvement in the investigation is necessary.

As suggested by the NPSF, selecting team members who were not involved in the event is preferred. Still, RCAs are sometimes conducted by those who were most closely associated with the event. This is often done to provide stakeholders with a sense of closure. It may also be done if the people in the organization with the most expertise in dealing with such situations are the staff involved in the event. In this model, interviews are completed before the RCA, with information and facts still forthcoming during the formal RCA. This also provides a forum for team members to state their concerns in front of peers, supervisors, and administration. This can be both emotional and cathartic. An argument for this model is that it provides closure and transparency. An argument against is that it can be subjective and driven by emotion. When standardization and effectiveness are key to the RCA, the risks of this model outweigh the benefits.

 If the staff involved in the incident are not a part of the RCA team, it's critical to ensure that the RCA is an objective review, with all information presented logically and credibly. This calls for intense skills and credibility on the part of the RCA team leader.

STEP 5: IDENTIFYING ROOT CAUSES

Many events have several root causes. Root causes are those conditions that precede the event. They are triggering factors that started upstream of the event. As noted, swatting mosquitoes does not eradicate the swamp that produced them.

One failure of many investigations is to avoid digging deeply to find the root causes. Jens Rasmussen (1990) concluded that often, people stop an investigation when they find a cause that is familiar or acceptable to them or a problem with a known "cure." For example, many health-care investigations stop at provider issues because remediating issues with a provider is known, familiar, and, for the most part, acceptable. Consequently, in one study that examined RCAs in New York (Deeter and Rantanen, 2012), leadership and organizational factors were frequently left out as root causes—perhaps because this is an area people are less comfortable addressing. An effective RCA must be able to identify unfamiliar problems that may or may not have a known solution.

The easiest way to identify root causes in an RCA is to progressively ask why and to then map the answers to these questions into a cause-and-effect map such as a fishbone diagram. One method, the Five Whys, can be very effective (Vidyasager, 2015). Consider a case in which a patient on a mental-health hold was allowed to access his personal belongings. This patient got dressed and walked out of the emergency department without anyone seeing him. The Five Whys method starts at the adverse outcome and asks why until the system issues emerge (see Figure 7.3). Without this method, the organization might have stopped on the second why and counseled or disciplined the employee deemed responsible without noticing the proverbial "swamp," or system issue, that was the root cause of the event.

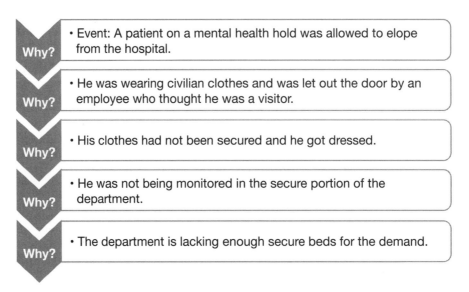

Why? • Event: A patient on a mental health hold was allowed to elope from the hospital.

Why? • He was wearing civilian clothes and was let out the door by an employee who thought he was a visitor.

Why? • His clothes had not been secured and he got dressed.

Why? • He was not being monitored in the secure portion of the department.

Why? • The department is lacking enough secure beds for the demand.

Figure 7.3   Using the Five Whys.

The Five Whys method can be very effective. It forces people to keep asking questions beyond what is a comfortable or familiar cause, such as human error. However, some situations may not have a logical "why," so it is important to frame the questions effectively. The outcome of asking "why" five times should be to arrive at a system issue that, if removed or corrected, would have prevented the event.

The NPSF report states that each root cause must adhere to the five rules of causation (2015). These rules are as follows:

- **Rule 1:** Clearly show the cause-and-effect relationship.

- **Rule 2:** Use specific and accurate descriptors for what occurred rather than negative and vague words.

- **Rule 3:** Human errors must have a preceding cause.

- **Rule 4:** Violations of procedures are not root causes but must have a preceding cause.

- **Rule 5:** Failure to act is only causal when there is a pre-existing duty to act.

Table 7.3 applies these five rules to the aforementioned mental-health patient.

TABLE 7.3   THE FIVE RULES OF CAUSATION APPLIED TO THE PATIENT-ELOPEMENT EXAMPLE

Rule Number	Rule Description	Application to Example
1	Clearly show the cause-and-effect relationship.	The patient eloped because he was not in a secure location and his clothes were accessible.
2	Use specific and accurate descriptors for what occurred rather than negative and vague words.	The patient could not be distinguished from a visitor because he was dressed in his own clothes.
3	Human errors must have a preceding cause.	The employee let the patient out the door because he thought the patient was a visitor because he was wearing civilian clothes.
4	Violations of procedures are not root causes but must have a preceding cause.	Procedure for securing clothes was not followed because the patient was not in the designated secured area of the emergency department.
5	Failure to act is only causal when there is a pre-existing duty to act.	The employee did not stop the patient from leaving because he did not know he was on a hold.

After asking the Five Whys and arriving at the root causes for a problem, you can plot these root causes into a fishbone diagram to visualize how they contributed to the event. *Fishbone analysis,* or the *Ishiwaka diagram,* is a method to study root causes by examining the categories of causes that led to an event. A fishbone analysis enables you to organize causes into similar categories that cover different aspects of the system, such as patient factors, human factors, culture, resources, information, and environment. For an example of and template for a fishbone diagram, see http:// www.isixsigma.com/tools-templates/cause-effect/cause-and-effect-aka-fishbone-diagram/. Figure 7.4 shows a fishbone diagram for the mental health–elopement example.

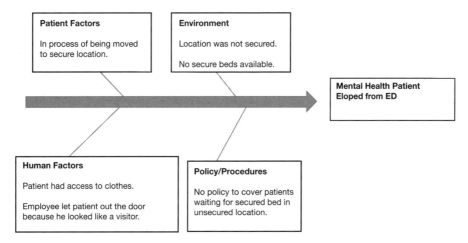

Figure 7.4   Example of a fishbone diagram.

STEP 6: IDENTIFYING ACTIONS

Action planning is the most important step in an RCA (NPSF, 2015). The failure of an RCA to drive change is often caused by action planning that:

- Did not match the root cause

- Relied on weak methods of intervention

- Did not have responsibilities and timelines attached

- Did not include accountability and follow-up

- Did not include measurable outcomes

Action planning should be robust. It should be clear as to what is to be done, who is responsible, how it will be measured, and the timing of follow-up (NPSF, 2015). Table 7.4 illustrates one root cause of an incident wherein a tracheostomy tube became dislodged during mobilization.

TABLE 7.4   ROOT CAUSE ACTION PLANNING SHEET

Root Cause	Action	Who	When	Measure
Lack of specific orders for tracheostomy stabilization during mobility	Order set revision	Physician group	November 1, 2015	Completion
				Compliance with use
				# of dislodgements after placement

Many RCAs fail to produce results due to weak interventions aimed at training or policy change. Often, we fall back on training or retraining staff after an event or error. Although training is sometimes necessary, human-factors research tells us that training without also addressing system issues is not likely to sustain a change for long. Without a system change, the condition that caused the error will likely surface again due to the human factor (Carayon et al., 2014). Moreover, training does not reach all staff—particularly new staff or floating staff. The strongest intervention is system-based forced functions that direct staff to safety instead of letting them drift away from it without realizing it. Table 7.5 shows the strength of different interventions for various problems.

TABLE 7.5   STRENGTH OF INTERVENTIONS

Problem	Weak	Intermediate	Strong
Infusing antibiotics too fast	Train all staff on appropriate rates.	Require staff to double-check rate prior to infusion.	Apply hard limits on pumps to prevent infusion above a certain rate.
Tube feeding hooked up through an IV line	Label tubing with "For Enteral Use Only."	Display alert on computer screen that reads "For Enteral Use Only."	Install incompatible connections so that equipment can be connected only to the correct tube or site.
Non-escalation of patient deterioration	Encourage escalation by staff members.	Standardize a communication tool to accurately relay urgency.	Automate a call to an emergency response team to respond and assess a patient based on vital sign parameters.

STEP 7: MEASURING SUCCESS

The actions identified in the RCA action plan should have measurable criteria. The structure, process, outcome (SPO) (Donabedian, 1988) model is a framework for use:

- Structural measures include changes to the physical environment of the facility such as breakaway doorknobs to prevent inpatient suicide.

- Process measures include the general practice of how things are done. An example of a process measure is performing a standardized assessment of suicide risk on each patient and implementing interventions tailored to high-risk patients.

- Outcome measures are "big picture" indicators that reflect the goal of care. In the suicide example, the outcome would be inpatient suicides or attempts. Outcome measures can also include items such as cost or provider issues—for example, nurse turnover.

General recommendations include a process and/or structural and outcome measure for each problem identified in the RCA. The process/structural measure is usually the action planned, and the outcome measure shows how effective the action is (NPSF, 2015). (See Figure 7.5.)

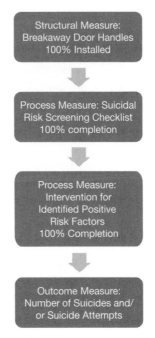

Figure 7.5 SPO measurement example.

Quality improvement measurement does not have to be as rigorous as research but does require rigor. Poor implementation of RCA actions is sometimes due to a lack of documentation of metrics that prove the work has been done and has affected the outcome. Each metric should have a clear plan for measurement that includes what to measure, the goal of the metric, frequency of measurement during the improvement period, and how to measure sustainability.

STEP 8: DISSEMINATING FINDINGS

The final step is the dissemination of results, although it is sometimes left out. There are two main types of dissemination:

- **Internal dissemination:** This refers to the dissemination of results to hospital staff and leadership. Staff involved in the event need to know the outcome of and changes from the RCA. You must also share the results in higher-level meetings to reflect on other areas where the findings might apply. For example, suppose a computerized order set contains a default to an adult dose of narcotic, which can be mistakenly used on a child. It is important to share this information not only with the area where it occurred but with other areas as well. Ask the question, "What order sets do you use on children and adults, and are there areas of potential risk there?" Finally, results should be disseminated to the hospital's leadership and board. Many interventions are made stronger simply by their support. A well-explained RCA case study can highlight identified risks within the system that, if not mitigated, could be easily replicated. When made aware of these risks, it is difficult for a board or executive leadership to *not* call for action.

- **External dissemination:** This moves the RCA to an examination of the bigger picture, with lessons learned from many RCAs being published or presented as a descriptive or analytical study of causes and effects. Taitz et al. (2010) stated that aggregating RCA results at a system level can lead to better and stronger interventions because of the resources available and the magnification of the event.

AVOIDING BIAS: THE PERILS OF JUDGING HUMAN BEHAVIOR

One of the biggest challenges in an RCA investigation is avoiding bias. Errors almost always involve a human factor. RCA groups include professionals with experience and expertise in the subject matter. Unfortunately, expertise and experience often lead to judgment. This is especially true when the expert, looking at the event with the benefit of hindsight, has more information than the person who was involved with the error had at the time. This may cause the placement of blame on the person who committed the error rather than an examination of system issues that caused the person to commit the error.

 The purpose of an RCA is to find root causes upstream within the system that led to the error so those issues can be addressed. If the real cause was just one person, there would be no need for an RCA.

Many types of bias can occur during an RCA. Two types of bias are discussed here:

- Hindsight bias
- Outcome bias

HINDSIGHT BIAS

Hindsight bias occurs when one looks back at events with information that fits the outcome and believes that the outcome was predictable from the onset (Dekker, 2011). The problem with looking back is that the information available afterward was often not available at the time of the event. Typical hindsight bias responses from patient safety events include thinking that the people involved should have known better. For example:

- "They should have seen the symptoms of high potassium before they gave that supplement."
- "They should have read the label more closely before they gave the wrong medication."

- ■ "They should have checked the trend of blood pressure before they gave that beta blocker."

- ■ "They should have turned up the alarms before they left the room."

- ■ "They should never have given that medication based on a verbal order."

The study of hindsight bias, also called *creeping determinism*, originated with psychologist Baruch Fischhoff in the 1970s (Fischhoff, 1975). Fischhoff found that when people know what happens, they often think the event was predictable. For example, if you watch a movie for a second time, you will see little clues that support the ending—which you already know—that you didn't see the first time you watched it. Therefore, you conclude from information gleaned after the fact that the ending was predictable from the information given beforehand.

Sidney Dekker (2011) describes hindsight bias as a person standing outside and on top of a tunnel who can see the whole tunnel from beginning to end. A person inside the tunnel does not have that view and can only see what is inside the tunnel—not what is around it or lying at the end. Dekker states that to avoid hindsight bias, we must "…try to guard ourselves against mixing our reality with the reality of the people whose performance we are trying to under-stand" (p. 50). Avoiding hindsight bias can be difficult, however—especially in light of how often it occurs. The ultimate outcome of hindsight bias in an RCA group is that it leads the group to stop looking for system causes that led to the failure and rest the case on human error. Most accidents in our complex system are not that simple, however. Resting the case on an individual is the easy way out—and is also the path that will lead to further errors. You must dig deeper to find the systems that contributed to the situation.

OUTCOME BIAS

Outcome bias is similar to hindsight bias but is different because it involves bias based on the severity of the outcome (Henriksen and Kaplan, 2003). Outcome bias is commonly known as the "no harm no foul" rule. Outcome bias occurs when judgment of a situation is made dependent on the outcome, not the decision-making or the process behind the outcome. For example, in healthcare, we rarely investigate events that lead to a positive outcome, regardless of whether the decision-making, structure, or process behind the outcome was faulty. However, if the same events lead to a bad outcome, we always investigate. Harsher judgments are often made when an outcome is bad, becoming even harsher depending on the severity (Dekker, 2011). The problem with outcome bias is that it results in judgments being made about and blame being assigned to an individual instead of an examination of system issues.

CONTROLLING BIAS

Outcome and hindsight bias are difficult to control. In the book *Of Ants and Men* (2014), David Green notes that human beings, as complex as they are, still want things to be simple and to feel that they have some control over situations. When bad events can be reduced to a single cause, humans feel in control of the situation. If you simply punish the bad person who caused the event, control is restored. The fact is, however, that the world is complex. However hard we try, it cannot be controlled. Still, this is not a notion that we humans want to entertain. If the world can't be controlled, then we are simply victims. For this reason, when judging human beings and events that occur at the "sharp end," you will always need to recognize and manage bias.

You can use the following strategies to help avoid bias during an RCA:

- Create a goal for the RCA investigation to consider local rationality and try to understand why actions made sense at the time (Dekker, 2011).

- Attempt to understand how culture and accepted group norms contributed to actions.

- Call out bias during the RCA. Recognize phrases that suggest hindsight bias, such as "They should have" or "I would have." Ask, "Would you have seen that if you were in the same situation under the same circumstances?"

SUMMARY

The RCA is a powerful tool not only to investigate events but also to prevent events from reaching patients if used proactively with near misses. An effective RCA:

- Considers system issues as causes and human errors as effects

- Considers many root causes

- Involves objective team members to avoid bias

- Results in strong, actionable, timed interventions and outcome measures that address the root causes found

- Is supported and resourced by the highest leadership levels of the organization

The RCA is a strong tool for HROs and can be made even stronger by higher use, more standardization, and stronger interventions. The use of RCA in this manner advances safety that will be sustained in an HRO.

KEY POINTS

- Use the RCA not only for severe outcomes but also for near misses and close calls.

- Invest in strong interventions that allow for the detection of adverse events and adaptive mechanisms to avoid errors.

- Invest in training for RCA facilitators and all staff who participate on an RCA team.

- Identify all system issues that led to the human error.

- Use the Five Whys method to get to root cause.

- Ensure that suggested actions are associated with strong timelines and follow-up.

- Discuss real work situations and how they affect the staff's ability to deliver safe patient care.

- Recognize and discuss sources of bias affecting the RCA process.

REFERENCES

Andersen, B., and Fagerhaug, T. (2006). *Root cause analysis: Simplified tools and techniques* (2nd ed.). Milwaukee, WI: ASQ Quality Press.

Carayon, P., Wetterneck, T. B., Rivera-Rodriguez, A. J., Hundt, A. S., Hoonakker, P., Holden, R., and Gurses, A. P. (2014). Human factors systems approach to healthcare quality and patient safety. *Applied Ergonomics, 45*(1), pp. 14–25.

Chassin, M. R., and Loeb, J. M. (2013). High-reliability health care: Getting there from here. *The Milbank Quarterly, 91*(3), pp. 459–490.

Cook, R. I., and Woods, D. D. (1994). Operating at the sharp end: The complexity of human error. In M. S. Bogner (Ed.), *Human error in medicine* (pp. 255–310). Hillsdale, NJ: Erlbaum and Associates.

Deeter, J., and Rantanen, E. (2012). Human reliability analysis in healthcare. 2012 Symposium on Human Factors and Ergonomics in Health Care.

Dekker, S. (2002). Reconstructing human contributions to accidents: The new view on error and performance. *Journal of Safety Research, 33(3)*, pp. 371–385.

Dekker, S. (2011). *Patient safety: A human factors approach*. Boca Raton, FL: CRC Press, Taylor and Francis Group.

Dekker, S. (2012). *Just culture: Balancing safety and accountability* (2nd ed.). Burlington, VT: Ashgate.

Dekker, S., Cilliers, P., and Hofmyer, J. H. (2011). The complexity of failure: Implications of complexity theory for safety investigations. *Safety Science, 49*(6), pp. 939–945.

Department of Veterans Affairs. (2011). VHA National Patient Safety Handbook. Retrieved from http://www.va.gov/vhapublications/ViewPublication.asp?pub_ID=2389

Donabedian, A. (1988). The quality of care. How can it be assessed? *Journal of the American Medical Association, 260*(12), pp. 1743–1748.

Fatima, A. (2015). How has the root cause analysis evolved since inception? Retrieved from http://www.brighthubpm.com/risk-management/123244-how-has-the-root-cause-analysis-evolved-since-inception/

Fischhoff, B. (1975). Hindsight ≠ foresight: The effect of outcome knowledge on judgment under uncertainty. *Journal of Experimental Psychology: Human Perception and Performance, 1*(3), pp. 288–299.

Green, D. G. (2014). *Of ants and men: The unexpected side effects of complexity in society*. New York, NY: Copernicus.

Henriksen, K., Dayton, E., Keyes, M. A., Carayon, P., and Hughes, R. G. (2008). Understanding adverse events: A human factors framework. In R. G. Hughes (Ed.), *Patient safety and quality: An evidence-based handbook for nurses*, chapter 5. Rockville, MD: Agency for Healthcare Research and Quality. Publication No. 08-0043.

Henriksen, K., and Kaplan, H. (2003). Hindsight bias, outcome knowledge, and adaptive learning. *Quality and Safety in Health Care*, *12*(Suppl. II), pp. ii46–ii50.

Hughes, R. G. (2008). Nurses at the "sharp end" of patient care. In R. G. Hughes (Ed.), *Patient safety and quality: An evidence-based handbook for nurses*, chapter 2. Rockville, MD: Agency for Healthcare Research and Quality. Publication No. 08-0043.

Institute of Medicine. (1999). To err is human: Building a safer health system. Washington, DC: The National Academies Press.

The Joint Commission (2015). Sentinel events. Retrieved from http://www.jointcommission.org/assets/1/6/CAMH_24_SE_all_CURRENT.pdf

National Patient Safety Foundation (2015). RCA²: Improving root cause analyses and actions to prevent harm. Retrieved from http://www.npsf.org/?page=RCA2

Percarpio, K. B., and Watts, B. V. (2013). A cross-sectional study on the relationship between utilization of root cause analysis and patient safety at 139 Department of Veterans Affairs medical centers. *The Joint Commission Journal on Quality and Patient Safety*, *39*(1), pp. 32–37.

Percarpio, K. B., Watts, B. V., and Weeks, W. B. (2008). The effectiveness of root cause analysis: What does the literature tell us? *The Joint Commission Journal on Quality and Patient Safety*, *34*(7), pp. 391–398.

Rasmussen, J. (2003). The role of error in organizing behavior. *Quality and Safety in Healthcare*, *12(5)*, pp. 377–383.

Reason, J. (1990). *Human error*. Cambridge, England: Cambridge University Press.

Reason, J. (2000). Human error: Models and management. *British Medical Journal*, *320*(7237), pp. 768–770.

Taitz, J., Genn, K., Brooks, V., Ross, D., Ryan, K., Shumack, B., … NSW RCA Review Committee. (2010). System-wide learning from root cause analysis: A report from the New South Wales Root Cause Analysis Review Committee. *Quality & Safety in Health Care*, *19*(6), p. e63. doi: 10.1136/qshc.2008.032144

Vidyasager, A. (2015). The art of root cause analysis. Retrieved from http://asq.org/quality-progress/2015/02/back-to-basics/the-art-of-root-cause-analysis.html

Weick, K. E., and Sutcliffe, K. M. (2007). *Managing the unexpected: Assuring high performance in an age of complexity* (2nd ed.). New York, NY: Jossey-Bass.

Woods, D. (1988). Coping with complexity: The psychology of human behaviour in complex systems. In J. Goodstein, H. Anderson, and B. Olsen (Eds.), *Tasks, errors and mental models* (pp. 128–148). London, England: Taylor and Francis.

Woods, D. D., Dekker, S., Cook, R., Johannesen, L., and Sarter, N. (2012). *Behind human error* (2nd ed.). Burlington, VT: Ashgate.

Wu, A. W., Lipshutz, A. K. M., and Pronovost, P. J. (2008). Effectiveness and efficiency of root cause analysis in medicine. *The Journal of the American Medical Association*, *299*(6), pp. 685–687.

CHAPTER 8

JUST CULTURE AND THE IMPACT ON HIGH RELIABILITY

Patricia A. Patrician, PhD, RN, FAAN

Gwendolyn Cherese Godlock, MS-PSL, RN, CPHQ, CMSRN

Apryl Shenae Lewis, MSN, RN, CCTN

Rebecca S. Miltner, PhD, RN, CNL, NEA-BC

> "I saw and experienced all the artifacts of a ceaseless striving for perfection: an obsession with detail in every aspect of everyday tasks that was more intense than anything that I have ever experienced before; a seemingly genuine desire, if not passion, to help others; and a real discouragement and even depression when interventions refused to yield the intended help.
>
> —Dr. Charles L. Bosk

This quote by Dr. Charles L. Bosk, professor of sociology at the University of Pennsylvania, comes from the preface of the second edition of his book, *Forgive and Remember: Managing Medical Failure.* This book was originally published in 1979, long before the Institute of Medicine's (IOM's) 1999 report "To Err Is Human" called medical errors to our attention. After countless hours observing surgical resident training, Bosk noted that striving for perfection is common in healthcare settings, where providers frequently feel a calling to do this difficult and demanding work. In other words, with very few exceptions, healthcare workers go to work every day to help those entrusted to their care. Yet mistakes do happen. We are all human, and humans make mistakes. Bosk took particular note of residents in training, who make mistakes because of their inexperience. In such cases, the error is acknowledged, forgiven, and remembered so that it does not happen again. Other mistakes are not so easily forgiven. Many more can be debated as to whether they are even errors (Bosk, 2003).

Switching gears from surgical residents to nurses in hospitals, one does not have to dive too deeply into the literature to find stories of legal retribution, moral retribution, and self-retribution for committing and even reporting errors. Nurses in Texas, for example, were fired from their hospital for reporting what they perceived to be an unsafe physician (Gorski, 2010). A nurse committed suicide following a fatal error after being fired from her job (Aleccia, 2011). These events and many others like them have sounded the call for "blameless" cultures where the system, not the individual, is considered to be at fault. Yet this poses a problem, too. What about the small percentage of healthcare providers who *do* intentionally cause harm? What action should a manager take when the same individual repeatedly causes errors in the workplace?

Clearly, the balance lies somewhere between a culture of "no blame" and holding individuals completely accountable for all errors. This middle point is where Just Culture resides. A *Just Culture* is defined as "an environment where professionals believe they will receive fair treatment if they are involved in an adverse event and trust the organization to treat each event as an opportunity for improving safety" (Petschonek et al., 2013, p. 192).

The purpose of this chapter is to discuss the history, theory, and challenges of implementing Just Culture in current practice. It begins with a brief discussion of the origin of the concept of Just Culture and why it is an essential element of high reliability organizations (HROs). It then explores the concept in terms of its differentiating features, antecedents, and consequences or outcomes. Measurement strategies for quantifying Just Culture are reviewed. Next, it turns to the most difficult parts: implementing a Just Culture in practice and educating the next generations of healthcare providers about Just Culture. The chapter offers tips and techniques for clinicians and educators. Finally, the end of the chapter presents and explores three case studies of Just Culture—its absence contrasted with its presence.

BACKGROUND

In 1997, James Reason documented the benefits of a Just Culture: promoting a climate of trust, empowering people, and rewarding people for reporting patient safety–related events. Just Culture is very particular when it comes to differentiating behavioral choices and just methods of accountability. That said, a Just Culture resides comfortably between patient safety and safety culture (American Nurses Association [ANA], 2010).

The IOM report "To Err Is Human" (1999) profoundly changed the way many healthcare professionals thought and talked about medical errors. This report initiated the conversation about medical errors and their consequences (Leape and Berwick, 2005). Interestingly, 10 years before the release of this report, no one spoke openly and honestly about quality and patient safety (Wachter, 2010). The term "safety culture" originated outside healthcare, in studies of HROs—that is, organizations that routinely decrease adverse events despite working in complex and hazardous environments.

In 2001, David Marx first reported the Just Culture model and its accompanying algorithm to use when seeking to differentiate human error from blameworthy acts (Wachter, 2010). Rather than just assume that an adverse outcome had a bad person associated with it, the Just Culture model focused on the differences among human error, at-risk behavior, and reckless behavior (Griffith, 2009). Human errors are inadvertent actions; at-risk behavior increases risk when risks go unrecognized; and reckless behavior involves choices that consciously disregard a substantial and unjustifiable risk. Administering justice based on the quality of the person's choice is an essential component of creating a culture of safety (Griffith, 2009). Just Culture fosters an environment where employees hunger for knowledge and for the early detection of risk—that is, near misses—so that learning can occur even before accidents happen.

Although many organizations have tried to adopt portions of a Just Culture, the fundamental concepts are often misapplied. Some have adopted a "blame-free" model of accountability, hoping a "softer, kinder" approach will reduce adverse events or raise their patient safety survey scores. The Just Culture model focuses on a balanced method of applying punishment and considering the front-line worker's perception when punishment is used within our healthcare system. The concept of perfection does not exist in this model because humans are destined to make mistakes. Human errors and adverse events are outcomes that require measuring and monitoring, with the goal of mitigating and decreasing patient harm (Marx, 2001).

Just Culture promotes openness and fairness, which facilitates efficient and honest reporting within safe systems (Griffith, 2009). Just Culture serves as a principal component in the creation of a culture of safety. When the organizational vision and goals are clearly defined and straightforward at all system levels, then buy-in to a culture of safety becomes easier.

Establishing a culture of safety using the Just Culture model is a critical step in achieving high reliability. HROs in healthcare maintain a high commitment to patient safety at all levels of the healthcare system. This commitment encompasses key features synonymous with the Just Culture model—for example, promoting a blame-free environment where members of the organization are comfortable reporting errors or near misses without fear of reprisal. HROs chronicle an environment of "collective mindfulness" in which every system level actively seeks and reports minor errors or near misses before these events negatively affect the organization (Chassin and Loeb, 2011).

The aviation industry is well-known for its ability to maintain and sustain highly reliable status. The industry has put systems in place that empower airplane mechanics, crew members, and pilots to report all mechanical problems before takeoff, even if it causes passenger delays. The industry recognized this critical safety concept because it has a duty to itself and its passengers to mitigate the risk of error, consistently preventing serious accidents. The aviation industry is no different from the healthcare industry in that it carries out intrinsically complex and hazardous work. Early detection, reporting, and collaboration across all system levels improve overall quality in both industries.

HROs in healthcare pride themselves on providing collaborative care across the healthcare continuum. This concept is built on trust, an essential characteristic in Just Culture, ultimately producing better patient outcomes. Working in an environment that incorporates Just Culture principles creates endless opportunities for improved care through communication and teamwork.

SBAR provides an effective, efficient, and standardized method to communicate critical information during transitions in care. The Joint Commission (TJC), the Institute for Healthcare Improvement (IHI), the World Health Organization (WHO), Team Strategies and Tools to Enhance Performance and Patient Safety (TeamSTEPPS), and the Advisory Board Company all promote the SBAR model. The successful application of communication tools such as SBAR supports transparency, structure, and synergy. The four key elements of the SBAR model are as follows:

- **Situation (S):** What is the acute problem and/or concern?

- **Background (B):** What is the pertinent background information related to the concern?

- **Assessment (A):** What are the objective and subjective signs or symptoms?

- **Recommendation (R):** What is recommended to improve the situation?

DESCRIBING AND MEASURING JUST CULTURE

Organizations that seek to numerically define components of their safety culture so as to improve that culture have long used the Agency for Healthcare Research and Quality (AHRQ) Hospital Survey for Patient Safety Culture (Sorra and Dyer, 2010). Although this survey contains ratings of many dimensions of patient safety culture, it does not specifically measure Just Culture. Petschonek et al. (2013) conducted a review of the literature to explore the concept of Just Culture and to better define its dimensions. From the literature, they identified six dimensions of Just Culture:

- Balance with respect to fair treatment of individuals involved in an error

- Trust in the organization and supervisors

- Openness to communication up the chain of command about errors and their solutions

- Quality of the event-reporting process, from the mechanics of reporting to the resources required to report

- Feedback and communication about events and their outcomes

- An overall goal of continuous improvement within the organization

From these subcomponents, Petschonek et al. created and tested the Just Culture Assessment Tool (JCAT) to specifically measure Just Culture (2013). For a new instrument, the JCAT performed well. Although the authors recommend further testing for the purposes of refinement, this tool is the first step in measuring Just Culture and could be used to determine how effectively an organization is moving toward Just Culture.

CHALLENGES IN IMPLEMENTING JUST CULTURE

Creating a fair and Just Culture indicates an organization's willingness to be transparent about weaknesses and using information to improve (Frankel, Leonard, and Denham, 2006). Equal effort toward creating an impartial Just Culture must also be given to safety activities such as safety walk rounds and training for teamwork and effective communication.

A number of barriers exist when working to create a fair and Just Culture (Frankel et al., 2006; Lazarus, 2011; Schelbred and Nord, 2007; Vogus, Sutcliffe, and Weick, 2010; Wu, 2000). These barriers include the following:

- **Lack of concern with failure:** An organization attempting to foster a fair and Just Culture must have a preoccupation with failure (Frankel et al., 2006). All staff from the chief officer to the janitor must take patient care seriously and commit to striving for zero defects. Although there is no such thing as a perfect organization, fair and Just Cultures do set a high bar for themselves with regard to quality and safety. An organization can expect this type of barrier if it does not have "collective mindfulness" staff—one that is constantly on the lookout for any size problem or unsafe condition and is never satisfied with only small, measured amounts of safety (Chassin and Loeb, 2011). An organization that does not reward and recognize staff for pointing out errors and safety concerns can expect to experience this barrier.

- **Little or no accountability from leadership and staff:** This barrier can be expected if there is not a sense that every person in the organization is an owner of patient quality and safety (Frankel et al., 2006). Each person must be clear on his or her own and others' accountability. Each employee assumes accountability and the associated risk of knowingly and unknowingly not following set rules and standards. If someone violates set rules and standards intentionally rather than inadvertently, the leader must respond accordingly. Diminished awareness of safety and quality gaps among leaders or an unwillingness to address them also affects accountability (Lazarus, 2011). Failing to enforce a level of accountability in which everyone can evaluate each other's work regardless of rank and position creates barriers to changing the culture. In addition, the organization must improve accountability by partnering with regulatory and accrediting agencies to create a fair and Just Culture and work toward the common goal of improved safety (Gorzeman, 2008).

- **Absence of transparency:** If barriers were prioritized, lack of transparency in an organization might rank toward the top. This barrier simply means people in the organization do not feel safe or comfortable in reporting potentially dangerous actions or practices (Frankel et al., 2006). Having a safe mechanism in place to report errors and a culture in which reporting is rewarded are ways to overcome this barrier. One hospital in the Midwest almost doubled the number of errors and safety concerns reported after it allowed reports to be submitted anonymously. This simple change caused continued increases in error reporting for years after its implementation. There was also a commitment to annually communicate the importance of reporting errors (Lazarus, 2011).

- **No set agreed-upon safety commitment:** Having no pre-set safety commitment and standard on which all team members agree poses a barrier (Frankel et al., 2006). Partnership among leadership across disciplines as well as staff participation in setting safety commitments and standards are crucial. You can overcome this barrier by having a written document that lists the commitment and a regular recommitment as well as daily upholding of the principles set.

- **Lack of action toward improvement:** Expect this barrier if there is all talk and no action. Part of becoming a fair and Just Culture lies not only in the preoccupation with failure but also in leadership and staff at all levels making the commitment to improve and also taking active steps to create change. Measured progress and use of outcomes-based initiatives and strategies to improve upon safety and quality gaps are ways to overcome this barrier.

- **Assumption that all staff are on board with safety commitments:** This is a common barrier. In fact, staff have varying levels of commitment. Although the organization may have set a standard, staff and leaders may not act according to the principles set. Having a clear sense of who is committed and who is not is key to overcoming this barrier. You must encourage those who are living the safety commitment and push those who do not show signs of being dedicated to either commit…or be let go.

- **Complexity of healthcare delivery:** The intrinsic complexity that exists in healthcare delivery creates barriers with respect to Just Culture. When safe care is delivered, it is often invisible—difficult to identify or visualize. Because safety is not something one can touch or feel, it can be hard to enforce—until it is violated (Vogus et al., 2010). Complexity of disease, medically fragile patients, and the release of patients from healthcare settings sooner than they may feel comfortable are common occurrences in healthcare. The combination of complexity and time pressures does not always make it easy for clinicians to choose the safest practice. Specialization in healthcare often makes it hard for multiple providers to agree on appropriate care and intervention, which may make it difficult to respond to and correct or prevent future errors. Finally, the use of workarounds for routine failures and hard-to-follow processes does not always coincide with doing the right thing (Vogus et al., 2010).

■ **No support for the person who committed the error:** The "blame and shame" of individuals for errors is traditionally how errors are handled in healthcare. When this occurs, there is no initiative to support the person who committed the error (Vogus et al., 2010). A Just Culture cannot be cultivated in organizations where this type of response is prevalent. Guilt, judgment, fear of making the mistake again, and fear of what their peers may feel are individual perceptions that perpetuate this barrier (Wu, 2000). Healthcare organizations must move past blaming individuals and support those who are the unfortunate "second victim" of a medical error.

An exploratory descriptive study of 10 hospital nurses in 2003 revealed that nurses experienced both a personal and a professional impact from the medical errors they made (Schelbred and Nord, 2007). Two ways to offer support are crisis-intervention support and manager support. Giving the person who made the mistake the ability to talk about it helps him or her to get past it. Practicing forgiveness for the mistake may also make the family more forgiving.

Organizations must take these barriers into consideration to determine how to respond to them and possibly proactively avoid them. Time and energy are needed to build a fair and Just Culture. Considering these barriers can help organizations save both. Working toward a fair and Just Culture is no small feat. It takes patience, will, commitment, and determination. Knowing the potential barriers may lead to quicker success and transformation toward a fair and Just Culture.

THE APPLICATION OF JUST CULTURE TO CLINICAL PRACTICE AND MANAGEMENT

The application of Just Culture concepts to clinical practice and management must be driven from the top down. Effective strategies include the following:

■ Leadership rounding

■ Employee recognition programs

■ Transparent communication about reported patient safety events

■ Mentoring and coaching of employees

■ Fair and just accountability principles

■ Gathering feedback from employees

These are just a few ways to ensure successful implementation.

Organizations that practice open communication to promote safe quality care are often referred to as Just Culture organizations. Just Cultures also incorporate aspects of organizational learning. Increasing the ability to learn from adverse events is likely to decrease the number of adverse events over time. An organization's ability to learn from adverse events depends on its identifying, reporting, and investigating structure.

There are various methods to integrate Just Culture into clinical practice and management. Khatri, Brown, and Hicks (2009) identified two premises for transitioning from a blame culture to a Just Culture. The first premise emphasizes focusing on the organization's culture rather than improvement strategies as a more sustainable technique. The second premise emphasizes the idea that organizations must be supported by a human resource (HR) department with the aptitude to implement a set of consistent HR practices designed to proliferate the new and desired form of culture (Khatri et al., 2009).

Most organizations have developed management philosophies. However, an early distinction is key to successful integration. Khatri et al. (2009) define two types of management philosophies:

- **Control based:** Control-based management philosophies speculate that employees are inept at managing their behaviors and require consistent monitoring and guidance. This type of management philosophy has a vertical hierarchical structure, and communication is driven from the top down. Employees tend to follow instructions or do what they're told, leaving little room for creativity at the front line. Over time, employees tend to leave organizations with this type of management philosophy, and absenteeism is chronically high.

- **Commitment based:** The commitment-based management philosophy is composed of two notions. First, employees are capable of managing their behaviors. Second, when employees are trusted, given autonomy, and fully committed to the organization, they perform very well (Khatri et al., 2009). This management philosophy comes highly recommended because it cultivates teamwork, synergy, and front-line engagement. It is an essential component in implementing and sustaining a Just Culture. It produces a learning effect by encouraging reporting of all patient safety–related events and investigating causal factors in a transparent manner. It also produces a motivation effect. That is, these types of organizations are composed of highly motivated employees actively pursuing opportunities to provide high-quality patient care.

Tucker, Nembhard, and Edmondson (2007) highlight two processes for the successful implementation of new practices:

- **Learn how:** Learn-how activities are aimed at the discovery of evidence-based practices (EBP) with the goal of operationalizing in a particular organization. These activities are very complicated, and not all organizations can implement them successfully.

■ **Learn what:** Learn-what activities are aimed at identifying best practices from existing knowledge.

Tucker et al. (2007) contend that learn-how versus learn-what activities play a vital role in implementation success.

Operationalizing Just Culture concepts within HROs requires leadership engagement very early on. Approximately 80% of all initiatives that require behavior changes fail due to lack of leadership engagement (McChesney, Covey, and Huling, 2012). Leadership-engagement strategies should take into consideration the impact the change will have on the organization—specifically, physicians and front-line staff. It's highly recommended that leaders analyze the organization's culture of safety assessment data as a baseline to help establish strategic aims and goals. After the data has been analyzed, Just Culture EBPs can drive implementation through front-line education, marketing, time, and resources. Aligning the organization's vision, mission, and values with Just Culture concepts will help pave the road to high reliability.

Coaching is vital to ensuring conversations among leaders and front-line staff yield desired outcomes and foster just relationships. Creating opportunities for positive interactions—for example, executive rounding, unit practice councils, and monthly town hall sessions—can help to achieve this. Creating patient safety coach teams that are well versed in Just Culture enables organizations to provide just-in-time peer-to-peer coaching, which has proven to be a valuable integration strategy. Overall, successful integration of Just Culture is contingent upon innovative marketing, leader transparency, open dialogue, and mutual support.

TEACHING JUST CULTURE

As discussed, Just Culture is a crucial but complex component of a high reliability system. It is critical to expose all health professions students to the concept and key principles in their professional curricula. There is no direct evidence of the best mechanisms for teaching Just Culture across health professional education levels. However, an examination of quality and patient safety education offers some recommendations for effective teaching about the topic.

WHO (2009) created a comprehensive curricular guide for medical education that includes a teacher's guide for embedding patient safety topics into the general medical school curriculum. It also includes an extensive topical outline of key patient safety topics, although there is no explicit mention of Just Culture. The teacher's guide suggests several mechanisms for including this content in the general curriculum, including standalone courses at predetermined times in the training process, standalone content embedded in multiple courses in the program, and content integrated with course content. The guide also outlines educational principles that are key to successful patient safety teaching and learning, including the importance of realistic examples within the local context and providing a safe learning environment.

Kirkman et al. (2015) completed a systematic review of 25 studies reporting patient safety education activities in graduate medical education. Common content included an overview of patient safety, communication and teamwork, systems-based analysis, and improvement principles. Most studies showed improved knowledge, skills, and attitudes for learners, but none showed any impact on patient outcomes. Courses generally used a mix of didactic and experiential learning activities, including lectures, small group discussion, Web-based learning, and project work. Case studies based on real scenarios were rarely used, although the authors suggest these have high value in patient safety education due to the popularity among learners and the opportunity to reflect and learn from a real event.

Tella et al. (2014) conducted an integrative review of 20 studies of patient safety education in prelicensure nursing education. The key elements of patient safety education in these studies were learning from errors, teamwork, patient safety–centered nursing, and complex environments (Tella et al., 2014). Teaching methods included lectures, readings, adverse events reporting systems, simulations, and clinical practice. These authors specifically state, "…a Just Culture is needed in nursing education, as it holds every individual accountable for their own actions" (Tella et al., 2014, p. 12).

These reviews of patient safety education and the international guidelines for teaching patient safety contain minimal references to the concept of Just Culture. However, they do provide some insight about best educational practices that may build the competencies—the knowledge, skills, and attitudes—needed to build, support, and practice within a Just Culture. Here are a few points to keep in mind:

- It is important for teachers to have deeper understanding of the characteristics of HROs, including the concepts of Just Culture and professional accountability.

- This content must be explicitly integrated into the curriculum in a more comprehensive manner than a one-time lecture or video. Some practices that show promise include student incident reporting systems for actual or near miss clinical and simulation errors. These systems provide opportunities for immediate reflection and learning by students and faculty as well as the ability to identify system problems that contribute to student error.

- The use of real case scenarios with small group discussion and analysis is more relevant to health professional students who fear making that first clinical error.

- It is important that educators create safe learning environments that allow open dialogue about this important and complex concept. Penn (2014) describes a successful policy change for student errors to align with Just Culture principles at one school of nursing. Integrating Just Culture principles as part of the school's values and structures can move this concept forward.

CASE STUDY 1

Tammy works the night shift and is assigned to four patients, one of whom is newly admitted. Medications for all of Tammy's patients are due at both 8 p.m. and 9 p.m. Tammy pulls the medications for all of her patients and keeps each patient's medications in separate plastic bags. Although the hospital medication policy directs nurses to pull medications for only one patient at a time, Tammy was taught to get all meds for all patients at the same time. She justifies her actions based on the traffic jam she has encountered with multiple nurses pulling medications for multiple patients, all at the same time.

Tammy enters the newly admitted patient's room and lists each medication she plans to administer to him. The patient acknowledges all the medications Tammy cites. However, right before administering a Lantus insulin injection, the patient states that he is not familiar with the medication. Tammy explains the purpose of the medication, its side effects, and how often the patient is to receive the medication. The patient says, "I am not a diabetic, and Lantus is not a medication I am prescribed." Tammy tells the patient, "Your physician has ordered the medication for you, and I am ordered to give it." The patient again states, "I am not ordered the Lantus, and I do not want to take the injection, as I believe I am not supposed to receive it." Tammy again says, "The doctor ordered the medication for you, and I am going to give you the medication." Tammy asks if the patient would like to receive the medication in his left arm or right arm. The patient states that he does not want to receive the medication. Tammy says, "Sir, I am giving you the medication you are ordered." She explains to him that she will need to wipe his arm with an alcohol prep pad before administering the medication. The patient has a look of frustration but lifts his left arm to receive the medication.

The next day on nursing leader rounds, the patient tells the nurse manager about the situation. The nurse manager starts the follow-up process. She reviews the patient's history and physical and sees no evidence of the patient having a diabetes diagnosis. She calls the attending physician to clarify why Lantus was ordered for the patient. The physician notes that Lantus was not ordered for the patient. Upon further review of the chart, the nurse manager sees that, in fact, Lantus is not on the patient profile.

The nurse manager calls Tammy to discuss what happened. Tammy says she gave the medication that was ordered and has done nothing wrong. The nurse manager reviews the investigation details with Tammy. She asks Tammy to apologize to the patient for making the mistake and for failing to listen to the patient when he repeatedly questioned Tammy's administration of the medication. Tammy refuses to apologize.

QUESTIONS

1. What should the nurse manager's first steps be in approaching the nurse with the medication error in a fair and just manner?

2. Should the nurse face any disciplinary action? If so, why?

3. What support and information can the nurse manager offer the nurse to encourage safe practice for future patients?

DISCUSSION

The nurse manager worked with Tammy to help her identify at what point in the situation the medication error could have been avoided. She then helped Tammy to understand the current process for medication administration. Next, she asked Tammy to identify steps in the process that she does not think work efficiently and that cause her to believe she must create a workaround to get her work done. Tammy was also asked to identify ways to find out whether other members of the unit nursing team have noted concerns with the process. Finally, the nurse manager encouraged Tammy to work with other team members in a systematic way, such as a unit practice council, to allow for the safe administration of medication as well as to obtain support in her efforts to comply with the medication administration steps.

Next, the nurse manager helped Tammy recognize the missed opportunity to listen to the patient and emphasized the importance of partnering with patients in their care. Patients take their medications every day and often manage their healthcare responsibilities independently or with help from others at home. The nurse manager asked Tammy to note what steps she might have done differently if she had listened to the patient. Would she have double-checked the rights of medication administration (right time, patient, route, reason, and date)? Would she have contacted the physician on call to clarify the order? Would she have double-checked the H&P and noted the lack of a diabetes diagnosis, labs, or other clinical data that would help support the patient's claim? Would she have consulted with the charge nurse to address the patient's concerns and set a plan of action together?

The final step was for the nurse manager to address Tammy's reluctance to apologize to the patient for the medication error. The nurse manager had a responsibility to help Tammy to see the situation from the patient's perspective. She must also adhere to the organization's culture regarding transparency with patients when mistakes occur as well as place a high priority on patient service and on ensuring patient concerns are heard and addressed.

The nurse manager had to carefully consider whether to take disciplinary action. She also had to fully evaluate the support needed for Tammy to practice safely. Was this the first time Tammy had made a mistake? In what way did Tammy violate hospital policy? How could Tammy be supported to follow the policy? How could the nurse manager help Tammy to understand why the steps of the process are necessary to achieving the highest level of patient safety? It was important for Tammy to understand the safety-related implications of listening to the patient, identifying problems she encounters with being compliant with processes, seeking out support early, and calling attention to processes that are broken.

To determine what support should be offered, the nurse manager asked Tammy to identify how she feels best supported. Support included helping Tammy practice safely as well as helping her to track and share when she comes across opportunities to listen to patients and how she is working on this important skill. The nurse manager also supplied resources related to careful listening, team coordination (to help identify ways for the nursing team to work together to practice safely), and safe practice.

CASE STUDY 2

In 2003, at Mandarian Hospital, a patient safety event occurred in the operating room (OR) when a piece of the drill used during the procedure broke off and another piece flew across the room. A fragment of the drill bit attached itself inside the patient's femur. Because of the chaos, no one noticed the drill bit fragment except the OR technician.

When the situation was under control, the OR technician attempted to notify the surgeon about the drill bit. The surgeon replied, "Be quiet so we can close. I don't have any more time to waste!" Unfortunately, the discovery of the drill bit was not made until the patient's MRI results were read post-surgery. The patient returned to the OR, and the foreign object was removed. This was reported to TJC as a sentinel event, and a root cause analysis (RCA) was launched.

QUESTIONS

1. What type of behavior did the surgeon display—human error, risky behavior, or reckless behavior?

2. What type of action is warranted based on the type of behavior displayed?

3. Were behavior expectations clear?

DISCUSSION

The RCA revealed that although there was an unexpected equipment failure, the surgeon also failed to create an environment that promoted open communication and transparency. The RCA focused on final time out, count before closure, and staff behavior. As a result of the investigation, the OR re-established safe processes and expectations for staff in each of these areas. In addition, all OR teams were required to attend TeamSTEPPS and Just Culture training. Surgeons were required to participate in a special training session on facilitating team behavior under stressful conditions and how to respond to junior members of the team when standard procedures are in jeopardy.

Creating a hostile work environment is problematic in healthcare settings and is a precursor to harm. In this case, it was found that the surgeon had a history of this type of behavior and was on a focused professional performance evaluation (FPPE) plan. The surgeon's blatant disregard for open communication and teamwork could be an example of reckless behavior, especially because he had been counseled before this incident. Lastly, equipment was not checked for serviceability—an example of risky behavior, assuming staff was required to follow a well-known policy and protocol with regard to maintaining equipment.

There is a tremendous amount of pressure to decrease errors, ensure patient safety, and achieve operational effectiveness within modern healthcare settings (Carmeli and Gittell, 2009). In a special commission of inquiry into public hospitals, Garling (2008) reported widespread bullying despite a zero tolerance policy. Garling (2008) expressed the need to address the absence of respect and the importance of developing a proper standard of behaviors as a method to deter bullying behaviors.

Prevention is the key. Therefore, organizations can employ strategies to encourage professional responsibility and accountability. Identifying workplace violence and crucial triggers early on can help an organization "muzzle" the activity before it can get out of hand. Resiliency training and support groups can serve as another viable tool for addressing workplace violence. Most importantly, providing a reliable, non-biased, and educated safety net for the staff is critical. Victims of workplace violence need to feel safe and protected. These two venues can provide healing, self-confidence, and an opportunity to communicate issues and concerns.

Consideration for others (COA) training and a conflict resolution counselor (CRC) are other ways an organization can help employees deal with workplace violence—not just the victim, but the perpetrator. They require counseling and support; however, this is on a case-by-case basis.

You must take care when differentiating among human error, risky behavior, and reckless behavior. Human error involves simple mistakes or lapses of memory but does not involve malicious intent. Risky behavior involves the failure to exercise the expected necessary precautions to mitigate risk for patient harm. Reckless behavior involves a conscious disregard of rules and risks associated with preventing patient harm.

CASE STUDY 3

Miss Nova is nearing the completion of her shift. Before she can leave, however, she must administer 10 units of regular insulin to her last patient.

The hospital has a policy that before the administration of certain high-risk medications, two licensed individuals must perform a check. In addition, the director of nursing services has noted that there have been several near misses involving regular insulin in both inpatient and outpatient units.

Staffing pattern usually calls for four registered nurses for 15 patients. Today, however, only three are on the floor due to a call out. This has caused an extra strain because there are fewer RNs available to verify Miss Nova's draw. In addition, Miss Nova needs to leave 5 minutes early because of a previously scheduled doctor's appointment. Miss Nova decides to administer the insulin without verifying the draw as per protocol. Five minutes after the administration, the patient begins to complain of feeling sluggish, dizzy, and faint. Miss Nova calls for help. Fortunately, the team is able to restore the patient to her normal baseline without any further progressing complications. It is revealed that the patient received 1 cc of insulin (which equates to 100 units) instead of 10 units.

QUESTIONS

1. What type of behavior did Miss Nova display—human error, risky behavior, or reckless behavior?

2. What type of action is warranted based on the type of behavior displayed?

3. Were behavior expectations clear?

DISCUSSION

The charge nurse called a huddle to discuss the incident and asked Miss Nova to recall the details leading up to the event. She also directed Miss Nova to perform the techniques used to draw the insulin. This revealed a process issue pertaining to the hospital's supply storage room. Insulin syringes were stocked in the wrong storage bin, and 3 cc syringes were stocked in their place. This was a system-related issue and was immediately corrected by the development of a color-coded insulin syringe storage system, which differentiated insulin syringe bins from all other syringe bins. Supply technicians were then educated on this new system.

Although a system issue contributed to the error, there is still accountability when applying Just Culture. Miss Nova possibly demonstrated reckless behavior by neglecting to verify a high-risk drug with another licensed provider because she knew the risk she was taking. However, this may have simply been risky behavior if she did not think the risk would result in an error. Miss Nova did state that she had neglected to verify insulin with another RN previously with no problems.

Miss Nova was directed to attend mandatory medication administration training and time management classes due to the behavioral choice made. All staff were also educated on the concept of normalization of deviance, or when unacceptable behavior becomes acceptable due to a lack of consequences. The hospital demonstrated accountability in attending to the system issues (storage of syringes and staffing) that contributed to the error and looked at the culture of the unit that made normalization of deviance possible.

Just Culture principles are multipurpose and are an essential component to supporting organizations in dealing with cultural issues, mainly to determine when to focus on the organization systems and when to focus on individual behaviors and accountability.

SUMMARY

Achieving a fair and Just Culture in healthcare organizations is not impossible but requires an investment of time and energy by leaders to create the changes that will foster and sustain this type of culture. This chapter offered a brief background on the origins of Just Culture, definitions and measurement strategies, and challenges to implementation. It offered tips for implementing Just Culture in clinical practice, management, and education. Case studies illustrated the concepts discussed in the chapter. Patient safety in healthcare organizations will not be achieved until the culture changes from one that blames individuals to one in which accountability resides within a system focused on improvement.

KEY POINTS

- A Just Culture is not a "blameless" culture; it is one that emphasizes fairness and balance in dealing with errors.

- If individuals believe they will be treated fairly, they are more likely to report errors and near misses.

- Reporting errors and near misses is critical to uncovering issues within a system—often before an actual error occurs.

- Front-line staff are in the best position to report errors. However, unless the culture is just and fair, they are the most vulnerable when an error occurs.

■ Leaders must invest the time and effort required for an organization to undergo a change in culture to a Just Culture.

REFERENCES

Aleccia, J. (2011). Nurse's suicide highlights twin tragedies of medical errors. Retrieved from http://www.nbcnews.com/id/43529641/ns/health-health_care/t/nurses-suicide-highlights-twin-tragedies-medical-errors#.VbqG803bJaQ

American Nurses Association. (2010). Just Culture position statement. Retrieved from http://nursingworld.org/psjustculture

Bosk, C. L. (2003). *Forgive and remember: Managing medical failure* (2nd ed.). Chicago, IL: The University of Chicago Press.

Carmeli, A., and Gittell, J. H. (2009). High-quality relationships, psychological safety, and learning from failures in work organizations. *Journal of Organizational Behavior, 30*(6), pp. 709–729.

Chassin, M. R., and Loeb, J. M. (2011). The ongoing quality improvement journey: Next stop, high reliability. *HealthAffairs, 30*(4), pp. 559–568.

Frankel, A. S., Leonard, M. W., and Denham, C. R. (2006). Fair and Just Culture, team behavior, and leadership engagement: The tools to achieve high reliability. *Health Services Research, 41*(4), pp. 1690–1709.

Garling, P. (2008). Final report of the Special Commission of Inquiry: Acute care services in NSW public hospitals. Retrieved from http://www.dpc.nsw.gov.au/__data/assets/pdf_file/0003/34194/Overview_-_Special_Commission_Of_Inquiry_Into_Acute_Care_Services_In_New_South_Wales_Public_Hospitals.pdf

Gorski, D. (2010). The legal establishment of Winkler County, Texas conspires to punish whistleblowing nurses. Retrieved from https://www.sciencebasedmedicine.org/the-medical-and-legal-establishment-of-winkler-county-texas-conspire-to-punish-whistle-blowing-nurses/

Gorzeman, J. (2008). Balancing Just Culture with regulatory standards. *Nursing Administration Quality, 32*(4), pp 308–311.

Griffith, K. S. (2009). Column: The growth of a Just Culture. *The Joint Commission Perspectives on Patient Safety, 9*(12), pp. 8–9.

Institute of Medicine (IOM). (1999). To err is human: Building a safer health system. Washington, DC: The National Academies Press.

Khatri, N., Brown, G. D., and Hicks, L. L. (2009). From a blame culture to a Just Culture in health care. *Health Care Management Review, 34*(4), pp. 312–322.

Kirkman, M. A., Sevdalis N., Arora, S., Baker, P., Vincent, C., and Ahmed, M. (2015). The outcomes of recent patient safety education interventions for trainee physicians and medical students: A systematic review. *BMJ Open, 5*(5), p. e007705. doi:10.1136/bmjopen-2015Choose Destination

Lazarus, I. R. (2011). On the road to find out...transparency and Just Culture offer significant return on investment. *Journal of Healthcare Management, 56*(4), pp. 223–227.

Leape, L. L., and Berwick, D. M. (2005). Five years after To Err Is Human: What have we learned? *Journal of the American Medical Association, 293*(19), pp. 2384–2390.

Marx, D. (2001). *Patient safety and the "Just Culture": A primer for health care executives*. New York, NY: Columbia University.

McChesney, C., Covey, S., and Huling, J. (2012). *The 4 disciplines of execution: Achieving your wildly important goals*. New York, NY: Free Press.

Penn, C. E. (2014). Integrating Just Culture into nursing student error policy. *Journal of Nursing Education, 53*(9 Suppl), pp. S107–S109.

Petschonek, S., Burlison, J., Cross, C., Martin, K., Laver, J., Landis, R. S., and Hoffman, J. M. (2013). Development of the Just Culture Assessment Tool: Measuring the perceptions of health-care professionals in hospitals. *Journal of Patient Safety, 9*(4), pp. 190–197.

Reason, J. (1997). *Managing the risks of organizational accidents*. Aldershot, UK: Ashgate Publishing Limited.

Schelbred, A. B., and Nord, R. (2007). Nurses' experiences of drug administration errors. *Journal of Advanced Nursing, 60*(3), pp. 317–324.

Sorra, J. S., and Dyer, N. (2010). Multilevel psychometric properties of the AHRQ hospital survey on patient safety culture. *BMC Health Services Research*, 10, p. 199.

Tella, S., Liukka, M., Jamookeeah, D., Smith, N. J., Partanen, P., and Turunen, H. (2014). What do nursing students learn about patient safety? An integrative literature review. *Journal of Nursing Education*, *53*(1), pp. 7–13.

Tucker, A. L., Nembhard, I. M., and Edmondson, A. C. (2007). Implementing new practices: An empirical study of organizational learning in hospital intensive care units. *Management Science*, *53*(6), pp. 894–907.

Vogus, T. J., Sutcliffe, K. M., and Weick, K. E. (2010). Doing no harm: Enabling, enacting, and elaborating a culture of safety. *Academy of Management Perspectives*, *24*(4), pp. 60–77.

Watcher, R. (2010). Patient safety at ten: Unmistakable progress, troubling gaps. *HealthAffairs*, *29*(1), pp. 165–173.

World Health Organization. (2009.) Patient safety curriculum guide for medical schools. Retrieved from http://www.who.int/patientsafety/education/curriculum/EN_PSP_Education_Medical_Curriculum/en/

Wu, A. W. (2000). Medical error: The second victim. *British Medical Journal*, *320*(7237), pp. 726–727.

PART 4

HRO CONCEPTS AND APPLICATION TO PRACTICE: SENSITIVITY TO OPERATIONS

ALARM SAFETY: WORKING SOLUTIONS

JoAnne Phillips, DNP, RN, CPPS

> Until you remove the noise, you are going to miss a lot of signals.
>
> —*Seth Godin*

The 21st century has brought dramatic changes to healthcare. Over the past three decades, the presence of technologically complex medical devices has increased significantly. In 1983, critical care units averaged six different types of clinical alarms. By 2011, that number had increased to 40 (Borowski et al., 2011; Chambrin, 2001; Cropp, Woods, Raney, and Bredle, 1994; Kerr and Hayes, 1983; Purbaugh, 2014; Sendelbach, 2012). Technology that was historically seen only in critical care units is now in general medical-surgical floors, labor and delivery suites, emergency departments, perioperative suites, skilled nursing units, and nursing homes, as well as used for home care. Alarms associated with these medical devices are designed to alert clinicians to either a change in the patient's physiologic condition or a failure of the equipment (Phillips, 2006; Sendelbach and Funk, 2013).

Although there is a focus in the literature on cardiac monitors, the concept of alarm safety applies broadly across all medical devices. In addition to cardiac monitors, there is a plethora of medical devices that generate alarms, including (but not limited to) mechanical ventilators, infusion pumps, pulse oximetry monitors, feeding pumps, bed exit devices, and sequential compression devices. Medical devices may also include monitoring devices, such as physiologic monitors; therapeutic devices, such as ventilators; and devices to deliver medications, such as intravenous smart pumps

(Imhoff and Kuhls, 2006). The source of most clinical alarms is physiologic monitors (Christensen, Dodds, Sauer, and Watts, 2014; Cvach, 2012; Sendelbach and Funk, 2013).

ECRI Institute, an independent nonprofit organization that researches the safety and efficacy of medical products and devices, has identified alarm hazards as the top technology hazard for the past 4 years (Sendelbach, Wahl, Anthony, and Shotts, 2015). The institute has addressed the risks associated with clinical alarms since the first report of alarm-related patient harm. In 1974, a patient experienced burns from a hypothermia machine that did not sound an alarm to notify staff of a problem (ACCE Healthcare Technology Foundation Task Force on Clinical Alarms, 2006; Sendelbach and Funk, 2013).

By 2002, The Joint Commission (TJC) had reviewed 23 reports in the Sentinel Event database of deaths or injuries experienced by patients on long-term ventilators. TJC announced the first National Patient Safety Goal (NPSG) addressing alarm safety in 2003–2004. The initial goal focused on regular preventive maintenance and proper audibility of alarms within a clinical environment (VA National Center for Patient Safety, 2002) but was retired after 2004 (TJC, 2013a). Although the goal was retired, the standards are still surveyed under Environment of Care (EC.02.04.01) and under provision of care, leadership, and patients' rights. The Centers for Medicare and Medicaid Services is also focusing on alarm safety, in conditions of participation 482.13, 482.23, and 482.41 (Association for the Advancement of Medical Instrumentation [AAMI], 2013; Sendelbach et al., 2015). Reports of patient harm continue to be reported to the Manufacturer and User Facility Device Experience (MAUDE) database and TJC's Sentinel Event database. High reliability organizations (HROs) recognize and act early on sources of risk (Chassin and Loeb, 2013). Alarm management has all the elements of high risk and potential for adverse events. This chapter focuses on how to manage alarms to control and contain that risk.

ALARM-RELATED HARM DATA

Multiple studies have shown that between 85 and 99% of clinical alarms are not clinically relevant and do not require intervention (Cvach, 2012; Feder and Funk, 2013; Graham and Cvach, 2010; Purbaugh, 2014; Sendelbach and Funk, 2013; Solet and Barach, 2012; Welch, 2012). Non-actionable alarms are a significant contributor to alarm fatigue, which is the most common cause of alarm-related sentinel events (TJC, 2013a). A *sentinel event* is "a patient safety event that reaches the patient and results in any of the following: death, permanent harm, severe temporary harm" (TJC, 2012, p. 1). Reporting sentinel events to The Joint Commission is voluntary; therefore, alarm-related sentinel events are likely to be underreported (TJC, 2013a; Sendelbach, 2012; Sendelbach and Funk, 2013; Whalen et al., 2014). Manufacturers, importers, and device users are required to report adverse patient safety events to the Manufacturer and User Facility Device Experience (MAUDE) database of the Food and Drug Administration (FDA). Alarm-related adverse events can result in temporary or permanent patient harm or in death.

MANUFACTURER AND USER FACILITY DEVICE EXPERIENCE

The MAUDE database contains adverse event reports submitted to the FDA by manufacturers, importers, and device users. Between 2005 and 2010, 566 reports of alarm-related deaths were submitted to the MAUDE database (Food and Drug Administration, 2015; TJC, 2013a; Whalen et al., 2014). Follow-up investigations often indicated that users were not familiar with how the monitoring equipment worked or had not checked the monitor's alarm status (Food and Drug Administration, 2015).

THE JOINT COMMISSION SENTINEL EVENT DATABASE

From 2009 to 2012, 98 alarm-related sentinel events were reported to TJC. The associated harm included 80 deaths, 13 patients with permanent loss of function, and 5 patients with unexpected additional care or extended stay (TJC, 2013a). As noted, experts believe that alarm-related sentinel events are likely to be underreported (TJC, 2013a; Sendelbach, 2012; Sendelbach and Funk, 2013; Whalen et al., 2014).

REGULATORY INFLUENCE

Accreditation by TJC reflects high standards of quality and patient safety. Approximately 79% of hospitals in the United States are accredited by TJC (TJC, 2015a). The National Patient Safety Goals are developed by the Patient Safety Advisory Council of TJC, through an analysis of patient safety trends and reports received in the sentinel event database. The development of the sentinel event alert and the National Patient Safety Goal on alarm safety reflects the ongoing concern of the Patient Safety Advisory Council for the issues related to alarm safety (TJC, 2015b).

SENTINEL EVENT ALERT

In response to ongoing patient harm and concerns from clinicians, TJC released a sentinel event alert on clinical alarm safety in April, 2013. The sentinel event alert highlighted a patient whose telemetry battery alarmed at a low level for 75 minutes, indicating that the battery needed to be replaced. The nursing staff did not recognize the alarm until it was a higher-level alarm, at which time it was too late. The delayed response led to the patient's death (Kowalczyk, 2011; Purbaugh, 2014; Sendelbach and Funk, 2013). To mitigate the potential for harm associated with clinical alarms, the sentinel event alert included recommendations from AAMI and ECRI Institute that served as the foundation for the National Patient Safety Goal to "improve the safety of clinical alarms" (TJC, 2013a).

NPSG 6.01.01: IMPROVE THE SAFETY OF CLINICAL ALARM SYSTEMS

In January 2014, National Patient Safety Goal (NPSG) 6.01.01, "improve the safety of clinical alarm systems," was introduced by TJC (see Table 9.1). The NPSG on alarm safety was designed to be phased in over a 2-year period. In 2014, hospitals were expected to establish alarm system safety as a hospital priority by engaging leadership and an interprofessional team to assess the organization's current state. The elements of performance required that organizations identify the most important alarm signals to manage by soliciting input from the medical staff and clinicians, assessing the risk to a patient if the alarm is not responded to, and whether specific alarms are needed or only contribute to alarm fatigue. *Alarm fatigue* is the "limited capacity to identify and prioritize alarm signals, which has led to delayed or failed alarm responses and deliberate alarm deactivations" (Ryherd, Okcu, Ackerman, Zimring, and Persson, 2012, p. 495). An assessment of internal incident history guided leaders to identify vulnerabilities within each organization. A search and synthesis of the literature provided guidance to the best available practices and guidelines (TJC, 2015).

TABLE 9.1   NATIONAL PATIENT SAFETY GOAL 6.01.01

Phase I 2014
Leaders establish alarm safety as a priority.
The most important alarm signals to manage are identified based on the following:
■ Input from the medical staff and clinical departments
■ Risk to patients if the alarm signal is not attended to or if it malfunctions
■ Whether specific alarm signals are needed or unnecessarily contribute to alarm noise and alarm fatigue
■ Potential for patient harm based on internal incident history
■ Published best practices and guidelines

Phase II 2016
Policies and procedures are established for managing alarms.

Policies and procedures that will cover at a minimum:

- Clinically appropriate settings for alarm signals

- When alarm parameters can be changed

- Who in the organization has the authority to set alarm parameters

- Who in the organization has the authority to change alarm parameters

- Who in the organization has the authority to set alarm parameters to "off"

- Monitoring and responding to alarm signals

- Checking individual alarm signals for accurate settings, proper operation, and detectability

Staff and licensed independent practitioners are educated about the purpose and proper operation of alarm systems for which they are responsible.

Adapted from TJC (2015c)

Phase II of the NPSG calls for a thorough review and revision of policies to ensure they address when alarm signals can be disabled and alarm parameters can be changed. The policies must also define who has the authority to set, change, or turn parameters to off. All disciplines that order, set, or respond to alarms must receive education on the proper operation of alarm systems (TJC, 2015c).

STRATEGIES FOR COMPLIANCE

There are several strategies to facilitate compliance with the elements of performance of the NPSG. To prioritize which alarms to manage, solicit feedback from front-line clinicians regarding which alarms cause the most concern. TJC suggests that organizations look within their own data to identify organizational vulnerabilities.

Failure Mode and Effects Analysis

One strategy to prioritize alarms is to assess equipment and alarms identified by staff through a failure mode and effects analysis (FMEA). An FMEA is a proactive risk-assessment tool that enables clinicians to identify practice areas of high risk. An interprofessional team conducts an FMEA by identifying the steps in a process, listing the potential failure modes, and noting the potential effects of the failure. For each potential failure mode, the team scores the severity, likelihood of occurrence, and detectability (see Figure 9.1). The overall criticality and risk priority number are calculated to determine the overall risk associated with each failure mode.

There are a number of medical devices with alarms that can result in an adverse event if not attended to in a timely fashion. An FMEA can help determine which equipment has the highest risk (Joint Commission Resources, 2013).

FAILURE MODE AND EFFECTS ANALYSIS (FMEA WORKSHEET)

Process/Product _____ FMEA Date (original) _____
Team Leader _____ FMEA Date (revision) _____
FMEA Focus _____ Prioritization of Level III alarms _____
Core Team _____ Alarm Safety Steering Committee _____ Key Date:_____ Page: ___ of ___

Column 1	Column 2	Column 3	C4	C5	C6	C7	C8
Step or Link in Process	List all potential Failure Modes	Potential Effect(s) of Failure (IF failure occurs, THEN what are the consequences	SEVERITY	LIKELIHOOD	DETECTABILITY	CRITICALITY C4 x C5	RPN C4 x C5 x C6
Cardiac Monitors	Alarm settings/parameters not congruent w pt. status	False alarms ↓	4	5	4	20	80
		Not appropriate notification of change in condition	3	4	4	12	48
	Nurse Occupied	Alarm unanswered	5	3	2	15	30
	Pt. not on the monitor	Undetected change in condition	5	2	2	10	20
	False (non-actionable) alarms	Alarm fatigue - response	4	5	5	20	100
		Disabling of alarms	5	2	4	10	40
		Incorrect analysis by monitor	5	3	2	15	30
	Volume of pager/alarm	Alarm unrecognized	4	2	5	8	40
Ventilators	Not actionable alarms	Alarm fatigue	4	4	2	16	32
		Alarm can reset	4	4	2	16	32
	No one answers	Pt. dies	5	4	1	20	20
		Pt. deteriorates	5	4	2	20	20
	Alarm silence	Alarms not answered	4	2	2	8	16

Pulse ox: Centrally monitored	Alarm turned off	Unrecognized deterioration	5	2	4	10	40
	Parameter not adjusted to patient	Alarm fatigue	5	5	2	25	50
	Probe placement loose/not correct		5	4	2	20	40
	Incorrect probe		5	2	4	10	40
	Poor pleth		5	4	1	20	20

Figure 9.1   Failure mode and effects analysis.

By identifying the potential failure modes and effects of failure, staff can prioritize the devices to manage. In one such FMEA, staff identified 15 different medical devices that may cause harm if the alarm is not responded to in a timely fashion. The list included devices used across many practice areas, such as cardiac monitors, mechanical ventilators, pulse oximetry, and bed exit alarms. They also identified devices that are used in focused practice areas, such as infant security tags, continuous renal replacement therapy, and ventricular assist devices. An all-day FMEA was conducted that included the review of each device by subject matter experts. The devices that had the highest risk priority numbers (RPNs) were those used in many practice areas—cardiac monitors, mechanical ventilators, pulse oximetry, and bed exit alarms. Although specific strategies were developed to manage these alarms, the structure is such that staff can apply the concepts to devices in focused practice areas.

Work Plan for NPSG

Working toward compliance with regulatory standards requires an organized systematic approach. An NPSG work plan designed by Hyman (2014) provides a structure for organizations to follow to establish timelines and accountabilities. (See Table 9.2.) The elements of performance associated with the NPSG on alarm safety are complex, requiring work by a committed interprofessional team. The work plan can be used to track tasks, success metrics, accountabilities, deadlines, and current status.

TABLE 9.2 ALARM SAFETY WORK PLAN

Part 1					
TJC Text	*Success Metric*	*Task*	*Accountable*	*Deadline*	*Status*
As of July, 2014 Leaders establish alarm safety as a hospital priority.	Establish interprofessional Alarm Safety Committee.	Establish committee, conduct stakeholder analysis. Present plan to Regulatory Readiness Committee. Present plan to Patient Safety Steering. Establish charter.			

Part 2					
TJC Text	*Success Metric*	*Task*	*Accountable*	*Deadline*	*Status*
During 2014 Identify the most important alarm signals to manage based on the following:					
1. Input from medical staff	Providers are part of the committee.	Establish committee with nurses, clinical engineers, providers, respiratory therapists, regulatory compliance specialists, and IS specialists.			

2. Risk to patients if not responded to appropriately	Define a list of which alarms will be the focus.	Conduct FMEA on alarms identified by committee members as having Level III alarms.
		
		Alarms to manage based on RPN:
		
		  ▪ Cardiac monitors
		
		  ▪ Ventilators
		
		  ▪ Pulse oximetry
		
		  ▪ Bed exit
		
		Establish workgroup:
		
		  ▪ Engage Nursing Practice Council and Nursing Quality Council.
		
		  ▪ Conduct gap analysis (Survey Monkey).
		
		  ▪ Conduct literature search.

3. Potential for harm based on organizational history	Review alarm event history:
	
	  ▪ Pager failure
	
	  ▪ Telemetry orders
	
	  ▪ Technology/ central station failure
	
	  ▪ Practice issues
		Use data from the review to confirm which alarms will be managed as part of the NPSG.

4. Whether specific alarm signals are needed or unnecessarily contribute to alarm noise and alarm fatigue	Establish a standard for notification (which alarms will be sent to the clinician and how).	Evaluate current practice around alarm notification (that is, which alarms go to pagers, how other Level III alarms are sent to clinicians, etc.).

continues

TABLE 9.2 ALARM SAFETY WORK PLAN (CONTINUED)

Part 2					
TJC Text	*Success Metric*	*Task*	*Accountable*	*Deadline*	*Status*
5. Decisions made based on published best practices	Put in place best practices/guidelines for alarm management.	Review the literature to assess best practices and guidelines for optimal alarm management.			

Part 3					
Clinical Policies					
TJC Text	*Success Metric*	*Task*	*Accountable*	*Deadline*	*Status*
By January 1, 2016 Establish clinically appropriate settings for alarm signals. ■ When alarm signals can be disabled or changed ■ Who in the organization has the authority to set/change alarm parameters ■ Who in the organization has the authority to set alarm parameters to "off"	Policies with Level III alarms identified in Part 2 will contain: ■ Guidelines for appropriate settings for alarms ■ Under what conditions alarms can be disabled or changed ■ Who in the organization has the authority to set/change the alarm parameter ■ Who in the organization has the authority to set alarm parameters to "off"	Determine whether all identified equipment will have the same approach. Determine who will decide what clinically appropriate alarm signals will be. Evaluate/modify policies associated with equipment with Level III alarms identified in Part 2. Revise policies to support decisions to meet elements of performance.			
Establish protocols for monitoring and responding to alarm signals.	An escalation process is defined in each policy for the equipment identified in Part 2.	Collaborate with clinicians managing identified equipment to establish an escalation process.			

Adapted from Hyman (2014)

ALARMS IN THE CLINICAL ENVIRONMENT

The increase in alarms in the environment is due not only to the increase in medical devices but also to the complexity of the alarms within each device. Kerr and Hayes described the six alarms in the ICU in 1983, noting that physiologic monitors had alarms for high and low heart rate and critical alarms such as ventricular fibrillation and asystole. Today's physiologic monitors not only have more parameters to monitor, but each parameter is more complex. As an example, today's physiologic monitors can sound alarms for premature ventricular contractions (PVCs) over a preset number, supraventricular tachycardia, atrial fibrillation, elevated ST segments, and other complex cardiac events. Monitors can differentiate critical or crisis alarms from less important alarms, sounding each alarm differently. Although the alarm sounds in response to the monitor's interpretation of the cardiac rhythm, clinicians must still interpret and synthesize the sounds of each alarm in the context of a potentially chaotic clinical environment.

SITUATIONAL AWARENESS

An important concept in alarm management is situational awareness. *Situational awareness* is the "ability of an individual to process information about the environment in which they are functioning" (Greig, Higham, and Nobre, 2014, p. 952). Situational awareness involves a three-step process:

1. The acquisition of relevant information

2. The integration or cognitive processing of the information

3. The use of the integrated information to make decisions

To apply that concept to clinical alarms, the nurse first needs to hear or see the alarm, which may be challenging in a clinical environment that is overwhelmed by other sensory stimuli. The next step is to integrate and interpret the information, including the priority of the alarm, the location, his or her accountability for responding to the alarm, and the risk if it goes unanswered. Finally, the nurse must decide how to respond to the alarm. Nurses respond to alarms based on the perceived reliability of the alarm. If nurses perceive that an alarm will require intervention 90% of the time, they will respond 90% of the time. If nurses perceive that an alarm will require intervention 10% of the time, they will respond 10% of the time (Bitan, Meyer, Shinar, and Zmora, 2004; Cvach, 2012; Sendelbach, 2012). The high number of false or non-actionable alarms can affect the nurse's perception of whether an alarm requires intervention and thus his or her decision on how to respond.

ALARM FATIGUE

Nurses and other clinicians can become overwhelmed by the sheer number of alarms in the clinical environment (Sendelbach, 2012). The complex cognitive burden associated with alarms is managed by an adaptive mechanism known as *alarm fatigue* (Gazarian, Carrier, Cohen, Schram, and Shiromani, 2015). Alarm fatigue is the most common factor contributing to alarm-related patient harm (TJC, 2013a) and is a significant risk to patient safety. Multiple studies have shown that between 85 and 99% of clinical alarms are not clinically relevant and do not require intervention (Cvach, 2012; Feder and Funk, 2013; Graham and Cvach, 2010; Purbaugh, 2014, Sendelbach and Funk, 2013; Solet and Barach, 2012; Welch, 2012). As clinicians synthesize the cognitive load created by nuisance alarms, important alarms may be missed (Guardia-LaBar, Scruth, Edworthy, Foss-Durant, and Burgoon, 2014; Drew et al., 2014; Solet and Barach, 2012).

Factors that contribute to alarm fatigue include the following:

- Alarms that are not customized to individual patients
- Inadequately trained staff
- Inadequate nurse staffing
- Alarms not integrated with other technology
- Equipment malfunction (TJC, 2013a; Sendelbach and Funk, 2013)

Nurses experiencing alarm fatigue may disable, silence, or ignore clinical alarms, placing the patient at risk for an adverse event (Cvach, 2012; Solet and Barach, 2012). Alarm response may occupy up to 35% of a nurse's time (Bitan et al., 2004).

ALARM MANAGEMENT

Non-actionable and nuisance alarms are key contributors to alarm fatigue. Non-actionable alarms are alarms that result from a violation of the alarm parameter that does not require patient therapeutic intervention. When a high number of non-actionable alarms occur, they are considered nuisance alarms (Welch, 2011; Welch 2012). (See Table 9.3.)

TABLE 9.3   ALARM DEFINITIONS

Actionable alarm	An alarm that requires a response to the bedside to avoid an adverse event
Non-actionable alarm	A true alarm that does not require patient therapeutic intervention or is a result of intentional actions

| False alarm | An alarm due to an artifact that produces false data |
| Nuisance alarm | A high occurrence of non-actionable alarms |

Adapted from Welch (2011)

Although non-actionable alarms are true alarms, they are often short and self-correcting. They can be caused by clinical interventions such as suctioning a patient on a ventilator or repositioning a patient in bed (Welch, 2012).

The goal of alarm management is to set actionable alarms. Alarm parameters should be customized so that alarms that do occur require clinical intervention. Customization of alarms involves critical thinking to ensure that the alarm that sounds is actionable and requires a clinical intervention. For example, if a patient has chronic atrial fibrillation, the alarm for atrial fibrillation and irregular rhythm do not require clinical interventions, and are thus non-actionable. To help staff understand options for customization, patient profiles associated with specific clinical environments can be developed. If a nurse is unsure about how to customize alarms, the patient profiles can provide examples based on unit-based standards. The following sections provide examples of patient profiles.

Patient Profile: COPD

Loretta Goldsmith is a 68-year-old female with chronic obstructive pulmonary disease (COPD) who was admitted for COPD exacerbation. If the alarms for this patient are not customized, the patient will alarm constantly, and an actionable alarm might be missed. (See Table 9.4.)

TABLE 9.4   COPD PATIENT PROFILE

Unit Defaults	Patient's Baseline	Monitor Customization
HR 50–120	95	None
RR 12–16	26	↑ to 30
SpO2 90%	82%	↓ to 80%

HR = heart rate; RR = respiratory rate; PVC = premature ventricular contractions; VT = ventricular tachycardia

Patient Profile: Heart Failure

Harold Preston is an 86-year-old man with New York Heart Association Class III heart failure. The discussion with the provider may include how many PVCs the provider would treat. The provider may need to understand that turning off the PVC alarm does NOT turn off the VT alarm. (See Table 9.5.)

TABLE 9.5   HEART FAILURE PATIENT PROFILE

Unit Defaults	Patient's Baseline	Monitor Customization
HR 50–120	74	None
RR 12–16	22	Evaluate need for continuous RR monitoring
SpO2 90%	94%	None
PVC rate: 10	14–18/min	↑ To 20/min or turn off

HR = heart rate; RR = respiratory rate; PVC = premature ventricular contractions; VT = ventricular tachycardia

Patient Profile: Marathon Runner:

Martin Glenn is a 42-year-old marathon runner who presented to the emergency department (ED) with chest pain. His EKG and cardiac biomarkers are normal, and his pain has resolved. The patient's baseline heart rate is 52. If the lower HR default is set at 50, the alarm is likely to sound constantly when he is asleep. (See Table 9.6.)

TABLE 9.6   MARATHON RUNNER PATIENT PROFILE

Unit Defaults	Patient's Baseline	Monitor Customization
HR 50–120	52	↓ 45
RR 12–16	14	Evaluate need for continuous RR monitoring
SpO2 90%	98%	Evaluate need for continuous pulse ox monitoring

HR = heart rate; RR = respiratory rate; PVC = premature ventricular contractions; VT = ventricular tachycardia

THE LIFE CYCLE OF AN ALARM

ECRI Institute has determined the life cycle of an alarm, no matter what the source device. The key steps in the life cycle of an alarm include the violation of a parameter, the sounding or the visualization of an alarm, the delivery of the alarm to the appropriate clinician, the interpretation of the criticality of the alarm by the clinician, and the appropriate response/resolution of the alarm condition by the clinician (see Figure 9.2). Interventions to improve the safety of alarm systems and mitigate alarm fatigue can occur at each step in the life cycle of an alarm.

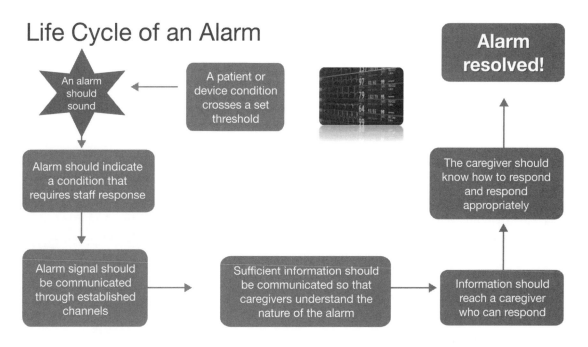

Figure 9.2 Life cycle of an alarm. Adapted with permission from ECRI Institute.

THE TENETS OF AN ALARM SAFETY PROGRAM

Alarm safety is a complex issue that requires a complex solution. An integrated alarm safety program is designed to decrease alarm fatigue and mitigate patient harm associated with alarms. The key tenets include leadership, technology and structure, policies, and education and practice. The foundation of success for such a complex initiative begins with leadership.

Leadership

Organizational leaders must demonstrate a commitment to patient safety and quality care. The role of leaders in alarm safety is to ensure that alarm management is a priority and that the resources necessary are committed to developing and supporting a program of alarm safety. This involves the following:

■ **Interprofessional alarm safety committee:** Alarm safety work requires participation and support from many disciplines. The creation of an interprofessional team is essential to creating an alarm-safe environment. Once the team is assembled, a stakeholder analysis should be conducted to ensure that all essential roles are represented on the team. One of the first actions of the interprofessional committee is to assess the current culture. The Healthcare Technology Foundation Survey "Perceptions, Issues, Improvements, and Priorities of Healthcare Professionals" (Healthcare Technology Foundation, n.d.) assessed the current state of attitudes and practice related to alarm safety, which can influence the alarm safety culture.

- **Organizational culture and incident history assessment:** Understanding organizational culture and incident history will help guide in the development of countermeasures to mitigate alarm safety risk. A review of previous incidents, root cause analyses, and action plans will provide the information needed to analyze organizational vulnerabilities. A review of alarm-related adverse events reported to ECRI Institute should include alarms that did not sound due to user error or technology failure, alarms not properly addressed, and alarm-related miscommunication, such as who was accountable to respond to the alarm (Addis, Cadet, and Graham, 2014).

- **Use of data to change practice:** Practice change begins with an understanding of the current state based on the data from the device. To affect alarm safety, you must extract data from the medical devices. There may be as many as 20 devices with alarms in an acute inpatient unit (Cvach, Currie, Sapirstein, Doyle, and Pronovost, 2013). The integration of different devices will affect the clinical engineer's ability to extract data from the medical devices. If the nurse call light, infusion pumps, and physiologic monitors are integrated into the nurse call light system, it may be easier for clinical engineers to extract the data. Data from the physiologic monitor will be used to identify vulnerabilities in individual clinical areas.

Table 9.7 summarizes the leadership requirements of an alarm safety program.

TABLE 9.7   ALARM MANAGEMENT PROGRAM: LEADERSHIP

Strategy	Assessment/Rationale/Intervention	Resource

Interprofessional alarm safety committee	A broad representation of clinicians is essential to address alarm-related issues at the organizational level. These include default settings, response algorithms, use of middleware, and recommendations for technology upgrades.
	
	Members may include the following:
	
	  ■ Administrative sponsor
	
	  ■ Medical staff
		Sendelbach and Jepson (2013)
		
		AAMI (2013)
		
		ECRI Institute (2014)
		
		Purbaugh (2014)
		
		Sendelbach and Funk (2012)

- Nursing staff

- Clinical engineering staff

- Information technology staff

- Patient safety officer/risk management

- Clinical nurse specialist/nurse manager

- Monitor technicians/monitor watcher

Organizational culture assessment	The Healthcare Technology Foundation survey "Perceptions, Issues, Improvements, and Priorities of Healthcare Professionals" is a survey designed to determine attitudes and practices related to clinical alarms. The survey contains 19 Likert scale questions. Participants are asked to prioritize nine alarm safety issues.	Korniewicz, Clark, and David (2008) Healthcare Technology Foundation (n.d.) Funk, Clark, Bauld, Ott, and Coss (2014)
Incident history assessment	1. Review organizational incident report history. 2. Review root cause analyses and associated action plans.	Sendelbach and Jepson (2013) ECRI Institute (2014)
Using data to change practice	1. Collaborate with clinical engineering to collect and analyze data from medical devices. 2. Data to analyze physiologic monitors may include the following (alarms/bed/day): - High-, medium-, and low-priority alarms - Average duration of alarms - Types of alarms	Cvach et al. (2013) TJC (2013b)

Technology and Structure

A clear understanding of technology is pivotal to providing safe care to patients with medical devices. The FDA analysis of alarm-related patient harm events demonstrated that nurses did not always understand the technology, which led to errors in management and adverse patient outcomes. The environmental structure of a clinical environment may influence how an alarm is heard and responded to. For example, if pulse oximeters or other equipment are not centrally monitored, staff must be cognizant of being able to hear the alarm. An understanding of the technology by all users and an environmental assessment are keys to safety alarm management:

■ **Environmental/architectural assessment:** An assessment of the physical layout of the environment will provide leadership with the information needed to make key decisions about structural or process changes, such as the addition of remote monitors at the end of a long hallway. It is important to understand alarm integration and the impact on alarm response. For example, are the telemetry, infusion pump, ventilator, or bed exit alarms integrated into the patient call system? How does that affect who responds to what alarm and the alarm escalation process? The physical layout of the unit can have an impact on the staff's ability to hear and respond to alarms and should be considered with renovation and new construction.

■ **Telemetry model:** Telemetry models vary across hospitals and sometimes even within hospitals. One popular model is the remote telemetry model, in which patients are monitored by a telemetry technician either down the hall or across town. In this model, communication from the telemetry technician must be clear and direct, without other caregivers or technology interrupting communication. In a second telemetry model, a local telemetry technician is in place on the unit. These technicians may have other duties as well, such as answering phones. A third popular model is the nurse accountability model, in which the nurse has total accountability for alarm setting and response.

■ **Alarm coverage:** Alarm coverage is affected by the physical layout of the unit, the placement of monitors and other medical devices, communication technology, and available staff. As noted in the discussion about the life cycle of an alarm (refer to Figure 9.2), when an alarm is activated, it must be communicated to the appropriate staff member for response. Clear and direct lines of communication and accountability prevent delays in responding to alarms. For example, on a floor with remote telemetry, the telemetry technician must have a direct method of communication with the clinician responsible for the patient. If not, a delay between alarm annunciation to alarm response may occur. If the identified clinician is not available, an established escalation process must be in place.

■ **Optimized technology:** Leaders must partner with vendors to articulate the need to optimize the safety options available on all technology. A pre-purchase collaboration with vendors is essential to ensure vendors are clear on organizational goals. Vendor standardization across the hospital will enable a focused approach to alarm safety by clinicians and clinical engineers. One option not available on all monitors is smart alarms. Smart alarms analyze data from multiple parameters before initiating an alarm (Graham and Cvach, 2010). For example, if the EKG senses asystole but the arterial line or pulse oximetry probe still shows that the patient has a pulse, an asystole alarm will not be initiated. Clinical leaders must understand not only the alarms that are created but also how they are annunciated, how they are sent to clinicians, and how clinicians need to respond to the alarms. Understanding the complexity of the alarms will enable clinical leaders to decide which alarms are necessary and which are superfluous. For example, if the monitoring system uses middleware that enables reminders to be sent to the clinicians, are the reminders necessary? How frequent and for how long should they be sent? Unnecessary reminders may play a role in alarm fatigue.

- **Multi-parameter monitors:** Bedside physiologic monitors provide the option of monitoring many different parameters, including electrocardiogram, invasive and non-invasive blood pressure, pulse oximetry, and respiratory rate, just to name a few. Not all patient populations require the continuous monitoring of all parameters, however. Clinicians must decide which parameters should be on by default (meaning they are automatically on when the monitor is turned on). Critical evaluation of parameter defaults will prevent many nuisance alarms.

- **Defaults:** Defaults—the monitor parameters set when the monitors are turned on—are set by the manufacturers but can be adjusted by clinical engineers in collaboration with clinicians. There is no research or clinical evidence to support specific alarm defaults. Alarms can and should be customized to individual patients. Expert review of alarms for a specific patient population should evaluate the most frequent alarms, duplicate alarms, and perceived nuisance alarms (Graham and Cvach, 2010). In a quality improvement project at Johns Hopkins Hospital, Graham and Cvach demonstrated a 43% reduction in critical physiologic monitor alarms through several small tests of change, including changes in cardiac monitor defaults (Graham and Cvach, 2010).

- **Delays:** Pulse oximetry false alarms are among the most common in clinical areas with continuous pulse oximetry (Graham and Cvach, 2010; Welch, 2011). Welch reported a predicted 32% decrease in pulse oximetry alarms by the addition of a 5-second delay. As most pulse oximetry alarms self-correct in a short period, longer delays may result in an even greater decrease in alarms—possibly up to 70% with a 15-second delay (Welch, 2011).

Table 9.8 summarizes the technology and structure requirements of an alarm safety program.

TABLE 9.8   ALARM MANAGEMENT PROGRAM: TECHNOLOGY AND STRUCTURE

Strategy	Assessment/Rationale/Intervention	Resource

Environmental/architectural assessment	1. Design of the space.
	
	    a. Assess the physical layout of the unit.
	
	2. What alarms are centrally monitored?
	
	3. What alarms are standalone?
	
	4. Can the alarms be heard from every location on the unit?
	
	5. Communication.
	
	    a. If phone calls will be received from telemetry technicians off site, how are they prioritized with other calls? Are they received on a separate line?
	
	6. Are there remote screens outside the central station?
	
	    a. If yes, do they allow for visual and/or audible notification of staff?
	
	7. What alarms are integrated into a central alarm system?
	
	    a. Bed exit alarms?
	
	    b. Infusion pumps?
	
	    c. Mechanical ventilators?	

Telemetry model	1. What telemetry model is in place?
	
	    a. Remote telemetry (telemetry technicians in a separate location)
	
	    b. Telemetry technicians on the unit
	
	    c. Nurse accountability model (nurses have full accountability, no telemetry technicians)
		Lazzara, Santos, Hellstedt, and Walter (2010)

Alarm coverage	1. Review/observe alarm coverage system. a. Who is accountable for each alarm (cardiac monitors, ventilators, call lights, IV pumps, etc.)? 2. Define the escalation process for alarms—if the primary clinician is not available, how does the alarm escalate to a second clinician?	Keller, Diefes, Graham, Meyers, and Pelczarski (2011)

Optimized technology	1. Change status or priority level of particular alarms.	Cvach, Frank, Doyle, and Stevens (2014)
	a. "Leads off" as a high-priority alarm	
	2. Single use sensors for continuous pulse oximetry.	ECRI Institute (2014, p. 30)
	3. Introduce and optimize smart alarms.	Keller et al. (2011)
	4. Use two-way communication for alarm response.	Welch (2011)
	5. Integrate alarm delays for pulse oximetry.	TJC (2013b)
	6. Identify which alarms are necessary.	Purbaugh (2014)
	7. Define the process for communication of an alarm to the clinician responsible for the patient.	Welch (2011)
	a. Clear and direct lines of communication to the responsible clinician	
Multi-parameter monitors	1. Evaluate necessity for each parameter.	Cvach et al. (2014)
	a. Does every patient need continuous pulse oximetry?	
	b. Does every patient need continuous respiratory rate?	
	c. Does every patient need continuous noninvasive blood pressure? What is the frequency set for?	
	i. Set for the least frequent vital signs time (every 2 hours; 4 hours)	
Defaults	There is no recognized science to support how alarm defaults should be set.	ECRI Institute (2014)
	1. Recommendations from alarm safety committee will facilitate adoption and spread of changes.	Graham and Cvach (2010)
	2. Defaults should be set for the population. For example, pediatric patients will have age-specific defaults.	Sendelbach and Funk (2013)
Delays	1. Majority of pulse oximetry alarms are false and self-correct.	Görges, Markewitz, and Westenskow (2009)
	2. Adding a 15-second delay may decrease false alarms by 70%.	Welch (2011)
	3. Overall ICU alarms may be decreased by 81% by adding a 19-second delay.	

Policies

The NPSG articulates specific policy requirements as part of the elements of performance (refer to Table 9.1). Policies for alarms identified as high risk if the alarm is not responded to must address each of the tenets of the element of performance (see Table 9.9). Policies are designed to support practice, thus the policy changes from TJC will support safe alarm practices.

TABLE 9.9 ALARM MANAGEMENT PROGRAM: POLICIES

Element of Performance	Recommendations to Meet the Elements of Performance	Source
Monitor only those who have an evidence-based indication for monitoring.	American Heart Association evidence-based practice (EBP) guidelines	Drew et al. (2004) Guardia-LaBar et al. (2014) Purbaugh (2014)

Identify clinically appropriate settings for alarm signals.
 	
Identify when alarm signals can be disabled.
 	
Identify when alarm parameters can be changed.
 	
Identify who has the authority to:
 	
  ■ Set alarm parameters
 	
  ■ Change alarm parameters
 	
  ■ Turn off alarm parameters
 	
Monitor and respond to alarm signals.
	Policies that cover the medical devices with alarms determined to be high risk if not responded to in a timely fashion should address each of these tenets.	ECRI Institute (2014)
		
		Guardia-LaBar et al. (2014)
		
		Purbaugh (2014)
		
		Sendelbach and Funk (2013)

Check individual alarm signals for accurate settings, proper operation, and detectability.	Ongoing clinical engineering assessment	

Education and Practice

To provide safe alarm management, the nurse must have the knowledge and understanding of what care needs to be provided. The foundation of that knowledge is provided through education. Education provides a framework for the nurse to deliver the highest standards of nursing practice:

■ **Education:** To support standards of practice, initial and ongoing standardized education is essential. Although the majority of alarms come from physiologic monitors, education must be provided as a foundation to support situational awareness for clinical alarms to all clinicians (TJC, 2013b; Guardia-LaBar et al., 2014; Purbaugh, 2014). To facilitate education on alarm safety—and in particular the NPSG—it can be helpful to design a template of which clinicians require what education (see Figure 9.3).

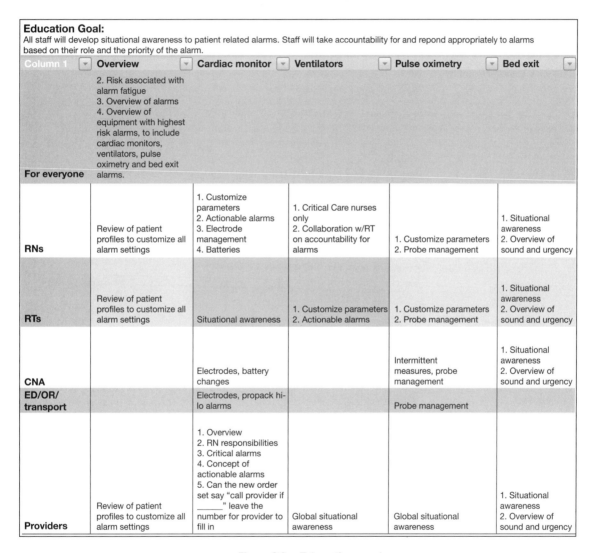

Education Goal:
All staff will develop situational awareness to patient related alarms. Staff will take accountability for and repond appropriately to alarms based on their role and the priority of the alarm.

Column 1	Overview	Cardiac monitor	Ventilators	Pulse oximetry	Bed exit
For everyone	2. Risk associated with alarm fatigue 3. Overview of alarms 4. Overview of equipment with highest risk alarms, to include cardiac monitors, ventilators, pulse oximetry and bed exit alarms.				
RNs	Review of patient profiles to customize all alarm settings	1. Customize parameters 2. Actionable alarms 3. Electrode management 4. Batteries	1. Critical Care nurses only 2. Collaboration w/RT on accountability for alarms	1. Customize parameters 2. Probe management	1. Situational awareness 2. Overview of sound and urgency
RTs	Review of patient profiles to customize all alarm settings	Situational awareness	1. Customize parameters 2. Actionable alarms	1. Customize parameters 2. Probe management	1. Situational awareness 2. Overview of sound and urgency
CNA		Electrodes, battery changes		Intermittent measures, probe management	1. Situational awareness 2. Overview of sound and urgency
ED/OR/ transport		Electrodes, propack hi-lo alarms		Probe management	
Providers	Review of patient profiles to customize all alarm settings	1. Overview 2. RN responsibilities 3. Critical alarms 4. Concept of actionable alarms 5. Can the new order set say "call provider if _____" leave the number for provider to fill in	Global situational awareness	Global situational awareness	1. Situational awareness 2. Overview of sound and urgency

Figure 9.3   Education goals.

■ **Practice:** Key best practices for alarm management include monitoring only patients with an evidence-based indication, daily electrode change with associated appropriate skin prep, and customization of alarms (Drew et al., 2004; Cvach, 2012; TJC 2013b; Guardia-LaBar et al., 2014; Purbaugh, 2014; Sendelbach and Funk, 2013). Staff who manage patients on medical devices that have high-risk alarms must have their competency assessed to ensure they have the cognitive and psychomotor skills necessary to safely manage the patients (TJC, 2013b; Allen, Hileman, and Ward, 2013).

Table 9.10 summarizes the education and practice requirements of an alarm safety program.

TABLE 9.10 ALARM MANAGEMENT PROGRAM: EDUCATION AND PRACTICE

Strategy	Assessment/Rationale/Intervention	Resource
Alarm management education	Initial and ongoing standardized education for each discipline (refer to Figure 9.3)	TJC (2013b) Guardia-LaBar et al. (2014) Purbaugh (2014)
Change electrodes daily	Clear protocol for how to prep the skin and care of the electrodes: ■ Remove chest hair that will interfere with the signal transmission. ■ Skin prep: soap and water. ■ Gently abrade the skin with dry gauze. ■ Change electrodes daily (or per manufacturer's guidelines). ■ Change telemetry box batteries every 24 hours.	Allen et al. (2013) Cvach (2012) Guardia-LaBar et al. (2014) Purbaugh (2014) Sendelbach and Funk (2012)
Customization	Alarms should be customized so that the violation should require clinical intervention (action). Patient profiles can be developed to help staff critically evaluate how to customize alarm settings for actionable alarms.	TJC (2013b) Cvach (2012) Purbaugh (2014) Sendelbach and Funk (2012)

Competency checklist	Cognitive and psychomotor critical elements of monitor alarm competency:	TJC (2013b)
		Allen et al. (2013, p. 8)
	■ Admit a patient to the cardiac monitoring system.	Phillips (2006)
	■ Explain the need for alarms to the patient and family.	
	■ Discharge a patient from the cardiac monitoring system.	
	■ Identify clinically significant alarms and demonstrate appropriate prioritization of alarm response.	
	■ Review alarm settings during handoff.	
	■ Customize alarm settings and document the settings in the EMR.	
	■ Properly perform skin prep and electrode placement on patient's chest.	
	■ Correctly load paper into the cardiac monitor central station.	
	■ Appropriately put patient in standby mode versus suspend mode.	
	■ Set monitors to correctly identify a patient with a permanent pacemaker.	

SUMMARY

Alarm safety is a complex issue that requires a complex solution. Excessive clinical alarms create noise and pull staff away from the care of their patients. The noise generated by alarms can be disruptive and anxiety-producing for staff, patients, and families, resulting in a syndrome referred to as *alarm fatigue*. Nurses experiencing alarm fatigue may disable, silence, or ignore clinical alarms, placing patients at risk (Cvach, 2012; Solet and Barach, 2012). To mitigate the risk associated with alarm fatigue, an integrated alarm management program must incorporate leadership, technology, culture, and safe practices (Addis et al., 2014). The work plans and examples in this chapter guide compliance with the NPSG on alarm safety, which in turn facilitates an alarm-safe environment for patients and staff.

KEY POINTS

■ An effective alarm safety program must be interprofessional and comprehensive, engaging participation from a broad spectrum of professionals, including clinical engineers, human factors engineers, providers, nurses, therapists, and administrators.

■ The impact of the complexity of clinical alarm systems on an organization's technology infrastructure and clinical practice must be appreciated to ensure the safety of patients, families, and care providers.

■ Compliance with the National Patient Safety Goal on Alarm Safety will guide organizations toward the culture necessary to create an alarm-safe environment.

REFERENCES

Addis, L. M., Cadet, V. N., and Graham, K. C. (2014). Sound the alarm. *Patient Safety and Quality Healthcare* (May/June). Retrieved from http://psqh.com/may-june-2014/sound-the-alarm

Allen, J. S., Hileman, K., and Ward, A. (2013). Simple solutions for improving patient safety in cardiac monitoring—eight critical elements to monitor alarm competency. *AAMI Foundation Safety Innovations*. Retrieved from http://www.aami.org/thefoundation/content.aspx?ItemNumber=1238

American College of Clinical Engineering Healthcare Technology Foundation Task Force on Clinical Alarms. (2006). Impact of clinical alarms on patient safety. Retrieved from http://thehtf.org/white%20paper.pdf

The Association for the Advancement of Medical Instrumentation (AAMI). (2013). The Joint Commission's national patient safety goal on alarm management: How do we get started? Retrieved from http://www.aami.org/thefoundation/content.aspx?ItemNumber=1498&navItemNumber=675#sthash.wZJWPWyN.dpuf

Bitan, Y., Meyer, J., Shinar, D., and Zmora, E. (2004). Nurses' reactions to alarms in a neonatal intensive care unit. *Cognition, Technology and Work*, *6*(4), pp. 239–246.

Borowski, M., Görges, M., Fried, R., Such, O., Wrede, C., and Imhoff, M. (2011). Medical device alarms. *Biomedizinische Technik*, *56*(2), pp. 73–83.

Chambrin, M. C. (2001). Alarms in the intensive care unit: How can the number of false alarms be reduced? *Critical Care*, *5*(4), 184–188.

Chassin, M. R., and Loeb, J. M. (2013). High-reliability health care: Getting there from here. *Milbank Quarterly*, *91*(3), pp. 459–490.

Christensen, M., Dodds, A., Sauer, J., and Watts, N. (2014). Alarm setting for the critically ill patient: A descriptive pilot survey of nurses' perceptions of current practice in an Australian regional critical care unit. *Intensive & Critical Care Nursing*, *30*(4), pp. 204–210.

Cropp, A. J., Woods, L. A., Raney, D., and Bredle, D. L. (1994). Name that tone. The proliferation of alarms in the intensive care unit. *Chest*, *105*(4), pp. 1217–1220.

Cvach, M. (2012). Monitor alarm fatigue: An integrative review. *Biomedical Instrumentation & Technology*, *46*(4), 268–277.

Cvach, M. M., Currie, A., Sapirstein, A., Doyle, P. A., and Pronovost, P. (2013). Managing clinical alarms: Using data to drive change. *Nursing Management*, *44*(11), pp. 8–12.

Cvach, M. M., Frank, R. J., Doyle, P., and Stevens, Z. K. (2014). Use of pagers with an alarm escalation system to reduce cardiac monitor alarm signals. *Journal of Nursing Care Quality*, *29*(1), pp. 9–18.

Drew, B. J., Califf, R. M., Funk, M., Kaufman, E. S., Krucoff, M. W., Laks, M. M., … Van Hare, G. F. (2004). Practice standards for electrocardiographic monitoring in hospital settings: An American Heart Association scientific statement from the Councils on Cardiovascular Nursing, Clinical Cardiology, and Cardiovascular Disease in the Young: Endorsed by the International Society of Computerized Electrocardiology and the American Association of Critical-Care Nurses. *Circulation*, *110*(17), pp. 2721–2746.

Drew, B. J., Harris, P., Zègre-Hemsey, J. K., Mammone, T., Schindler, D., Salas-Boni, R., ... Hu, X. (2014). Insights into the problem of alarm fatigue with physiologic monitor devices: A comprehensive observational study of consecutive intensive care unit patients. *PLoS One, 9*(10), e110274.

ECRI Institute. (2014). *Alarm Safety Handbook.* Plymouth Meeting, PA: ECRI Institute.

Feder, S., and Funk, M. (2013). Over-monitoring and alarm fatigue: For whom do the bells toll? *Heart & Lung: The Journal of Critical Care, 42*(6), pp. 395–396.

Food and Drug Administration. (2015). Medical device reporting. Retrieved from http://www.fda.gov/medicaldevices/safety/reportaproblem/default.htm

Funk, M., Clark, J. T., Bauld, T. J., Ott, J. C., and Coss, P. (2014). Attitudes and practices related to clinical alarms. *American Journal of Critical Care, 23*(3), pp. e9–e18.

Gazarian, P. K., Carrier, N., Cohen, R., Schram, H., and Shiromani, S. (2015). A description of nurses' decision-making in managing electrocardiographic monitor alarms. *Journal of Clinical Nursing, 24*(1–2), pp. 151–159.

Görges, M., Markewitz, B. A., and Westenkow, D. R. (2009). Improving alarm performance in the medical intensive care unit using delays and clinical context. *Anesthesia and Analgesia, 108*(5), pp. 1546–1552.

Graham, K. C., and Cvach, M. (2010). Monitor alarm fatigue: Standardizing use of physiological monitors and decreasing nuisance alarms. *American Journal of Critical Care, 19*(1), pp. 28–34.

Greig, P. R., Higham, H., and Nobre, A. C. (2014). Failure to perceive clinical events: An under-recognised source of error. *Resuscitation, 85*(7), pp. 952–956.

Guardia-LaBar, L. M., Scruth, E. A., Edworthy, J., Foss-Durant, A. M., and Burgoon, D. H. (2014). Alarm fatigue: The human-system interface. *Clinical Nurse Specialist, 28*(3), pp. 135–137.

Healthcare Technology Foundation. (n.d.). 2011 Alarms Survey Results. Retrieved from http://thehtf.org/alarms_survey2011.asp

Hyman, W. A. (2014). A work plan for the Joint Commission alarm national patient safety goal. *Journal of Clinical Engineering, 39*(1), pp. 23–27. doi: 10.1097/JCE.0000000000000011

Imhoff, M., and Kuhls, S. (2006). Alarm algorithms in critical care monitoring. *Anesthesia and Analgesia, 102*(5), pp. 1525–1537.

The Joint Commission. (2007). Improving America's hospitals: A report on quality and safety. Retrieved from http://www.jointcommission.org/assets/1/6/2006_Annual_Report.pdf

The Joint Commission. (2012). Sentinel event policy. Retrieved from http://www.jointcommission.org/assets/1/6/camh_2012_update2_24_se.pdf

The Joint Commission. (2013a). Sentinel Event alert issue 50: Medical device alarm safety in hospitals. Retrieved from http://www.jointcommission.org/sea_issue_50/

The Joint Commission. (2013b). Johns Hopkins improves clinical alarm safety with escalation algorithms. *The Source 11*(9) pp. 1–7.

The Joint Commission. (2015a). Facts about hospital accreditation. Retrieved from http://www.jointcommission.org/facts_about_hospital_accreditation/

The Joint Commission. (2015b). Facts about the National Patient Safety Goals. Retrieved from http://www.jointcommission.org/facts_about_the_national_patient_safety_goals/

The Joint Commission. (2015c). 2015 National Patient Safety Goals. Retrieved from http://www.jointcommission.org/standards_information/npsgs.aspx

Joint Commission Resources. (2013). Risky business: Conducting proactive risk assessments. Retrieved from http://www.jcrqsn.com/VA/2013_jcr3-VA.pdf

Keller, J. P., Diefes, R., Graham, K., Meyers, M., and Pelczarski, K. (2011). Why clinical alarms are a "top ten" hazard: How you can help reduce the risk. *Biomedical Instrumentation and Technology*, (suppl), pp. 17–23.

Kerr, J. H., and Hayes, B. (1983). An "alarming" situation in the intensive therapy unit. *Intensive Care Medicine, 9*(3), pp. 103–104.

Korniewicz, D. M., Clark, T., and David, Y. (2008). A national online survey on the effectiveness of clinical alarms. *American Journal of Critical Care, 17*(1), pp. 36–41.

Kowalczyk, L. (2011). Patient alarms often unheard, unheeded. *Boston Globe.* Retrieved from http://www.boston.com/lifestyle/health/articles/2011/02/13/patient_alarms_often_unheard_unheeded/

Lazzara, P. B., Santos, A. R., Hellstedt, L. F., and Walter, R. (2010). The evolution of a centralized telemetry program. *Nursing Management, 41*(11), pp. 51–54. doi: 10.1097/01.NUMA.0000388670.02663.b6

Phillips, J. (2006). Clinical alarms: Complexity and common sense. *Critical Care Nursing Clinics of North America, 18*(2), pp. 145–156.

Purbaugh, T. (2014). Alarm fatigue: A roadmap for mitigating the cacophony of beeps. *Dimensions of Critical Care Nursing, 33*(1), pp. 4–7.

Ryherd, E. E., Okcu, S., Ackerman, J., Zimring, C., and Waye, K. P. (2012). Noise pollution in hospitals: Impacts on staff. *Journal of Clinical Outcomes Management, 19*(11), 491–500.

Sendelbach, S. (2012). Alarm fatigue. *Nursing Clinics of North America, 47*(3), pp. 375–382.

Sendelbach, S., and Funk, M. (2013). Alarm fatigue: A patient safety concern. *AACN Advanced Critical Care, 24*(4), pp. 378–386.

Sendelbach, S., and Jepsen, S. (2013). Alarm management. Retrieved from http://www.aacn.org/wd/practice/content/practicealerts/alarm-management-practice-alert.pcms?menu=practice

Sendelbach, S., Wahl, S., Anthony, A., and Shotts, P. (2015). Stop the noise: A quality improvement project to decrease electrocardiographic nuisance alarms. *Critical Care Nurse, 35*(4), pp. 15–22.

Solet, J. M., and Barach, P. R. (2012). Managing alarm fatigue in cardiac care. *Progress in Pediatric Cardiology, 33*(1), pp. 85–90.

VA National Center for Patient Safety. (2002). JCAHO patient safety goals 2003. Retrieved from http://www.patientsafety.va.gov/docs/TIPS/TIPSDec02.pdf

Welch, J. (2011). An evidence-based approach to reduce nuisance alarms and alarm fatigue. *Biomedical Instrumentation & Technology*, (suppl), pp. 46–52.

Welch, J. (2012). Alarm fatigue hazards: The sirens are calling. Retrieved from http://psqh.com/alarm-fatigue-hazards-the-sirens-are-calling

Whalen, D. A., Covelle, P. M., Piepenbrink, J. C., Villanova, K. L., Cuneo, C. L., and Awtry, E. H. (2014). Novel approach to cardiac alarm management on telemetry units. *The Journal of Cardiovascular Nursing, 29*(5), pp. E13–22. doi: 10.1097/JCN.0000000000000114

CHAPTER **10**

INNOVATIVE TECHNOLOGY, STANDARDIZATION, AND THE IMPACT ON HIGH RELIABILITY

Jane Englebright, PhD, RN, CENP, FAAN

Kelly Aldrich, DNP, RN-BC

Highly reliable operational processes are necessary to drive consistent results. In healthcare, most processes are carried out by human beings (caregivers) for other human beings (patients). This introduces variability. Magnify that variability by the number of team members contributing to the around-the-clock care of a hospitalized patient or by the number of specialty teams coordinating care across settings for a patient with chronic disease, and the achievement of high reliability and consistent results can seem impossible.

Technology and standardization offer the promise of "hard-wiring" processes of care across caregivers and settings, driving out variability and increasing consistency of results. However, patients are not mass-produced consumer products on an assembly line. They are highly variable in needs, wants, and preferences. Standardization must be balanced with flexibility to meet individual patient circumstances. Technology is a tool that can support both

> The key to optimizing patient safety is to design systems that prevent the inevitability of human error from reaching the patient.
>
> —Leotsakos et al.

standardization and individualization within processes of care. This chapter examines why technology can be so effective in hard-wiring care processes, using examples from clinical practice.

FRAMEWORK

Improving outcomes often starts with identifying a best process and finding ways to hard-wire that process within a specific care setting. There are several approaches for hard-wiring, or making a process highly reliable, and many are discussed in this book. The approaches vary from simple (such as posting a checklist on the wall) to complex (for example, re-engineering workflow and technology).

The approaches also vary in effectiveness. The Institute for Safe Medication Practices (ISMP) has proposed a hierarchy of effectiveness of common approaches in achieving reliability (ISMP, 1999). (See Figure 10.1.) Technology, automation, and forcing functions are the most effective approaches identified in this hierarchy.

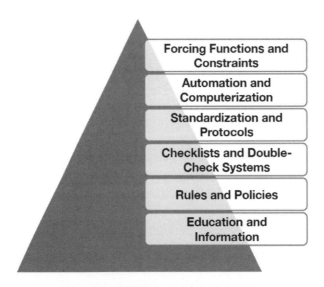

Figure 10.1   Institute for Safe Medication Practices hierarchy of reliability (ISMP, 1999).

The ISMP hierarchy contains the following levels:

- **Education and information:** The most basic level of the ISMP hierarchy of reliability (ISMP, 1999) is education. While education is a critical element of most change efforts in healthcare, this hierarchy suggests it is the least effective in driving consistent processes.

EDUCATION AND INFORMATION EXAMPLE

An upgrade to the nurse call system seemed very straightforward to the nurse manager. The week before turning on the new software, staff members were asked to view an educational video and to review the updated policy describing the "No Passing Zone" response to call lights. When the big day came, the manager noticed an increase in call light alarms and delays in response times. In a debrief with staff, the manager learned that some staff interpreted the "No Passing Zone" to mean they should not respond over the intercom but should get up and go to the patient's room. Other staff misunderstood how to use the intercom so the patients could not hear the response and were activating the call bell multiple times for the same request.

- **Rules and policies:** The second level of the ISMP hierarchy (ISMP, 1999) is rules and policies. In a highly regulated field, such as healthcare, there are lots of policies and standards. The policies may or may not reflect actual care processes. By themselves, they are ineffective in driving consistent practices. Both education and policies still rely on individual clinicians attending to the information and applying it in their interactions with patients. The challenge is getting each clinician to understand and act on the information in the same way to achieve highly reliable performance and outcomes.

- **Checklists and double-check systems:** The third level of the ISMP hierarchy (ISMP, 1999) is checklists and double-check systems. This strategy has demonstrated effectiveness in several high-risk areas. However, a checklist or double-check process still allows for significant variation.

CHECKLISTS AND DOUBLE-CHECK SYSTEMS EXAMPLE

When preparing to implement barcoded verification technology for medication administration, a group of nurses described the double-check process used to verify insulin doses. All were performing double-checks for this high-alert medication, but there was tremendous variation in the process used.

- Some insisted the double-check process be done at the bedside, others in the medication room, and still others said it could be done anywhere.
- Some insisted that reviewing the patient's glucose level was a component of the double-check while others did not review lab values.
- Some checked only the amount of insulin in the syringe while others verified type of insulin and expiration date.

■ **Standardization and protocols:** The fourth level of the ISMP hierarchy of reliability (ISMP, 1999) is standardization and protocols. Protocols are well-known in the healthcare environment. They are powerful tools for eliminating errors of omission, improving timeliness of response to changes in patient condition and ensuring all team members are aware of the patient's treatment plan. Protocols and standardization are effective strategies for reducing variation. Standardization of both processes and technology to reduce variation is discussed in more detail in the next section.

■ **Automation and computerization:** Automation (ISMP, 1999) is a powerful tool for reducing variation. Automation is common in laboratory and pharmacy operations within a healthcare system. Automated systems effectively hard-wire processes by removing some of the variability that accompanies human intervention. Automation is also entering the direct care environment. One of the most prevalent examples is automated vital signs monitors. These portable machines automate various components of vital sign measurement, eliminating variability from differences in human hearing capacity in some (but not all) aspect of technique. The simplicity and consistency of these machines have enabled support personnel to assume responsibility for this task, which was once reserved for physicians and nurses. Computerization (ISMP, 1999), with or without automation, is effective in driving consistency and preventing errors of omission. Standard data-entry screens drive consistency in patient assessment and information storage. Computerized reminders for scheduled or timed events alert clinicians to critical care activities.

 Both automation and computerization are discussed in more detail in this chapter.

AUTOMATION AND COMPUTERIZATION EXAMPLE

The electronic medication administration record (eMAR) provides a schedule of the medication profile for a patient. The eMAR alerts nurses to the next medication due and to any late medications. When giving medications that require data input, such as a heart rate for each dose of digoxin, the eMAR provides a reminder to document heart rate in a specific place, using a specific data format.

■ **Forcing functions and constraints:** Forcing functions and constraints, the top level in the ISMP hierarchy (ISMP, 1999), provide a single path to accomplish tasks, precluding variation and driving consistent practice. An example of a forcing function in healthcare is the fittings on oxygen and nitrous oxide. It is nearly impossible for a distracted or novice anesthesia provider to attach oxygen tubing to an anesthesia gas source. They simply don't fit. Climbing the hierarchy of reliability is one way to systematically eliminate human factors that often contribute to error. Forcing functions essentially eliminate human variation from a process. Every driver must engage the brakes on a car before putting that car into reverse. This technology requires this type of action. In contrast, although a stop sign signals a need to stop, it does not force a driver to do so.

The goal of high reliability strategies is to make it easier to do the right thing and harder to do the wrong thing. This increases the likelihood that distracted, busy, and fallible humans will consistently do the right thing. Airlines have used this approach to encourage passengers to lock the bathroom door; locking the door turns on the light, thereby eliminating many disruptive events! Similarly, in healthcare, putting all the products necessary for a procedure in a kit increases the likelihood that the clinician will go to the bedside with everything needed to safely perform the procedure and limits the need for improvisation and shortcuts (Leonard, Frankel, and Simmonds, 2004).

STANDARDIZATION

Standardization reduces variability. This chapter previously discussed the variability that often exists among caregivers. There is also variability in care processes, equipment, supplies, and the environment. Technology itself can introduce variability in data capture, transmission, and storage. For technology to be most effective in improving safety and efficiency, standardization is required.

This raises the question: Where do you begin the task of standardizing? The answer is, you start where you are. Technology operates within care processes, and care processes operate within an organizational culture (see Figure 10.2). Disrupting any of these elements affects all of them. Adding new technology changes work processes, and new work processes change organizational culture. Understanding these relationships is important to orchestrating a successful technology integration.

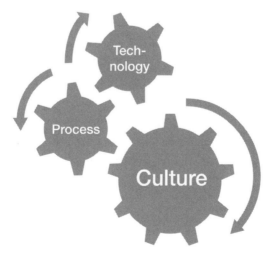

Figure 10.2 The culture-process-technology approach.

The culture of an organization is defined by the way its people think and act (Connors and Smith, 2011). The culture reflects values and beliefs. Culture can be an enabler or a barrier to standardized work processes and the effective use of technology. A culture that values innovation, for example, may be very accepting of new technology. But a culture that values autonomy may be very resistant to the standardizing processes necessary for the new technology to be effective. This paradox explains why the staff in a critical care unit easily adapt to a new intra-aortic balloon pump but actively resist a computerized documentation system that standardizes patient assessment components.

Linking change to a commonly held value within the culture is an effective strategy in change management. For example, when implementing a standard medication administration process using barcode verification technology, emphasizing the common value of patient safety can be effective in persuading nurses and pharmacists to adopt it.

Assessing organizational culture and aligning improvement efforts with deeply held cultural beliefs is key to a successful change effort. Change efforts can start with changing the culture or they can start with changing the process or technology. The systematic adoption of new processes and technologies does affect culture. For example, a leadership process of generating daily safe practice adherence reports and following up with staff individually on discrepancies will affect the staff's perception of how the organization values safety—that is, its culture of safety.

Process standardization begins with determining the best or ideal process that is most likely to produce the desired outcome. This can be derived from the research literature or from observing top performers. A common misconception is that technology should be adapted to fit all the different variations on workflow that exist within an organization. Rather, technology should be configured to support the best or ideal workflow. When the ideal process is defined, gaps between current processes and the ideal process may be assessed. Care processes should be adjusted to the ideal process before or in conjunction with the introduction of the technology. The technology then acts as a stent, reinforcing the desired process and providing feedback to clinicians and managers who are monitoring and supporting the process.

The demand for real-time data at the point of care to support clinical decision-making is growing. Answering this demand requires several layers of standardization. Data elements that will be used in the decision-support algorithm must be labeled in a standard way and stored in a standard place for the algorithm to find them. There must be a standard place or places for the decision support to display within the workflow at a time in which it is actionable. Failing to address these areas of standardization can result in non–value added or nuisance alerts and notifications that actually interfere with efficient and effective care processes.

STANDARDIZATION EXAMPLE

Designing clinical decision support and analytics to improve patient restraint management started with articulating the organization's value for patient safety and patient rights. The goal was to create processes and tools for maintaining patient safety and minimizing the use of restraints. The ideal process included key steps such as assessing potential for harm, using alternatives to restraint, obtaining second opinions, safe application of restraints, frequent monitoring of patients in restraints, management, and oversight processes.

The resulting solution included the following:

- Standard staff education on the goal of a restraint-free environment
- Standard patient-assessment elements in the electronic health record
- Standard double-check processes for all decisions to use restraint, triggered by the patient-assessment findings
- A standard monitoring process with standard documentation elements and time-based reminders in the electronic health record
- Standard management reports derived from electronic documentation data that generated a list of patients in restraints for daily review
- Standard trended usage reports that aggregated restraint documentation elements for each nursing unit, allowing executives to compare performance, identify best performers, establish benchmarks, and drive improvement

In the preceding restraint example, simple decision support was added to the documentation screens to aid decision-making. This included adding the definition for restraint types—behavioral and safety—to assist the nurse in selecting the appropriate type of restraint for the situation. This selection then triggered a more complex decision-support tool, a protocol. A different protocol was attached to each restraint type. The protocol provided automated reminders for the frequency of monitoring, the documentation requirements, and the review time frames required for each restraint type.

We often think of technology as the electronic health record. In the restraint example, the electronic health record was an important part of the standardization and automation strategy. Other types of information systems may also be used to drive standardization in clinical processes, however. In the restraint example, the organization also eliminated leather and vest restraints from their supply inventory. This was effectively a forcing function that eliminated the types of restraints that pose the most significant risks to patient safety. Clinical technologies, supplies, and equipment can also be used to reduce variation and introduce standardization in clinical processes.

The bundle approach to reducing central line–associated blood stream infection (CLABSI) is a great example of using education, procedures, protocols, and checklists to drive consistency in clinical practice (The Joint Commission [TJC], 2013). The bundle is a tool for reducing variation in the clinical process. The bundle includes education, policies, checklists, and protocols. Variation can be reduced even further by leveraging clinical technology and the electronic health record (EHR). Standardizing the contents of the central line insertion kits available in the institution to contain only those options identified in the bundle improves adherence to the bundle. Building standard documentation elements related to central line insertion, maintenance, and monitoring puts reminders in front of the staff in the midst of their workflow, increasing adherence to the bundle. The data derived from the standard documentation elements can be used to automate reminders to review the need for the central line each day. The data may also be used to generate reminders and alerts to the care team, the quality team, and managers. Finally, the data can be aggregated to evaluate adherence to the bundle at the unit or at the individual caregiver level. These reports equip leaders with powerful tools for reducing variability and creating highly reliable processes. (See Figure 10.3.)

Central Line Insertion Checklist – Template

Patient Name/ID#: _____ Unit: _____ Room/Bed: _____

Date: _____ Start time: _____ End time: _____

Procedure Location: (Operating Room / Radiology / Intensive Care Unit / Other: _____)

Person Inserting Line: _____ Person Completing Form: _____

Catheter Type: (Dialysis / Tunneled / Non-tunneled / Implanted / Non-implanted / Peripherally Inserted Central Catheter)

Impregnated: (Yes/No) _____ Number of Lumens: (1, 2, 3, 4) _____ Catheter Lot Number: _____

Insertion Site: (Jugular / Chest / Subclavian / Femoral / Scalp / Umbilical) _____ Side of Body: (Left / Right) _____

Reason for Insertion: (New indication / Malfunction / Routine Replacement / Emergent) _____ Guide Wire Used: (Yes/No) ___

Critical Steps	Yes	Yes with Reminder	No*	n/a	Comments
BEFORE the procedure:					
Patient is educated about the need for and implications of the central line as well as the processes of insertion and maintenance					
Patient's latex/adhesive allergy assessed (modify supplies)					
Patient's infection risk assessed. If at greater risk, why?					
Patient's anticoagulation therapy status assessed					
Consent form and other relevant documents complete and in chart (Exception: Emergent Procedure)					
Operator and Assistant used appropriate hand hygiene immediately					
Equipment assembled and verified—materials, medications, syringes, dressings, and labels					
Placement confirmation method readied					
Patient identified with 2 sources of identification					
Procedural time-out performed					
Site assessed and marked					
Patient positioned for procedure					
Skin prep performed with alcoholic chlorhexidine greater than 0.5% (unless under 2 months of age) or tincture of iodine or an iodophor or alcohol					
Skin prep allowed to dry prior to puncture					
Patient's body covered by sterile drape from head to toe					
All those performing procedure using sterile gloves, sterile gown, hat/cap, mask, and eye protection/shield					
Others in room wearing mask					
Catheter preflushed and all lumens clamped					
Local anesthetic and /or sedation used _____					
DURING the procedure: If 'No' for any 'DURING the procedure' critical items, end the procedure.					

Confirmation of venous placement PRIOR TO dilatation of vein by: ultrasound/ transesophageal echocardiogram / pressure transducer / manometry method / fluoroscopy				
Blood aspirated from each lumen (intravascular placement assessed)				
Type and Dosage (mL/units) of flush _____				
Catheter caps placed on lumens				
All lumens clamped (should not be done with neutral or positive displacement connectors)				
Catheter secured (sutured /stapled /steri-stripped)				
Tip position confirmation via fluoroscopy OR chest X-ray				
Sterile field maintained				
Lumens were not cut				
Qualified second operator obtained after 3 unsuccessful sticks				
Blood cleaned from site				
Sterile dressing applied (gauze, transparent dressing, gauze and transparent dressing, antimicrobial foam disc)				
AFTER the procedure:				
Dressing dated				
Verify placement by x-ray				
"Approved for use" writing on dressing after confirmation				
If a femoral line placed, elective PIC placement ordered				
Central line (maintenance) order placed				
Patient is educated about maintenance as needed				

* **Procedure Deviation:** If there is a deviation from process, immediately notify the operator and stop the procedure until corrected.
Procedure Notes/Comments: _____

Catheter Measurements: External length _____ Internal length _____

Distribution Instructions: Please return the completed form to the designated person in your area.

Central Line Insertion Care Team Checklist Instructions

Operator Requirements:
- Specify minimum requirements. For example:
   - A minimum of 5 supervised successful procedures in both the chest and femoral sites is required (10 total). If a physician successfully performs the 5 supervised lines in one site, they are independent for that site only. Please note that in the absence of contraindications, a chest site is preferred over the femoral due to a lower incidence of mechanical and infectious complications.
   - A total of 3 supervised rewires is required prior to performing a rewire independently.
   - Obtain a qualified second operator after 3 unsuccessful sticks (unless emergent).

Roles:
- Operator Role: Person inserting the line
- Assistant Role: RN, ClinTech, Physician, NP, PA (responsible for completing checklist)

Patient Positioned for Procedure:
- For Femoral/ Peripherally Inserted Central Catheter: Place supine.
- For Chest/External Jugular: Use Trendelenburg (HOB < 0 degrees) unless contraindicated.

Sterile Field:
- Patient full body drape
   - Long sterile may need to be added to commercially prepared kits.
- Sterile tray and all equipment for the procedure
- Ultrasound probe

Prep Procedure:
- Scrub back and forth with chlorhexidine with friction for 30 seconds, allow to air dry completely before puncturing site. Do not wipe, fan, or blot. (Groin prep: Scrub 2 minutes and allow to dry for 2 minutes to prevent infection.)
   - Chlorhexidine/alcohol applicator used; Dry Technique: 30-second scrub + 30-second dry time
   - Chlorhexidine/alcohol applicator used; Wet Technique: 2-minute scrub + 1-minute dry time

Guide Wire:
- Do *not* cut the guide wire due to the increased risk of losing the guide wire in the patient.

Figure 10.3 TJC central line bundle.

© The Joint Commission, 2015. Reprinted with permission.

You can also create your own bundles. Standard documentation elements for central line insertion might include the following:

- Date
- Time
- Catheter type
- Catheter size
- Catheter distance to hub

Standard documentation elements for central line maintenance might include the following:

- Date
- Time
- Dressing change
- Tubing change
- Site appearance

Standard documentation elements for central line discontinuance might include the following:

- Date
- Time
- Site appearance

INNOVATIVE TECHNOLOGY

Innovative technology is continuously emerging to address gaps in clinical care environments and to support the clinical care team in new ways. Integrating these innovations into the clinical environment requires a systematic approach and a platform of standardization to achieve high reliability. Each day, the bedside care team identifies the need for technology solutions that may be used to support them in the care process. If a tool doesn't exist or doesn't meet their requirements, workaround solutions often develop. Clinicians are seeking tools that are easy to use and highly reliable—meaning that the technology works…all of the time. Providing the right technology to the right person at the right time creates a highly reliable solution that contributes to highly reliable processes and predictable outcomes.

WORKAROUNDS: REVEALING GAPS IN SAFE PRACTICE

Workarounds often point to failure points or opportunities to improve a solution. Barcode verification technologies offer proven techniques for improving the accuracy of medication and blood product administration and specimen collection within healthcare settings (Perry, Shah, and Englebright, 2007). Part of sustaining the use of these technologies is monitoring utilization or scanning percentages. Sudden changes in scanning percentages may indicate that workarounds have developed and point to gaps in safe practices. Here are a few examples of workarounds that reveal gaps in safe practice:

- **Workaround:** Nurses are scanning chart labels instead of patient armbands.
  - **Gap:** Patient armbands are applied with elements of the barcode obscured.
- **Workaround:** Nurses are not scanning multivitamins.
  - **Gap:** The pharmacy changed from One-A-Day to Centrum but didn't update the file on the computer, causing all the medication scans to generate a "wrong medication" warning.
- **Workaround:** The fifth floor has had a marked decrease in scanning percentages, and the mobile devices are noted to be in the "home" location more frequently.
  - **Gap:** Wireless access has been disrupted on one hallway of the fifth floor due to construction.

The Affordable Care Act (ACA) has rapidly advanced the presence and utilization of electronic health records across the nation. Much of the emphasis now is on integrating other technologies within the care environment into the electronic health record. For example, integrating data from monitoring devices, medication delivery devices, and even patient beds directly into the EHR improves both accuracy and efficiency. Integrating disparate systems, however, has been difficult in healthcare because of the lack of standards for interoperability and data exchange. There is mounting pressure within the industry to enforce both technical interoperability standards and data standards across a multitude of technology vendors to enable integrated technology solutions.

One way integrated solutions offer the potential for both efficiency and error reduction is by removing the clinician from the role of data transcriber between technologies. The VitalsNow solution described in the following case study is an example of how this type of technology can be used to create a highly reliable process for patient surveillance, early detection of deterioration, and rapid response to patient needs.

CASE STUDY: VITALSNOW

VitalsNow illustrates the innovative use of technology to address inefficiency and unreliability in a critical clinical process: patient surveillance. The VitalsNow project integrated an innovative technology into the point-of-care process of vital signs monitoring to decrease labor-intensive tasks such as repetitive documentation and to improve the timeliness and reliability of communication and access to information.

The solution entails attaching a mini-computer to mobile electronic vital signs monitors. The patient is positively identified by barcode association. Vital signs are taken using the mobile monitor, and the results are sent to the mini-computer. The staff member interacts with the mini-computer to enter modifiers, such as left arm, and data not captured by the monitor, such as respiratory rate and level of consciousness.

After a complete set of vital signs for that patient is entered and verified at the point of care, the data is wirelessly transmitted to the EHR. Within seconds, the data is available for other care team members to use as information elements for safe, efficient, effective care delivery. In the transmission process, clinical decision support is applied to the data, calculating a modified early warning score (MEWS). Algorithms within the EHR send alerts to identified team members when the MEWS score meets the alerting parameters.

Traditionally, manual documentation of vital signs occurs in many steps. Here is a summary:

1. Identify the patient.
2. Take the vital signs using the mobile monitor.
3. Transcribe vital sign values from the mobile monitor onto a clipboard.
4. Add modifiers or missing data elements to the clipboard.
5. After data from all patients is collected, transcribe clipboard data into the EHR.

Observations undertaken before the VitalsNow project found that this process often resulted in vital signs not being available in the EHR until 4 hours after the measurement was taken, creating significant delays in patient care. Equally important, the two layers of transcription introduced two opportunities for incorrect data to enter the EHR and the clinical decision-making process.

The ease of data collection and accessibility of information resulting from VitalsNow have led most units to increase the frequency of vital sign monitoring. The availability of near–real-time data and clinical decision support provided an opportunity to improve patient surveillance, increase rapid response team activations, and decrease resuscitation events. The increased efficiency of the process was a significant enabler to increasing the frequency of surveillance activities.

Innovation is also occurring outside the EHR. In fact, innovative technologies in other aspects of the care environment are enabling data transmission and care coordination to occur outside the constraints of the EHR infrastructure. Some of these innovative technologies are being added to existing structures in the care environment, such as the advent of "smart" hospital beds and "smart" monitors in the home. Some innovative technologies are repurposed from other industries, such as patient kiosks for registration similar to airline check-in and interactive television services for patient entertainment and education.

Telehealth solutions are a great example of innovative technologies repurposed from other industries. The simplicity and efficiency of drive-thru banking and eating has developed into a robust set of virtual communication services that can connect clinicians with patients and with other clinicians. These exciting technologies are improving access to specialty care for underserved patient populations. This includes neurosurgical evaluation of stroke patients in the emergency department and remote assessment and diagnosis of retinopathy of prematurity in the neonatal ICU. Technologies are also reaching into the home setting with virtual appointments and remote monitoring.

A consistent theme in emerging technologies is mobility. Nurses and other members of the care team are mobile knowledge workers. Many innovative technologies are being developed to provide information at the point of care and to enable clinicians to communicate on the go. In the hospital environment, this often entails integrating mobile technology with more traditional hospital systems. iMobile is an example of this type of innovation.

CASE STUDY: iMOBILE

iMobile is a care team communication solution that entails equipping every member of the care team with a smartphone and integrating staff assignments with the phone numbers and patient call system. The solution requires ubiquitous wireless access, advanced nurse call system capabilities, and advanced phone system capabilities within the organization. These foundational functions enable care team members to use a smartphone to identify team members associated with each patient and communicate directly with individuals on the team or the entire team using voice or text capabilities.

The impact of asynchronous communication in the form of secure text messaging has been significant. It has decreased interruptions in care activities and patient interactions, improving both safety and satisfaction. The technology has also improved staff efficiency and enabled more frequent communication among team members.

> iMobile has altered patterns of communication among the team, allowing for messages and alerts to go directly to the intended staff member. For instance, patient requests for pain medication go directly to the registered nurse, while patient requests for an extra blanket go first to the nurse assistant. Alerts from patient care monitors or equipment go noiselessly to the phones instead of adding noise to the environment. This new communication technology has eliminated overhead paging, waiting for staff to come to the desk for phone calls, and searching for the name and number of the team member needed to address a patient issue.

A critical component of achieving the return on investment for innovative technologies is retiring old systems. This includes eliminating the support activities associated with these systems. This often requires reworking clinical processes reliant on the obsolete systems. Failure to do this can allow clinicians to go back to the old, more comfortable way of doing things.

In the iMobile example, eliminating the cost of the old beeper system was part of the return on investment calculation for the project. To be sure beepers could not be used as a workaround or alternative to adopting the new process and technology, the beeper network needed to be removed. This required reworking on-call team notification processes to allow the entire infrastructure to be removed. Before removing the technology, the beeper devices were collected, and the beeper network was turned off. The implementation team quickly learned that hospital volunteers were using that same beeper infrastructure in the waiting rooms for family members. A new process involving text messages to families on their personal phones was quickly devised so the removal of the beeper infrastructure could continue.

> Removing old technology usually represents a cost savings but can also be a forcing function, preventing staff from slipping back into more familiar work patterns or technology.

A word of caution about removing old systems: Sometimes these systems are being used in ways that people don't remember. In the preceding example, the facility canvassed all the departments of the hospital to identify all the areas using beepers. They neglected to canvass the volunteers who staffed the surgical waiting room, however. Removing the beeper infrastructure caused major disruption to the communication processes in the waiting room. A better strategy is to turn the old system off for a defined period of time rather than removing it and see if anyone notices or complains!

Innovative technologies that improve efficiency while advancing quality and safety are essential to achieving leadership support and staff adoption. A clinician's readiness and acceptance to use innovative technologies are a prerequisite for successful technology implementation. Approaches for implementing technology into the care environment require careful consideration of appropriateness. Factors to consider include the caregivers' environments, technology ease of use, and staff satisfaction.

BLENDING EDUCATION, LEADERSHIP, AND TECHNOLOGY

Developing, implementing, and maintaining innovative technologies requires a significant financial commitment from the organization. Ensuring widespread and appropriate use of the technology is critical to achieving highly reliable results and to realizing the return on investment in the technology. Achieving this level of reliability requires both leadership engagement and targeted education addressing technology utilization.

The blending of education, leadership, and technology (BELT) approach merges education models and technology acceptance models to drive meaningful adoption and utilization of innovative technology in the clinical environment (Aldrich, 2009). BELT is another application of the culture-process-technology framework. Attention to all three elements is essential for success.

Leadership sets the culture of the organization, the willingness of staff to embrace or change, and technology. Leadership engagement in defining and communicating goals, monitoring progress toward goals, and driving staff utilization of the technology is essential for achieving and maintaining consistent processes, use of the technology, and highly reliable outcomes.

Equally important is the process used to introduce the technology to the staff. The building blocks of an effective education process are an emphasis on the reason for change, training on the use of the technology within the clinical workflow, support during the learning process, and ongoing feedback on performance.

Finally, the characteristics of the technology itself are critical to adoption. Characteristics such as ease of use, integration with other systems, and similarity to other systems greatly affect user adoption. Blending education and leadership strategies supports consistent implementation and ongoing utilization of technology that are necessary to achieve highly reliable processes and outcomes.

Achieving meaningful adoption and utilization of the VitalsNow solution included strategies directed at leadership engagement and staff education. Leaders established the goals related to improved efficiency of data availability, transcription error elimination, patient outcome improvement, and technology utilization rates. A key component of the VitalsNow project was developing a management tool that enabled leaders to have daily review of progress toward these goals. Education for VitalsNow included establishing the need for change, potential advantages of the technology, and the ease of use of the solution. Need for change and potential advantages of the technology included the following:

- Improve overall patient-centered care and safety.
- Provide seamless work environment.

- Reduce redundancy and improve accuracy of documentation.

- Improve timeliness of care team communication.

With regard to ease of use, the following occurred:

- Ease of use was demonstrated in a simulated environment.

- Staff was asked to participate in a "See One, Do One, Teach One" exercise.

The adoption of technology is often viewed as an easy way to change clinical processes and introduce high reliability principles. However, effective understanding and application of technology adoption are essential to achieving the best possible outcomes, realizing the return on the investment, and achieving high reliability.

CAUTIONARY NOTES

Technology and standardization are highly effective tools in improving reliability of care processes, but they can also introduce new vulnerabilities into a system. Integrating technology into clinical care processes requires a systematic approach that addresses culture and process in relation to the technology and actively looks for intended and unintended consequences with each perturbation of the system.

The early years of safety technology were punctuated with specific solutions targeting specific problems. Barcode medication administration (BCMA) technologies, for example, sought to solve the problem of errors in medication administration. As more of the clinical workflow becomes digital, new strategies are emerging to coalesce clinical data to create closed-loop processes, generate insights into care, and create decision support. These new technology solutions require healthcare organizations to take a systematic approach to innovation to realize the full benefit of each incremental advance.

One systematic approach is the life cycle of innovation (Chassin and Loeb, 2013). This life cycle is as follows:

- **Why:** Identify the gap for which a solution could contribute to an improved care environment.

- **What:** Define the discrete elements from a system's thoughtflow and workflow perspective.

- **How:** Implement slowly, examining each use case before spreading.

- **Optimize:** Plan for refinement of the technology and process after clinicians have gained experience, impact metrics are collected, and patient outcomes are evidenced.

■ **Iterate:** Repeat this cycle with each technology in the care environment on a regular basis and whenever a new technology is added.

This type of cycle is essential to becoming a learning health system in which information from care processes is harvested. This information is then aggregated and analyzed to derive learning. This learning drives organizations to create or search out innovative solutions. When implemented into care processes, these innovative solutions generate additional information, and the cycle continues (Platt, Huang, and Perlin, 2013).

In this cycle, innovators need to remain open to the idea that a solution in its end form may not be what was intended and accept its failure as a point from which to launch another attempt to innovate. Therefore, if the solution is found to have not provided the outcomes intended, proper leadership should be practical to recognize and re-identify where the system falls short.

SUMMARY

The ISMP hierarchy of reliability (ISMP, 1999) provides a valuable framework for reducing variation and improving consistency of outcomes. The framework can be used both retrospectively to understand why high reliability has not been achieved and prospectively in designing new initiatives to improve reliability. The rate of technology innovation in healthcare will continue to accelerate as new technologies are created or adapted for the healthcare environment. Successful integration of these technologies requires a systematic approach, grounded in a commitment to patient safety, to achieve highly reliable performance.

KEY POINTS

■ Highly reliable operational processes are necessary to drive consistent healthcare results.

■ Technology, automation, and forcing functions are the most effective approaches to hard-wiring, or making a process highly reliable, within care environments.

■ Technology can support both standardization and individualization within processes of care when thoughtfully configured to support the best or ideal workflow.

■ Standardization reduces variability in care processes and the environment of things but must be balanced with flexibility to meet individual patient circumstances.

■ Standardization is linked to culture, process, and technology. All must be considered as equal contributors to success metrics.

■ Integrating innovative technology into the clinical environment requires a systematic approach and a platform of standardization to achieve high reliability and address gaps in clinical care environments.

■ Realizing a clinical return on investment requires blending education and leadership strategies to support consistent implementation and ongoing utilization of technology to achieve highly reliable processes and outcomes.

REFERENCES

Aldrich, K. (2009, unpublished). Putting technology into practice: An informatics educational model. Submitted in partial fulfillment of requirements for DNP, University of South Florida, Tampa.

Chassin, M. R., and Loeb, J. M. (2013). High-reliability health care: Getting there from here. The Joint Commission. Retrieved from http://www.jointcommission.org/assets/1/6/Chassin_and_Loeb_0913_final.pdf

Connors, R., and Smith, T. (2011). *Change the culture, change the game: The breakthrough strategy for energizing your organization and creating accountability for results.* New York, NY: Portfolio.

Institute for Safe Medication Practices (ISMP). (1999). Medication error prevention toolbox. Retrieved from http://www.ismp.org/newsletters/acutecare/articles/19990602.asp

The Joint Commission. (2013). CLABSI toolkit and monograph. Retrieved from http://www.jointcommission.org/topics/clabsi_toolkit.aspx

Leonard, M. S., Frankel, A., Simmonds, T., and Vega, K. B. (2004). *Achieving safe and reliable healthcare: Strategies and solutions.* Chicago, IL: Health Administration Press.

Leotsakos, A., Zheng, H., Croteau, R., Loeb, J. M., Sherman, H., Hoffman, C., … Munier, B. (2014). Standardization in patient safety: The WHO High 5s project. *International Journal for Quality in Health Care, 26*(2), pp. 109–116.

Perry, A., Shah, M., and Englebright, J. (2007). Improving safety with barcode-enabled medication administration. *Patient Safety and Quality Healthcare* (May/June), pp. 26–30.

Platt, R., Huang, S. S., and Perlin, J. (2013). A win for the learning health system. Retrieved from https://www.nihcollaboratory.org/Products/Platt_%20Win%20for%20Learning%20Health%20System_Commentary_IOM.pdf

PART 5

HRO CONCEPTS AND APPLICATION TO PRACTICE: DEFERENCE TO EXPERTISE

CHAPTER 11

INTERPROFESSIONAL COLLABORATION

Amy J. Barton, PhD, RN, FAAN

Gail E. Armstrong, DNP, ACNS-BC, CNE

Connie Valdez, PharmD, MSEd, BCPS

Increased focus on quality, safety, and efficiency in healthcare has placed greater attention on understanding the complexity of healthcare teams. The purpose of this chapter is to describe and explain interprofessional collaboration and teamwork in the context of high reliability organizations (HROs).

THE CURRENT NEED FOR INTERPROFESSIONAL COLLABORATIVE CARE AND TEAMWORK

Since the publication of "Crossing the Quality Chasm," in 2001, the Institute of Medicine (IOM) has inspired changes to healthcare delivery. Collaboration among healthcare professionals is encouraged to provide effective and efficient patient care. Increasing reliability in healthcare outcomes is connected to improving teamwork performance and interprofessional collaboration. Studies have shown positive outcomes such as increased patient satisfaction, reduced clinical error rates, improvement in rates of diabetes testing, and improved mental health practitioner competency using

> Coming together is a beginning. Keeping together is progress. Working together is success.
>
> —Henry Ford

an interprofessional approach compared with the traditional independent practitioner approach (Barr, 2002; Carlisle, Cooper, and Watkins, 2004; Cook, Gerrish, and Clarke, 2001; Reeves, Perrier, Goldman, Freeth, and Zwarenstein, 2013; Shunk, Dulay, Chou, Janson, and O'Brien, 2014). Additional benefits may include increased practitioner satisfaction and better adherence to standards of care when working in a team-oriented environment (Cox and Naylor, 2013).

When practitioners witness an increase in positive outcomes, it is likely they will feel a sense of satisfaction and pride. This is not surprising. It is a reflection of the accomplishments of the team, of which each individual is an active member. Furthermore, it is likely the practitioner will have a personal investment in further developing and/or expanding services and programs to ensure continual optimal patient care.

THE MANDATE FOR INTERPROFESSIONAL COLLABORATION IN HEALTHCARE

After publication of the IOM quality chasm series, a subsequent publication made this recommendation for health professions education: "All health professionals should be educated to deliver patient-centered care as members of an interdisciplinary team, emphasizing evidence-based practice, quality improvement approaches and informatics" (Greiner and Knebel, 2003, p. 45). Two subsequent international reports highlighted the evidence concerning the effects of team-based care to achieve quality patient outcomes.

The first report was from the World Health Organization (WHO) (2010). It described a model that identified a continuum in which interprofessional education can serve as an impetus to transform a fragmented health system into one strengthened by a collaborative, practice-ready workforce. "Interprofessional education occurs when students from two or more professions learn about, from and with each other to enable effective collaboration and improve health outcomes" (p. 10). When educational and clinical care systems align to facilitate collaborative practice, a system of optimal health services can lead to improved health outcomes. In health agencies, the following actions are recommended:

- Develop processes that promote shared decision-making, regular communication, and community involvement.

- Design a built environment that promotes, fosters, and extends interprofessional collaborative practice, both within and across service agencies.

- Develop personnel policies that recognize and support collaborative practice and offer fair and equitable remuneration models.

- Develop a delivery model that allows adequate time and space for staff to focus on interprofessional collaboration and delivery of care.

■ Develop governance models that establish teamwork and shared responsibility for health-care service delivery between team members as the normative practice (p. 30).

A second report, in the *Lancet*, provided this vision: "All health professionals in all countries are educated to mobilize knowledge, and to engage in critical reasoning and ethical conduct, so that they are competent to participate in patient-centered and population-centered health systems as members of locally responsive and globally connected teams" (Frenk et al., 2010, p. 1951). Clearly, both reports highlight the need to shift from a discipline-specific to a person-centered approach to improve the care delivery process as well as patient outcomes.

A 2015 white paper from the Robert Wood Johnson Foundation (RWJF), "Lessons from the Field: Promising Interprofessional Collaboration Practices," also emphasized the urgent mandate for effective interprofessional teamwork in healthcare to improve patient outcomes. This white paper explored, explained, and disseminated some of the most useful practices for effective interprofessional collaboration. The six takeaways from RWJF's review of systems that are effectively growing interprofessional team capacity echo many of the core elements of HROs. They are as follows:

■ Put patients first.

■ Demonstrate leadership commitment to interprofessional collaboration as an organizational priority through words and actions.

■ Create a level playing field that enables team members to work at the top of their license, know their roles, and understand the value they contribute.

■ Cultivate effective team communication.

■ Explore the use of organized structure to hard-wire interprofessional practice.

■ Train different disciplines together so they learn how to work together.

COMPETENCIES FOR TEAMWORK AND COLLABORATION

Increasing the reliability of teams means including teamwork and collaboration education for all health profession students. Experts state that there is a need for interprofessional education to be introduced early within the specific program, before individuals have had time to develop their own personal identity or negative attitudes toward other health professions (Carlisle, Cooper, and Watkins, 2004). Studies have highlighted the importance of uniting professions early in the educational process to increase awareness of roles and decrease the risk for problems concerning professional boundaries and tension in the future (Barr, 2002). Educating future professionals with a focus on interprofessional collaboration and team orientation has become the focus of academic health centers across the United States.

QUALITY AND SAFETY EDUCATION FOR NURSES

One of the first efforts to define competencies for teamwork among health professionals occurred as part of the Quality and Safety Education for Nurses (QSEN) initiative. For the QSEN initiative, leaders used the IOM recommendations to develop specific competencies as well as knowledge, skill, and attitude attributes for each of the recommended domains. The competency for teamwork and collaboration is "Function effectively within nursing and inter-professional teams, fostering open communication, mutual respect, and shared decision-making to achieve quality patient care" (Cronenwett et al., 2007, p. 125). Table 11.1 lists salient knowledge, skills, and attitudes (KSAs) that shape the operational elements of this competency.

TABLE 11.1 KNOWLEDGE, SKILLS, AND ATTITUDES THAT OPERATIONALIZE TEAMWORK AND COLLABORATION IN QSEN

Domain	Attributes
Knowledge	Describe strategies for identifying and managing overlaps in team member roles and accountabilities.
	Describe impact of own communication style on others.
	Examine strategies for improving systems to support team functioning.
Skills	Clarify roles and accountabilities under conditions of potential overlap in team member functioning.
	Integrate the contributions of others who play a role in helping the patient and family achieve health goals.
	Choose communication styles that diminish the risks associated with authority gradients among team members.
Attitudes	Value different styles of communication used by patients, families, and healthcare providers.
	Contribute to resolution of conflict and disagreement.
	Appreciate the risks associated with handoffs among providers and across transitions in care.

 An inclusive list of KSAs for all six QSEN competencies is available at the QSEN website (http://qsen.org).

INTERPROFESSIONAL EDUCATION COLLABORATIVE (IPEC)

More recently, a consortium of health profession educational organizations collaborated to create competencies for interprofessional education. They identified the importance of teamwork in "cooperating in the patient-centered delivery of care; coordinating one's care with other health professionals so that gaps, redundancies, and errors are avoided; and collaborating with others through shared problem-solving and shared decision making, especially in circumstances of uncertainty" (IPEC, 2011, p. 30). The general competency statement for teams and teamwork is to "apply relationship-building values and the principles of team dynamics to perform effectively in different team roles to plan and deliver patient-/population-centered care that is safe, timely, efficient, effective, and equitable" (p. 31).

CHARACTERISTICS OF EFFECTIVE TEAMS

Clear identification of five common characteristics of effective HROs has benefited the emerging understanding of successful teams. Baker, Day, and Salas (2006) identified effective teamwork as a core component of successful HROs and named the following characteristics necessary for effective teams:

- Team leadership
- Backup behavior
- Mutual performance monitoring
- Communication adaptability
- Shared mental models
- Mutual trust
- Team orientation

TEAM LEADERSHIP

Reliability is challenging for many teams. It is even more difficult when teams operate in complex, dynamic work environments, such as healthcare. Effective leadership on healthcare teams is vital to help teams navigate the dynamic fluidity of the complex work environment. Team leadership "denotes the ability to coordinate team members' activities, ensure that tasks are distributed appropriately, evaluate performance, provide feedback, enhance the team's ability to perform, and inspire the drive for high-level performance" (Leasure et al., 2013, p. 586).

Characteristics of effective team leadership include the following:

- Established culture where members feel the leader cares about them
- Clear, common purpose
- Clear but flexible role definitions
- Appropriate members involved in decision-making
- Effective meetings
- Work assigned and distributed thoughtfully
- Team goals and plans established and revised (Baker et al., 2006)

Effective leadership shares responsibilities, facilitates collaboration, and effectively addresses the work at hand. Consistently clarifying the goals of the group and reminding members that each profession brings a different area of expertise to patient care strengthens the team's sense of priorities and can aid in the development of situation monitoring.

MUTUAL SUPPORT

Mutual support is sometimes called *backup behavior* because it allows teams members to know that their colleagues offer support and assistance when needed. An important part of mutual support is task assistance. Task assistance is a discrete skill that includes both asking for assistance when needed and offering assistance when an opportunity arises. Task assistance is guided by situational monitoring because situation awareness enables team members to effectively identify when they or other team members need support (Agency for Healthcare Research and Quality [AHRQ], 2014a). The following clinical example illustrates how mutual support can enhance patient outcomes.

CLINICAL EXAMPLE

A patient presented to clinic with uncontrolled diabetes. The patient's high blood sugar values and high hemoglobin A1C values were attributed to the patient not taking the necessary medication for her diabetes because of financial constraints. Upon further investigation by the social work intern, it was found that there was an important contributing cause to the patient's situation that had initially been missed. Not only was her diabetes not controlled, but the patient was suffering from severe depression, even stating that she would rather die than take her medications. The patient was not engaging in treating her diabetes as a result of her depression. A clinical situation such as this demonstrates that there may be underlying issues, such as depression, which may affect a patient's ability to be engaged with her chronic illness, which a social worker can best uncover.

TEAM AWARENESS

Reliability on teams results from effective and ongoing team training. One widely used initiative for effective team training to improve team reliability in healthcare is Team Strategies and Tools to Enhance Performance and Patient Safety (TeamSTEPPS). TeamSTEPPS is an evidence-based initiative developed by the Department of Defense with the Agency for Healthcare Research and Quality (AHRQ). It was designed to improve quality and safety in healthcare and is based on strategies found to be effective from research in high-stress, high-risk industries, such as military aviation. The tools and strategies from TeamSTEPPS are available online at http://teamstepps.ahrq.gov and can be customized for various care settings.

The TeamSTEPPS model features a trifecta model of team awareness. This trifecta is composed of the following:

- Situation monitoring

- Situation awareness

- A shared mental model

Situation Monitoring

Situation monitoring is an individual skill that involves four areas of constant scanning for all team members:

- **The status of the patient:** Team members are taught to continuously check the status of the patient (for example, the patient history, vital signs, medications, physical exam, plan of care, and psychosocial condition).

- **The status of other team members:** Awareness of other team members focuses on fatigue level, workload, task performance, skill level, and stress level.

- **The environment:** Monitoring of the care environment teaches team members to be aware of new information regarding triage acuity or equipment status.

- **Team progress toward the goal:** Awareness of the team's progress toward specific goals promotes focus on the status of the team's patients, goals of the team, tasks/actions completed or that need to be completed, and continued appropriateness of the plan. When team members incorporate team monitoring into their daily work, situational awareness results for all team members.

With effective situation monitoring continuously running in the background of all team members, there is an individual awareness of the larger context of care. Shifting information and fluctuating conditions can be more effectively managed. Situation monitoring can be foundational for effective support of fellow team members. Situation monitoring is an individual skill that enables all team members to be responsive to shifting information.

Situation Awareness

Successful mastery of the individual skill of situation monitoring leads to the individual outcome of situation awareness. Situation awareness is a concept developed in the aviation industry that reflects a pilot's simultaneous awareness of the immediate dynamic elements of a situation in the context of the larger aviation system model, with special ability to anticipate what might occur next (Adams, Tenney, and Pew, 1995). Within healthcare, situational awareness means the following:

- Knowing the current conditions affecting the team's work
- Knowing the status of a particular event
- Knowing the status of the team's members
- Understanding the operational issues affecting the team
- Maintaining mindfulness

Situation awareness teaches team members to be concurrently aware of their own work and the larger picture of what is occurring during the work of a team. Without situational awareness, team members easily blame colleagues for gaps in the system or ineffective work processes, as shown in the following clinical example.

CLINICAL EXAMPLE

A patient calls the clinic requesting results of his labs and leaves a message for the nurse. The nurse notices some of the lab values are out of normal limits, so she writes down the patient's results and leaves a message on the provider's desk. The medical assistant then places a small stack of non-urgent documents on top of the written message without realizing he is covering up the lab results and written message. Three days later, the patient calls back upset, as no one has returned his original call. The nurse states that she provided the message to the provider and knows that the provider received it, thus placing blame on the provider for not calling the patient back. The nurse then addresses the situation with the provider. The provider finds the message under a stack of papers and becomes upset. She feels the situation was the fault of the medical assistant, who placed non-urgent documents on top of the message. The provider also blames the nurse for not verbally telling her that she needed to review labs and call back the patient. Such widespread blame undermines trust and harms the development of team cohesion.

Shared Mental Model

System gaps are effectively addressed when a highly functioning team has a shared mental model. TeamSTEPPS identifies a shared mental model as a team outcome and as "the perception of, understanding of, or knowledge about a situation or process that is shared among team members through communication" (AHRQ, 2014b). Having a common understanding of priorities, plans, drivers, potential barriers, and team tools contributes to team effectiveness and team success. A shared mental model is reinforced and modified through continuous team communication. Continuous team communication strategies can be adjusted for a variety of healthcare team contexts.

The team outcome of effective situation monitoring and situation awareness is a shared mental model. See Figure 11.1 for the interconnection between these concepts in TeamSTEPPS.

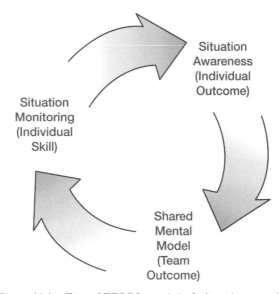

Figure 11.1   TeamSTEPPS model of situation monitoring.

Adapted from TeamSTEPPS 2.0 with permission from the Agency for Healthcare Research and Quality (AHRQ, 2014b).

TRUST ON TEAMS

A vital and complex dynamic in effective, reliable team function is trust among team members. Ring and van de Ven (p. 488, 1992) define trust as "confidence in another's goodwill," which emphasizes the role of cooperation and reliability on one's team members. Trust is difficult to measure but is often identified by the nature of one's behavior toward others. Adler (2001) describes three bases of trust:

- A calculated trust from an assessment of costs and benefits

- Trust from experience with continuing interaction

- Trust based on shared values and norms

A common model used to teach effective teamwork for health professions students is the Tuckman Model of Team Functioning. Tuckman and Jensen's (1977) stages of team development reflect the growth of trust among team members.

1. **Forming stage:** In this stage, team members get to know each other and their tasks and roles, and conflicts begin to arise.

2. **Storming stage:** Relationships are negotiated to fit the needs of the patients, the team, and the healthcare environment.

3. **Norming stage:** Team members get to know and trust each other, settle into patterns of interaction, and begin to resolve earlier differences.

4. **Performing stage:** Team members now have good working relationships and a positive sense of group identity.

5. **Adjourning stage:** Team members labor to conclude the work of the group on a positive note. This stage is the formal conclusion to a group's process.

A climate of trust and safety allows for innovation and creativity, which contribute to a team's growth and continued productivity. This trust also allows team members to voice disagreements and manage conflict in ways that strengthen rather than undermine the team (Jones and Jones, 2011).

Unfortunately, healthcare teams usually do not have the luxury of time and repeated exposure to progress through Tuckman's stages, yet they must develop trust among team members. Many teams in healthcare have consistently changing membership, physical separation between team members, and multiple concurrent demands on members' energy and time. Teams may form and disband on an as-needed basis, working together for only one shift or even one patient, such as a surgical case or a critical resuscitation. These teams often face especially complex tasks, with high-risk and high-stakes outcomes. They must perform at a high level, despite their lack of prior experience with one another.

Meyerson, Kramer, and Weick (1996) contend that teams under these circumstances must develop "swift" trust to function safely. Healthcare team members often have little data to support person-based interactions; they must rely instead on role-based interactions. These interactions reinforce the roles, which allows for less uncertainty and more facile development of trust. This trust is further developed by having a salient, high-stakes purpose, such as occurs in many healthcare settings. Consider the following example.

CLINICAL EXAMPLE

A patient with hyperglycemia presented to the clinic with a blood glucose of 473. It was determined that the patient had run out of insulin 8 days before her clinic visit, and her blood sugars had been running very high for the past week. The nurse practitioner (NP) did not feel comfortable treating the patient's hyperglycemia in the clinic, as she was afraid the patient might become hypoglycemic and be unable to drive home safely. The NP suggested that the patient pick up her insulin and inject her dose at home but did not fully explain the clinical rationale behind this suggestion. To the patient, it appeared as though the team disregarded her concern because the NP did not wish to treat the patient in the clinic. In reality, because of incomplete communication, the team never understood the NP's concern of the patient becoming hypoglycemic while driving and thought the NP was suggesting that the patient did not deserve to be treated in the clinic because of her recent noncompliance with her insulin.

Ultimately, the group decided to treat the patient with rapid-acting insulin in the clinic setting. When that happened, the NP was upset because she believed her clinical concerns were being ignored. Feeling offended, the NP did not try to readdress her concerns because she felt as though she had no choice than to comply with the team. The patient was treated with rapid-acting insulin in the clinic and in fact did end up becoming hypoglycemic while driving home. As a result, she got into an accident. The NP, who did not want to treat the hyperglycemia in clinic, was very upset about the outcome. She felt it was unfair to be asked to accept share of the blame because she did not agree with the original plan. The silent NP was loath to participate fully in future team decisions because of her fear that her voice would not be heard in the case of a similar situation. Clearly, an interruption in collegial trust can impact future ability of a team to effectively collaborate.

The most effective models of reliable care and reliable teams in healthcare include the patient and family. Therefore, the patient and family team members must also develop swift trust. Because patients and families have traditionally been excluded from the care team, they may not expect or even realize that they have a role on the team. As discussed, swift trust is often initially based on role interactions. Clinical care providers can facilitate swift trust by explicitly designating patients and family as team members and by identifying the role expectations for all members of the team. For example, a family member's role might be to report any slight changes he or she notices in a patient's clinical condition that might be overlooked by clinical staff. A patient's role might include taking responsibility for an outpatient medication regimen and reporting any symptoms that might be adverse side effects of a medication.

Similarly, clinical care providers must trust the patient and family members to maximize their contributions to the team. Again, clarifying role expectations up front is a key to developing swift trust. Issues that might obscure trust, such as HIPAA concerns, or perceived conflicts of interest among family members must be addressed directly with the entire team as early as possible.

TEAM ORIENTATION

Team orientation provides the foundation of an interprofessional approach where members work together on projects and prefer not to work as individuals. Effective teams:

- Select new members who value teamwork
- Have a strong belief in the ability of the collective team to succeed (Baker et al., 2006)

Unfortunately, despite the clear benefits, multiple barriers may exist that hinder the growth of an efficient interprofessional, team-oriented environment. The first is a misunderstanding or lack of education about other professionals who provide healthcare to patients. A disconnect may exist in understanding the roles and responsibilities of each clinician, leading to an inefficient use of his or her knowledge and skills.

Reliability is based on all team members valuing cooperation and collaboration and sharing a commitment to grow in these skill sets. However, an overly introverted personality with a mindset of constantly "working alone" can have a strong negative impact on such a team. To foster an efficient team-oriented environment, each member must make an effort and work together toward the collective goal of improving patient care. Allowing individuals with varying areas of expertise to see the patient allows for a more comprehensive workup of each patient, making it possible to address problems from social to behavioral to physical. It is also common to fix one problem, only to have it affect another—even when they are seemingly unrelated. Consider the following clinical example.

CLINICAL EXAMPLE

A new physician assistant (PA) who is not team-oriented is hired to work at a busy primary care clinic that serves Native Americans. The new PA not only prefers to work independently but is also concerned about his liability, so his behavior suggests that he values having complete control over his patients. He does not request consults from other team members, which suggests that he does not want input from them and does not value their clinical expertise. This new PA's omission could be construed as arrogance. Furthermore, his office is located away from the other team members, which further contributes to his isolation and limits impromptu communication.

The perceived lack of team orientation from this PA ripples across the clinic, disrupting the operational flow, resulting in uncoordinated patient care. Historically, this clinic was one of the top-performing Native American health clinics, managing patients with diabetes. However, with the addition of this new PA, coordination among providers is lost. Because of his isolation, the PA does not refer his patients to the diabetes group visit program and does not use the independent diabetes patient visit workup by clinical pharmacy, where the patient's drug therapy is evaluated for appropriateness based on current guidelines and patient-specific factors. Without team involvement, the patients of this PA are not screened for immunizations, do not receive an annual foot exam, do not receive a dilated eye exam, are not screened for depression, do not receive biannual dental exams, and do not receive annual bloodwork and labs (for example, TSH, CMP, CBC, and urine albumin). The patients of this PA are missing the input of other clinical team members who can assist with protocol-based patient management or the prescribing/renewing of medications. Furthermore, this PA does not ask for recommendations or consults by other practitioners. Although the PA is maintaining his perceived control of the care of his patients, the quality of the actual care received by his patients is significantly diminished.

Finally, the environment may also become a literal barrier. While open communication is key to an efficiently functioning team orientation, burdensome layouts may hinder access to communication. A study performed in the United Kingdom found that information transaction was enhanced by geographical proximity of team members (Cook et al., 2001). Additional effort is required on behalf of team members if all members work in separate offices with closed doors as opposed to an open area for individuals to consult with each other when necessary.

GROUP DECISION-MAKING AND PROBLEM-SOLVING

The requirement for efficient group decision-making lies in the communication among the members of the group. As patients become more engaged with the care process, they participate in shared decision-making. Légaré and colleagues (2011) conceptualized the shared decision-making process as involving six stages:

1. Sharing knowledge

2. Information exchange

3. Values clarification

4. Feasibility

5. Actual decision

6. Ongoing support

A challenge of shared decision-making is that one group member may dominate the communication among the team. This seeming authority affects the processes and outcomes of group decision-making and ultimately may lead to a group decision that is more extreme than desired

(Cook et al., 2001). Often, members may disagree with the group's decision but fail to speak up due to fear of rejection or deterioration of relationships among group members. This reluctance can lead to a phenomenon referred to as *pluralistic ignorance* in which the fear of disrupting the unity of the group's decision causes the member to avoid speaking up, only to discover later that other members of the group had similar thoughts as well (Rosenstein and O'Daniel, 2005).

Because the efficacy of group decision-making is directly affected by the strength of the communication in the group, fostering an open and safe environment for discussion is optimal. When brainstorming ideas, it is ideal to be clear how "one is questioning the ideas rather than attacking the source of them" to maintain a "congenial climate" for all the group members to adequately provide their opinions and thoughts (Institute for Safe Medication Practices, 2004). This approach provides the group with a safe environment in which members do not have to be concerned with an increased tension with their peers.

The major benefit of working as an interprofessional team in healthcare is achieving a common goal: "a recognition by the professions that they have an inescapable responsibility to work together to improve the health and well-being of individuals, families and communities" (Barr, 2002, p. 188). Simply expressed, all team members work toward the collective goal of optimizing patient care.

SHARING RESPONSIBILITY

When an interprofessional environment is created where effective, reliable teamwork is the basis of practice, work tends to be rewarding and fun. Practitioners and staff enjoy working with each other and respect one another, which can improve morale, patient care, and clinical outcomes. However, teamwork is based on the relationships of the practitioners and staff, and like any relationship, these relationships may break down if all team members do not take accountability for their actions and share responsibility.

It is important to distinguish accountability from responsibility. Accountability can be assigned to individual team members. It involves an agreement to complete a task and produce results. Responsibility, however, is a personal feeling of ownership that is generated by the individual. Responsibility means the individual owns the results of the situation. Shared responsibility is an extension of this concept, where team members feel ownership as a unit and share the results of all team actions, beneficial and deleterious. Unfortunately, shared responsibility on teams is rare in the clinical setting. Rather than sharing responsibility, shifting blame at individual team members is usually the norm. Not only does this ineffective strategy impede patient care, but it deteriorates morale of a team. The lack of communication, teamwork, and respect is a common occurrence throughout today's healthcare system.

A vital step in developing high-functioning teams is making an accurate assessment of a team's strengths and weaknesses. Table 11.2 provides a comprehensive resource for evidence-based tools that support teams in assessing the current state to best identify short-term goals for improving team function.

TABLE 11.2 TOOLS FOR INTERPROFESSIONAL HEALTHCARE TEAMS

Team Characteristic/Assessment Questions	Tool and Description	Link to Tool
Leadership		
Does your organization have recurring data to support the need for improving specific areas (for example, adverse event and near-miss reports, root cause analyses or failure modes and effects analyses, administering the AHRQ Patient Safety Culture Survey, surveys of patient or staff satisfaction, unit- or site-specific process and outcome measures, and so on)? Will building a stronger safety culture specific to teamwork address your institution's needs?	**TeamSTEPPS Teamwork Perceptions Questionnaire (T-TPQ) and Teamwork Attitudes Questionnaire (T-TAQ)** T-TPQ assesses health professionals' perceptions of interprofessional teamwork within an organization and group-level team skills and behavior. T-TAQ measures how individuals approach team-related issues and assesses the impact of interprofessional education on health professionals' attitudes, knowledge, and team skills.	https://nexusipe.org/resource-exchange/teamstepps%C2%AE-teamwork-perceptions-questionnaire-t-tpq-and-teamwork-attitudes#sthash.pY0MIwsS.dpuf
When a mistake occurs, does your organization use the resulting data as an opportunity for learning (for example, discussing the process that contributed to the errors and how the error could have been prevented)? When transferring patient care to another colleague (for example, giving report), is time spent discussing patient-specific considerations (for example, atypical signs and symptoms that the patient has presented with and to watch out for, identifying situations that have exacerbated the patient's condition, and so on)? When a unique critical situation occurs, does your organization defer to expertise and take advantage of the unique skills and collective expertise to resolve it?	**Safety Organizing Scale (SOS)** This tool enhances the understanding of behaviors that contribute to an effective safety culture.	https://nexusipe.org/resource-exchange/safety-organizing-scale#sthash.MOTOYPoV.dpuf

continues

TABLE 11.2   TOOLS FOR INTERPROFESSIONAL HEALTHCARE TEAMS   (CONTINUED)

Team Characteristic/Assessment Questions	Tool and Description	Link to Tool
Leadership		
Is recurring tension among clinicians and staff a common barrier to effective teamwork? Are decisions made "from the top," with little input from those working with patients? Do your teams defer to expertise, despite hierarchy? Does the practice setting seem stressful or chaotic?	**Survey of Organizational Attributes of Primary Care (SOAPC)** This tool assesses healthcare professionals' perceptions of the organizational resources for change required in primary care settings and measures organizational attributes of practice teams as providers of quality of care.	https://nexusipe.org/resource-exchange/soapc-survey-organizational-attributes-primary-care#sthash.NvHza6OQ.dpuf
Mutual Performance Monitoring		
Are team members familiar with each other's role? At your primary care practice site, are you considered to be an integrated team member who helps provide medication-related services? If yes, how frequently do you take the "lead role," "shared lead role," "supportive role," "minor role," and "no role" when performing medication-related processes in primary care (for example, selecting drug regimen, monitoring for safety and effectiveness, documenting medication-related information in the chart, teaching medical students and residents about drug therapy, identifying errors, and so on)?	**Medication Use Processes Matrix (MUPM)** This tool measures how primary healthcare professionals' perceive their own and others' contributions to medication-related processes.	https://nexusipe.org/resource-exchange/mupm-medication-use-processes-matrix-#sthash.Cqe8wG7R.dpuf

Do team members have a good understanding of patient care treatment goals and plans?

Do team members respect others' roles and expertise?

Does your leadership clearly define roles and responsibilities of team members?

Do your providers usually ask other team members for opinions about patient care?

Do your team members share responsibility and accountability for team decisions and outcomes?

When meeting with your team, do processes encourage an open, comfortable, safe place to discuss concerns?

Does your team share community resource information?

Collaborative Practice Assessment Tool (CPAT)

This tool assesses levels of collaboration intended to assist clinical teams in identifying strengths and weaknesses in their collaborative practice, thereby providing opportunities for focused educational interventions.

https://nexusipe.org/resource-exchange/cpat-collaborative-practice-assessment-tool#sthash.jyaEqsu1.dpuf

Do you feel there are often disruptions in giving or receiving information?

Does your organization expect team members to develop conflict-resolution skills on their own?

Do delays, errors, and redundancies result in reducing the quality, safety, and efficiency of patient care?

Relational Coordination Scale (RCS)

This tool measures the quality of teamwork between unbounded teams and the quality of interprofessional interaction by looking at four areas of communication (frequency, timeliness, accuracy, and problem-solving) and three areas of relationships (shared goals, shared knowledge, and mutual respect).

https://nexusipe.org/resource-exchange/relational-coordination-scale-rcs#sthash.6txq8YeG.dpuf

continues

TABLE 11.2   TOOLS FOR INTERPROFESSIONAL HEALTHCARE TEAMS   (CONTINUED)

Team Characteristic/Assessment Questions	Tool and Description	Link to Tool
Backup Behavior		
Are surgical time-outs used regularly and correctly? Before surgery, is your team asked if all team members are prepared to begin the operation? Does the surgeon enhance timing of instrument exchange by giving prior notification to the scrub nurse? Are instructions and explanations provided to assistants? Do team members monitor various aspects of the operation (for example, patient condition, table positioning, position of team members, and so on)?	**Observational Teamwork Assessment for Surgery (OTAS)** This tool measures the quality of teamwork and interactions in the operating room.	https://nexusipe.org/resource-exchange/otas-observational-teamwork-assessment-surgery#sthash.PjndwgXq.dpuf
Do you feel that your professional colleagues often lack openness and have little appreciation of interprofessional groups? Does frustration among individuals within interprofessional groups occur often? Is it difficult to get interprofessional groups to work well because different professionals have different priorities?	**Perception of Interprofessional Collaboration Model Questionnaire (PINCOM-Q)** This tool measures perceptions and behavior between professionals in the interprofessional collaboration process on an individual, group, and organizational level.	https://nexusipe.org/resource-exchange/pincom-q-perception-interprofessional-collaboration-model-questionnaire#sthash.85Ta-CI3S.dpuf
Does the team decision process help you consistently make efficacious recommendations for all patients? Does the team decision process help you become more competent? Does the team decision process help you effectively solve problems?	**Team Decision Making Questionnaire (TDMQ)** This tool assesses the quality of interprofessional teams and helps to evaluate clinical staff's perceptions of decision-making.	https://nexusipe.org/resource-exchange/tdmq-team-decision-making-questionnaire#sthash.6qUx-u8QG.dpuf

Team Orientation

Are your team members informed of events that happened on other shifts? Does your leader explain standards of excellence to you and other team members? Do your team members effectively address conflict when disagreement occurs? Do you look forward to working each day with your team? When taking care of patients, does your team have safe, quality outcomes?	**Interdisciplinary Team Performance Scale (ITPS)** This tool assesses interdisciplinary team performance in long-term care settings and to measure performance in the Program of All-Inclusive Care for the Elderly (PACE).	https://nexusipe.org/resource-exchange/itps-interdisciplinary-team-performance-scale#sthash.9spSgjYF.dpuf
When transferring a patient, are all team members' concerns considered regarding the patient's needs? When transferring a patient, is there collaboration among all team members in making this decision? How satisfied are you with the process your team employs for decisions (for example, transferring a patient)?	**Collaboration and Satisfaction About Care (CSACD)** This tool assesses the quality of interactions in making care decisions and satisfaction with the decision-making process in the health setting.	https://nexusipe.org/resource-exchange/csacd-collaboration-and-satisfaction-about-care-decisions#sthash.2JNJJ5sf.dpuf
Are there opportunities for you to consistently give feedback to your colleagues in your practice setting? Do you perceive that teamwork with professionals from other disciplines is important to your ability to care for patients? Do your colleagues from other disciplines defer to you frequently?	**Index for Interdisciplinary Collaboration (IIC)** This tool measures the self-reported level of collaboration among professionals.	https://nexusipe.org/resource-exchange/iic-index-interdisciplinary-collaboration#sthash.9Uv3xGJO.dpuf

continues

TABLE 11.2 TOOLS FOR INTERPROFESSIONAL HEALTHCARE TEAMS (CONTINUED)

Team Characteristic/Assessment Questions	Tool and Description	Link to Tool
Team Orientation		
Do you and your colleagues respect and trust each other? Are all of your team members committed to the goals identified by the team? Does your team encourage and support open communication, including patients in the discussions?	**Assessment of Interprofessional Team Collaboration Scale (AITCS)** This tool measures collaboration within teams and when patients are included as team members.	https://nexusipe.org/resource-exchange/assessment-interprofessional-team-collaboration-scale#sthash.eqqVfOdT.dpuf
Do the healthcare providers and staff on your unit work as a high-functioning team? Do the staff members you work with contribute to important decisions about patient care? Does your unit work well with other departments in the hospital? If you have an idea about how to make things better on your unit, are the managers, providers, and staff willing to implement your idea?	**Healthcare Team Vitality Instrument (HTVI)** This tool assesses team collaboration and patient safety, with a specific emphasis on team vitality.	https://nexusipe.org/resource-exchange/htvi-healthcare-team-vitality-instrument#sthash.QXj5407d.dpuf

TEAM TRAINING

TeamSTEPPS offers specific tools and strategies that can be modified for a variety of healthcare contexts. The communication strategies in TeamSTEPPS emphasize the importance of a shared mental model on teams, so that information can be freely exchanged and understood.

Specific strategies for feedback are offered in the TeamSTEPPS toolkit. Feedback is a discrete skill that contributes to mutual support. Feedback is information provided for the purpose of improving team performance. Teams require outcome data to engage in continuous improvement. Feedback can be given by any team member at any time to foster improvement in the team culture, to meet the team's need for growth, to promote healthy working relationships, and to help the team set goals for ongoing improvement. A shared mental model is reinforced and modified through continuous team communication, known as *closed-loop communication*. See Figure 11.2 for the TeamSTEPPS model of closed-loop communication.

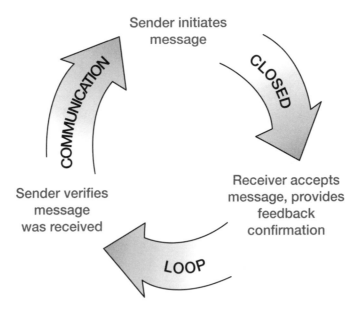

Figure 11.2 TeamSTEPPS closed-loop communication.

Adapted from TeamSTEPPS 2.0 with permission from the Agency for Healthcare Research and Quality (AHRQ, 2014c).

In the support of team shared mental models, TeamSTEPPS teaches teams the utility of abbreviated team check-ins throughout the course of care in the following forms:

- **Briefs:** Briefs are short team communications that occur at the start of the shift and bring everyone up to speed on the plan for the day. In some environments, leadership rounding or interdisciplinary rounding is used as a form of team briefing to be sure all team members are up to date in their information. TeamSTEPPS suggests that briefs cover essential team foci, such as team members and roles (who is on the team and who is the designated leader), clinical status of the team's patients (current condition, diagnosis and status), plan of care for each of the team's patients (what is to be accomplished, what the expected outcomes are, and who is to carry out team tasks) and issues affecting operations (resources normally available that may be restricted).

- **Huddles:** Huddles occur while care is being provided. These are ad-hoc meetings that any team member can call to touch base, regain situational awareness, discuss critical issues, or address emerging events. Team members can also call a huddle in the case of a safety concern.

- **Debriefs:** Debriefs are a way to finish the work of a team, with an emphasis on a shared mental model. TeamSTEPPS offers a debrief checklist that focuses on the recounting of key events, analysis of why an event occurred, what was effective and what did not work, lessons learned and how a team improved a plan, and reinforcement of what went well and how a team can repeat that behavior. Teams that debrief effectively build shared understanding and perform 40% better. They also improve performance through self-critique and problem-solving. Finally, they are more effective in uncovering and identifying problems earlier than other teams (Smith-Jentsch, Cannon-Bowers, Tannenbaum, and Salas, 2008).

TeamSTEPPS training includes a variety of teachable skills to increase team members' awareness of their own roles and functions and those of their team members. Because of the complexity of healthcare teams, which continuously change from shift to shift, from setting to setting, and over time, it is important that team members are aware of the work and roles of other members of the team.

TeamSTEPPS training emphasizes how task assistance contributes to healthy team culture. The risk of errors is increased when people are under stress, in high-risk situations, and feel unable to ask for assistance. Assistance should be actively given and offered whenever there is a concern for patient safety.

Standardization of some communication techniques to operationalize mutual support is one of the notable strengths of TeamSTEPPS training. These standardized communication techniques help contribute to a team culture of predictability around communication and tangible mutual support. Because of power hierarchies on teams, TeamSTEPPS offers specific strategies such as the following to standardize often-difficult aspects of team communication:

- The Two-Challenge Rule
- The CUS Technique
- The DESC Script

THE TWO-CHALLENGE RULE

The Two-Challenge Rule identifies every team member's responsibility to attempt to raise any patient advocacy concern with the team at least twice. The first challenge should be in the form of a question. The second challenge should provide some support for the concern. TeamSTEPPS training teaches that if a team member is challenged by another team member, it is the expectation that concerns will be acknowledged and addressed, not ignored.

THE CUS TECHNIQUE

The CUS Technique teaches team members to state their concern (C), to state why they are uncomfortable (U), and then state that there is a safety (S) issue. (See Figure 11.3.) It uses identifiable signal words such as "danger," "warning," and "caution," which are common and easily recognized. As in auto manufacturing plants, which are similarly complex work environments as healthcare, CUS serves as an effective tool to teach concerned team members that they have the ability to "stop the line" if they believe unsafe or erroneous care is being delivered.

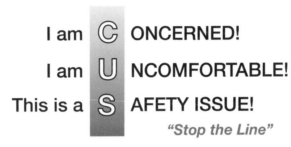

I am **C** ONCERNED!

I am **U** NCOMFORTABLE!

This is a **S** AFETY ISSUE!

"Stop the Line"

Figure 11.3 The acronym CUS from TeamSTEPPS.

Adapted from TeamSTEPPS 2.0 with permission from the Agency for Healthcare Research and Quality (AHRQ, 2014d).

THE DESC SCRIPT

The DESC Script is a technique for conflict resolution. It can be used to facilitate mutual support during all types of conflict. DESC is a mnemonic for the following:

- **D:** Describe the specific situation.
- **E:** Express your concerns about the action.
- **S:** Suggest other alternatives.
- **C:** Consequences should be stated.

Employment of standardized communication techniques during high-stress, high-pressure, uncomfortable team situations alerts all team members that an individual is uncomfortable and perhaps distracted (AHRQ, 2014c).

LINKING TEAM CHARACTERISTICS TO HROS

Characteristics essential for team functioning map to the key values of high reliability organizations, as illustrated in Table 11.3.

TABLE 11.3 THE LINK BETWEEN CHARACTERISTICS OF TEAMS AND HROS

Team Characteristics	Techniques and Strategies	Cross-Reference to HROs
Leadership	Error management	Preoccupation with failure
	Feedback	
	Team self-correction	
Mutual performance monitoring	Situation monitoring: the status of the patient, other team members, the environment, and team progress toward goal	Sensitivity to operations
	Standardized communication	
	Information exchange	
	Briefs, huddles, debriefs	
Backup behavior	Performance monitoring	Commitment to resilience
	Shared mental models	
	Task assistance; feedback	
Adaptability	Adaptability/flexibility	Reluctance to simplify
	Planning	
Team orientation	Assertiveness	Deference to expertise
	Collective orientation	
	Expertise	
	Swift trust	

Wilson, Burke, Priest, and Salas (2005)

The interprofessional nature of healthcare is becoming more complex while also more urgent to effectively address. A high-functioning team that incorporates these characteristics and values might be described as follows:

The Family Care Clinic has a team of practitioners, including primary care providers, nurses, a clinical pharmacist, a certified diabetic educator, behavioral health specialists, and health professions students. This team's hard-earned synergy is evidenced by the team's collaboration in developing several patient-centered programs. Over the years, this interprofessional group of clinicians has developed: (1) a diabetes group management program, (2) a comprehensive practice model to ensure patients are receiving appropriate standards of care, (3) protocols to allow clinical pharmacy and nursing services to assist the provider in managing patients who need more intensive management (for example, insulin titration, anticoagulation, thyroid replacement, and so on), (4) policies to allow other team members to assist with ensuring new prescriptions and refills are prescribed/renewed in a timely manner, and (5) consultation services where providers are able to seek advice from or refer to other team members (for example, medication consultations/recommendations, referrals to meet with the certified diabetic educator, behavioral health or clinical pharmacy practitioners). Part of this interprofessional team's success is due to its explicit goal of optimizing patient outcomes.

SUMMARY

This chapter outlined essential characteristics for team functioning and provided clinical examples to illustrate how they may be incorporated into the care environment. Team characteristics link closely to the values of HROs. Strategies useful for team training may assist in the transformation to an HRO.

KEY POINTS

- Reliability is complex with regard to interprofessional healthcare teams.

- Highly reliable teams in healthcare often share the explicit value of improving patient outcomes.

- Many macrosystem professional organizations in healthcare have made strong recommendations that interprofessional education and interprofessional training must be top priorities for healthcare teams.

- Effectively reliable healthcare teams exhibit lithe leadership that can adjust to complex situations, strong situation-monitoring skills, a commitment to mutual support, and an ability to swiftly develop trust among team members.

- Discrete communication skills can improve teams' abilities to effectively adjust to complex clinical demands in healthcare.

- Evidence-based tools exist to help teams assess their skill strengths and skill gaps and develop team training to improve their patient outcomes.

REFERENCES

Adams, M. J., Tenney, Y. J., and Pew, R. W. (1995). Situation awareness and the cognitive management of complex systems. *Human Factors*, *37*(1), pp. 85–104.

Adler, P. S. (2001). Market, hierarchy, and trust: The knowledge economy and the future of capitalism. *Organization Science 12*(2), pp. 215–234.

Agency for Healthcare Research and Quality (AHRQ). (2014a). TeamSTEPPS Essentials Course: Classroom slides (slide 23). Retrieved from http://www.ahrq.gov/professionals/education/curriculum-tools/teamstepps/instructor/essentials/slessentials.html#s23

Agency for Healthcare Research and Quality (AHRQ). (2014b). TeamSTEPPS Fundamentals Course: Module 3. Communication (slide 14). Retrieved from http://www.ahrq.gov/professionals/education/curriculum-tools/teamstepps/instructor/fundamentals/module3/slcommunication.html#sl14

Agency for Healthcare Research and Quality (AHRQ). (2014c). TeamSTEPPS Fundamentals Course: Module 5. Situation Monitoring (slide 5). Retrieved from http://www.ahrq.gov/professionals/education/curriculum-tools/teamstepps/instructor/fundamentals/module5/slsitmonitor.html#sl5

Agency for Healthcare Research and Quality (AHRQ). (2014d). TeamSTEPPS 2.0 Core Curriculum. Retrieved from http://www.ahrq.gov/professionals/education/curriculum-tools/teamstepps/instructor/index.html

Baker, D. P., Day, R., and Salas, E. (2006). Teamwork as an essential component of high-reliability organizations. *Health Services Research*, *41*(4), pp. 1576–1598.

Barr, H. (2002). Interprofessional education. In J. Dent and R. Harden (Eds.), *A practical guide for medical teachers* (3rd ed.) (pp. 187–192). London, England: Churchill Livingstone.

Carlisle, C., Cooper, H., and Watkins, C. (2004). "Do none of you talk to each other?" The challenges facing the implementation of interprofessional education. *Medical Teacher*, *26*(6), pp. 545–552.

Cook, G., Gerrish, K., and Clarke, C. (2001). Decision-making in teams: Issues arising from two UK evaluations. *Journal of Interprofessional Care*, *15*(2), pp. 141–151.

Cox, M., and Naylor, M. (Eds.). (2013). Transforming patient care: Aligning interprofessional education with clinical practice redesign. Retrieved from http://macyfoundation.org/docs/macy_pubs/TransformingPatientCare_ConferenceRec.pdf

Cronenwett, L., Sherwood, G., Barnsteiner, J., Disch, J., Johnson, J., Mitchell, P., … Warren, J. (2007). Quality and safety education for nurses. *Nursing Outlook*, *55*(3), pp. 122–131.

Frenk, J., Chen, L., Bhutta, Z. A., Cohen, J., Crisp, N., Evans, T. … Zurayk, H. (2010). Health professionals for a new century: Transforming education to strengthen health systems in an interdependent world. *The Lancet*, *376*(9756), pp. 1923–1958.

Greiner, A. C., and Knebel, E. (2003). *Health professions education: A bridge to quality*. Washington, DC: The National Academies Press.

Institute for Safe Medication Practices. (2004). Intimidation: Practitioners speak up about this unresolved problem (Part I). Retrieved from https://ismp.org/newsletters/acutecare/articles/20040311_2.asp

Institute of Medicine. (2001). *Crossing the quality chasm: A new health system for the 21st century*. Washington, DC: The National Academies Press.

Interprofessional Education Collaborative. (2011). Core competencies for interprofessional collaborative practice: Report of an expert panel. Retrieved from http://www.aacn.nche.edu/education-resources/ipecreport.pdf

Jones, A., and Jones, D. (2011). Improving teamwork, trust and safety: An ethnographic study of an interprofessional initiative. *Journal of Interprofessional Care*, *25*(3), pp. 175–181.

Leasure, E. L., Jones, R. R., Meade, L. B., Sanger, M. I., Thomas, K. G., Tilden, V. P., … Warm, E. J. (2013). There is no "I" in teamwork in the patient-centered medical home: Defining teamwork competencies for academic practice. *Academic Medicine*, *88*(5), pp. 585–592.

Légaré, F., Stacey, D., Pouliot, S., Gauvin, F. P., Desroches, S., Kryworuchko, J., … Graham, I. D. (2011). Interprofessionalism and shared decision-making in primary care: A stepwise approach towards a new model. *Journal of Interprofessional Care*, *25*(1), pp. 18–25.

Meyerson, D., Kramer, R. M., and Weick, K. (1996). Swift trust in temporary groups. In R. M. Kramer and T. R. Tyler (Eds.), *Trust in organizations: Frontiers of theory and research* (pp. 166–195). Thousand Oaks, CA: Sage Publications, Inc.

Reeves, S., Perrier, L., Goldman, J., Freeth, D., and Zwarenstein, M. (2013). Interprofessional education: Effects on professional practice and healthcare outcomes (update). *Cochrane Database of Systematic Reviews, 3.*

Ring, P. S., and Van de Ven, A. H. (1992). Structuring cooperative relationships between organizations. *Strategic Management Journal, 13*(7), pp. 483–498.

The Robert Wood Johnson Foundation. (2015). Lessons from the field: Promising interprofessional collaboration practices. Retrieved from http://www.rwjf.org/content/dam/farm/reports/reports/2015/rwjf418568

Rosenstein, A. H., and O'Daniel, M. (2005). Disruptive behavior and clinical outcomes: Perceptions of nurses and physicians. *American Journal of Nursing, 105*(1), pp. 54–64.

Shunk, R., Dulay, M., Chou, C. L., Janson, S., and O'Brien, B. C. (2014). Huddle-coaching: A dynamic intervention for trainees and staff to support team-based care. *Academic Medicine, 89*(2), pp. 244–250.

Smith-Jentsch, K. A., Cannon-Bowers, J. A., Tannenbaum, S. I., and Salas, E. (2008). Guided team self-correction: Impacts in team mental models, processes, and effectiveness. *Small Group Research, 39*(3), pp. 303–327.

Tuckman, B. W., and Jensen, M. A. C. (1977). Stages of small group development revisited. *Group Organization Management, 2*(4), pp. 419–427.

Wilson, K., Burke, C., Priest, H., and Salas, E. (2005). Promoting health care safety through training high reliability teams. *Quality and Safety in Health Care, 14*(4), pp. 303–309.

World Health Organization. (2010). Framework for action on interprofessional education and collaborative practice. Retrieved from http://whqlibdoc.who.int/hq/2010/WHO_HRH_HPN_10.3_eng.pdf

CHAPTER 12

NURSES CREATE RELIABLE CARE BY ADVANCING PATIENT ENGAGEMENT

Julianne Morath, MS, RN, CPPS

Jane S. Braaten, PhD, APRN, CNS, ANP, CPPS

This chapter focuses on the importance of the relationship between the nurse and the patient and family rather than on organizational strategies to engage patients and families, such as serving on advisory committees, rounding, populating design and safety committees, and other such structures. These structures are necessary and important but insufficient by themselves to produce engagement and reliable care. These structures often place the patient and family in a consultant or advisory role after the care episode. To ensure reliable, appropriate, and cost-effective healthcare, we must put less emphasis on what we can do *for* patients and more on what we can do *with* patients to improve quality in real time. In other words, we must flip or expand our thinking to incorporate the patient and his or her family as engaged, integral partners in the patient's care, and embrace the complex cultural, structural, and other changes in priority that this inclusion implies.

The focus of this discussion is not separating the nurse and the patient. The focus is on the space between them and

> The world as we have created it is a process of our thinking. It cannot be changed without changing our thinking.
>
> —*Albert Einstein*
>
> Change will not come if we wait for some other person, or if we wait for some other time. We are the ones we've been waiting for. We are the change that we seek.
>
> —*Barack Obama*

how we can fill it to produce reliable healthcare based on patient engagement. In a recent editorial, Karen Drenkard (2016) states that a major shift in thinking is needed and that we no longer can treat patients as guests who visit "our system." The focus should be on how we partner with them to collaborate and meet mutual goals, just as we would with any other discipline. We don't treat our multidisciplinary colleagues as though they are visitors to our system; we treat them as collaborators coming together to meet common goals. Why should it be different with our patients? This chapter explores where we are now, where we need to be, and how we can get there.

"NOTHING ABOUT ME WITHOUT ME"

At the 1998 Salzburg Global Seminar, "Through the Patient's Eyes: Collaboration Between Patient and Healthcare Professionals," an important breakthrough occurred. There, a new mantra was coined by a nurse midwife: "Nothing about me without me" (Billingham, 1998). This rallying cry caused nurses and organizations to view patients in a more active and inclusive way. We began to fully understand that patients and their families *must* be fully engaged as part of the system of care, not passive recipients of our clinical expertise. Since then, we have all moved forward from different starting points, at different speeds, and with different strategies based on our organizational culture, local leadership, and communities and populations served. It is therefore not surprising that we have wide variation and an unstable system of patient/family engagement. This wide variation and instability is contrary to the definition of high reliability.

In the seminal book *Through the Patient's Eyes*, we learned what was important to patients in their care (Gerteis, Edgman-Levitan, Daley, and Delbanco, 1993). Yet we have been painfully slow as an industry to incorporate these requirements into the system of care. As a result, we have created a patient experience that is inconsistent, compromised, and, in many cases, seemingly uncaring. The inability to codify specifications into reliable and standard work in care delivery has resulted in ambiguities and requires the nurse and care team to work with patients in a highly situational and variable (that is, unreliable) manner.

One integrated healthcare system analyzed the results from focus groups, satisfaction surveys, and consumer interviews and studies. The findings describe the care experience desired by patients and healthcare plan members in their own words:

- "I get what I need when I need it, easily."
- "I am a knowledgeable partner in my healthcare."
- "I am pleasantly surprised by my experience."
- "I believe the system and its staff are competent."
- "I am respected as an individual and treated with dignity."
- "I feel safe and secure." (Morath, 1998)

What if we developed minimum system specifications in which patients and families were partners in care? In a partnership, there is full transparency of the plan of care and ongoing analysis of its concordance with the beliefs, values, and wishes of the patient and family. This becomes central to the design of the system of care delivery and directs the behaviors of nurses and care teams to perform reliably to achieve this system property.

There is much use of the term *partnership*, but operationally and behaviorally, what does it mean and what would it look like? It's interesting to note the derivation of the term *partner* here. Merriam-Webster defines partner as two or more people, businesses, etc., that work together or do business together to create a common outcome. Partners bring different backgrounds to the challenge, yet all partners are essential to fulfilling the work. Another definition of partner is a wooden framework used to strengthen a ship's deck at the point where a mast or other structure passes through it. It allows the mast to remain stable as the sail fills with wind to chart a course of action forward (Merriam-Webster, 2016). The word *partner* is thus a metaphor for stability.

Such partnership and forward action is underway and is a priority in many of our hospitals. However, we may have been too focused on putting our internal systems in place—our workforce and system levels of quality control and continuous quality improvement models. While essential, these foundations do not completely get to the heart of the matter. The distinguishing feature of reliability in healthcare is that it brings the patient and family and communities *in* rather than solely getting a product *out*, such as physical care, surgical procedures, or diagnostic tests. In other words, we have been so focused on our own internal systems that we have overlooked the whole purpose for these systems: to serve people.

We recognize that teams of people with specialized knowledge and skills working together fare better than individual, autonomous people working in an asynchronous manner based on asynchronous communication with patients and families (Knox and Simpson, 2013). Shouldn't we assume that our patients also have specialized knowledge and skills about their own needs, desires, and preferences?

RELIABILITY AND RESILIENCE

As nurses, we work daily toward a standard of adherence to evidence-based practices to create reliable care. *Reliability* is defined as producing intended results, each time, in complex environments, and often under trying conditions. High reliability organizations (HROs) are organized to anticipate and manage the unexpected and exhibit these six basic principles:

- Preoccupation with failure
- Reluctance to simplify interpretations
- A sensitivity to operations

- A commitment to resilience

- A deference to expertise

- Learning from failure (Goldenhar, Brady, Sutcliffe, and Muething, 2013)

In addition, high reliability healthcare requires the following:

- Use of evidence

- Intentional design of the delivery system

- A culture of situational awareness and mindfulness

- Relentless pursuit of the elimination of abnormalities (defects) from the standard design of the work

- Transparency

- Teamwork

- Accountability

- A learning and improvement system

- Attention to operations to detect signals for improvement or redesign (Weick and Sutcliffe, 2007)

This requires awareness (that is, presence of mind or mindfulness), commitment, and discipline. It is not a brittle or inflexible adherence to routine. When confronted with unexpected or novel conditions, the ability to adapt and fine-tune as an interdependent care delivery team is the hallmark of resilience.

Reliability and *resilience* are opposite sides of the same coin. Both are required to achieve excellence in care delivery. Reliability requires standard work, where each team member knows who does what, when to do it, and how to do it, and has authority to ask, "Why do we do it that way?" Reliability also requires operations engineering—an end-to-end analysis of bottlenecks and opportunities for clinical and facility-wide process improvement. This includes an understanding of human factors science. Finally, reliability requires teamwork. This is engineering science and cognitive science applied to the complexity of healthcare. It is also the backbone of a safety culture and safe care delivery.

Resilience cannot exist without reliability. Reliability is the foundation for the improvisation and innovation required (resilience) when novel or unexpected conditions are present and cannot be addressed sufficiently by standard work. Most often, high reliability principles are applied to patient safety events. However, the same principles apply to patient engagement and are an essential component of care.

HIGHLY RELIABLE PATIENT ENGAGEMENT

At its heart, healthcare is people caring for people, and people are unpredictable, complex, and full of paradoxes—especially when we interact with each other and when we are sick, anxious, or confused (Smith, Hiatt, and Berwick, 1999). This is the challenge in healthcare—particularly nursing care, in which there are intimate caregiving relationships. An HRO not only realizes that high reliability is achieved through a safety culture that anticipates and mitigates error but also recognizes that partnerships and collaboration are imperative.

One of the tenets of high reliability is deference to expertise, or allowing those who are closest to the problem to make decisions regarding the problem (Weick and Sutcliffe, 2007). Who is closest to and most expert about their health? The patient.

Patient-centered care is not new. It has been discussed for many years. Various terms are used in association with patient-centered care, such as *patient engagement*, *patient experience*, and more recently *patient activation* (see Table 12.1). However, the concept has, for whatever reasons, almost universally fallen short of fully involving patients and families in their care decisions and participation in care to the extent they are able and willing. In recent years, work in patient-centeredness has matured.

TABLE 12.1 DEFINITIONS OF TERMS RELATED TO PATIENT ENGAGEMENT

Term	Definition
Patient-centered care	Care that is respectful of and responsive to individual patient preferences, needs, and values. Ensures that patient values guide all clinical decisions (Institute of Medicine [IOM], 2001).
Patient engagement	The actions individuals take to obtain the greatest benefit from the healthcare services available to them. Engagement focuses on actions taken by the individual rather than actions of clinicians and institutional polices (Center for Advancing Health, 2010).
Patient activation	The willingness and motivation to independently manage one's health (Hibbard and Greene, 2013).
Patient experience	"The sum of all interactions, shaped by an organization's culture, that influence patient perceptions across the continuum of care" (The Beryl Institute, n.d.).

A growing body of evidence directly relates patient and family engagement and experience to clinical outcomes (Simmons, Wolever, Bechard, and Snyderman, 2014) and patient safety outcomes (Doyle, Lennox, and Bell, 2013). Patient activation has been correlated with better patient outcomes and better patient experience (Hibbard and Greene, 2013). Furthermore, in one study, patients with high activation levels were more likely to do the following:

- Engage in healthy behaviors such as exercising or eating healthy foods
- Avoid unhealthy behaviors such as smoking or drug use
- Seek out health information
- Use preventative services
- Avoid hospitalizations
- Prepare questions to ask their healthcare provider (Greene and Hibbard, 2011)
- Have lower healthcare costs than those with lower activation scores (Hibbard, Greene, and Overton, 2013)

Thus, we will not reach our goal of high reliability without fully partnering with and knowing the engagement capacities of our patients. Three important building blocks to high reliability are as follows:

- A commitment to improvement
- Robust process improvement methods, which include standard work
- A culture of constant questioning

Framing patient engagement in these building blocks is an important factor in building the culture that will support the needed change.

COMMITMENT TO IMPROVEMENT: DIGNITY AND RESPECT ARE CORE VALUES

Dignity and respect for the patient and family are considered preconditions to achieve reliability in the care delivery process and require a shared commitment from the whole organization.

- **Dignity:** Dignity is defined as the state or quality of being worthy of honor or respect.
- **Respect:** Respect is defined as a feeling of deep admiration for someone or something elicited by the person's abilities, qualities, or achievements. (Merriam-Webster, 2016)

For instance, instead of being referred to as "the hip fracture in room 1106," patients are introduced during rounds or handovers in care in a more humanized, dignified way. Here's an example:

> *Mrs. Jones is a retired teacher and active community member. She suffered a fractured hip 2 days ago, requiring this admission. She has two daughters and three grandchildren who may be visiting during her stay.*

The patient is now established as a person and brought into the care process. Instead of telling Mr. Smith, a gentleman with diabetes, "You've got to manage your hemoglobin A1C values" (perhaps a meaningless command to him), the message might be personalized to reflect his goal of seeing his grandson graduate. The dialogue could start with something like the following:

> *Mr. Smith, by following your diet and exercising, you can help keep your diabetes in check and be able to achieve your goal of seeing your grandson graduate from high school. We can help you realize this very important goal.*

This way, education and care planning starts with respecting what is important and valued to the patient. Isn't this the way it should always be? What if we considered insults to dignity and respects as a "never event" and committed to zero violations?

EXAMPLE: TREATING INSULTS TO DIGNITY AND RESPECT AS AVOIDABLE HARM

A commitment to highly reliable patient engagement means defining any violation of respect and dignity as reported by a patient, family member, or any member of the care team as harm. This triggers an event analysis as would be used for any physical harm, such as a fall, infection, or pressure ulcer.

Emotionally harmful events include insults to dignity and respect. These events are often reported as complaints or grievances by the patient with an apology or other means of service recovery given to the patient as an outcome. However, there is generally a lower level of improvement attention given to these events than to events that cause physical harm because the harm is not as visible or considered as important.

Beth Israel Deaconess Medical Center (BIDMC) in Boston is blazing the trail to define emotional harm and treat it in the same way as physical harm (Sokol-Hessner, Folcarelli, and Sands, 2015). BIDMC asserts that these events are just as harmful and perhaps cause longer-lasting effects than physical harm and should be treated as such using the same reporting and investigative rigor.

BIDMC has begun a program of research that seeks to do the following:

- Capture emotional harm events through the occurrence reporting system.

- Categorize emotional harm events. Category examples include communication, privacy, property, and end-of-life care.

- Quantify the severity of emotional harm with a harm scale.

- Define a culture of individual and system accountability for emotional harm.

- Investigate emotional harm with the same tools used to assess physical harm, such as event reviews and root cause analysis.

This places reliable patient engagement in the same spotlight of attention as use of the Andon cord for process abnormality and analysis to remedy the situation. An *Andon cord* is a cord that hangs near employees on an assembly line. When an employee spots a defect or needs assistance, the cord is pulled, and the problem-solving team comes together to address the issue in real time. It does not pass a problem or defect along (Morath and Turnball, 2010). This raises questions of whether a highly intimate relationship of care can be standardized to a reliable process, and if such reliability at the very point of care between nurse and patient will accelerate high reliability performance in healthcare.

INCORPORATE STANDARD WORK

Just as standard work in patient safety is a mainstay of high reliability, so should standard work in patient engagement. Failure to codify specifications into standard work in the domain of patient engagement results in ambiguities. In addition, it places the burden solely on the nurse and care team to satisfy patient and family expectations based on uniquely individual interpretations of the nurse, which may be subject to bias—most specifically, confirmation bias. *Confirmation bias* is a continuum of incidents and fallacies that can occur during and after patient care, including the following:

- Preselecting segments of the seen and generalizing to the unseen

- Seeking certainty and missing the nuance

- Retrospective distortion in conforming and confirming what we do know (Taleb, 2007)

 Confirmation bias can have a major impact on experience and outcome when we impose our bias on patient experience without fully understanding it.

We understand the importance of building patient and family participation and preferences into our care delivery systems. Yet we have been going about it backward—or at least inconsistently. Seeking patient and family feedback through satisfaction surveys after the fact falls short of engaging patients and families. Perhaps standard work includes measuring and assessing the level of engagement to affect care in real time? Many facilities nationally and internationally focus on standard work such as nurse and leader rounding, but how many have built-in standard work that allows for time at the bedside to understand the values, beliefs, and attitudes of patients?

QUESTIONING THE STATUS QUO

Curiosity is a characteristic of those on the road to high reliability. When dealing with the subject of reliability through patient engagement, we are confronted with several complex issues:

- How do we convert data to knowledge and understanding about a patient and family, and their values, beliefs, and wishes for care and for health?

- How do we identify and close gaps in communication?

- How do we design systems that allow for the vulnerabilities of humans as patients, nurses, and care teams?

- How do we identify the barriers that isolate patients and their families when interacting with the care team and healthcare system?

Some interesting studies are grappling with such questions. Much like we determined that bloodstream infections are not an inevitable byproduct of complex care, we are questioning whether objectification and lack of respect and dignity are inevitable byproducts of being a hospitalized patient. In today's healthcare environment, the myth that the "doctor or nurse knows best" has been shattered. The patient's voice must be heard loud and clear if we are to transform care reliability into an effective patient-engagement model. An example of questioning the status quo is the work with experience-based design at Virginia Mason Medical Center.

EXAMPLE: EXPERIENCE-BASED DESIGN AT VIRGINIA MASON MEDICAL CENTER

A relatively new term emerging in healthcare is *experience-based design.* Bate and Glenn (2006) describe experience-based design as user-focused and as a collaboration between the user and the designer. The authors discuss a concept called the *continuum of patient influence* that describes a journey to true patient engagement. The journey starts out viewing patients as issuers of complaints, evolves to seeing patients as consultants (patient and family advisory councils), and finally sees patients as co-designers of their experience and as full partners with the clinicians involved in their care (Bate and Glenn, 2006).

Virginia Mason Medical Center has led the field in co-designing care experience with patients. Experience-based design at Virginia Mason is defined as a philosophy and set of tools and methods focused on understanding the experiences and emotions of those who are involved in receiving and delivering healthcare services—striving to understand what people *naturally do and feel* (Haufe, 2014). Experience-based care includes three components of good design:

- **Experience/aesthetics of experience (usability/comfort):** How does the interaction with the service feel? What emotions does the experience bring forth?
- **Performance (functionality):** How well does the service do the job?
- **Engineering (reliability/safety):** How safe and reliable is the design of the service? (Bate and Glenn, 2006)

At Virginia Mason, patient and family engagement and a posture of constant curiosity are the mainstays of improvement using the philosophy, tools, and methods of the Virginia Mason Production System (adopted from Toyota). Any failure in patient-family engagement and experience is made visible and analyzed to remove the defect and to learn how to improve performance. At the broad organization level, experience-based design includes patient/family participation through the following:

- **Observations:** Observing and shadowing patients as they go through the process of care and transitions
- **Interviews:** Intentionally collecting stories from patients about their experience
- **Experience questionnaires:** Providing a visual depiction of the process to customers, enabling customers to select illustrations that depict emotions they felt at each touch point
- **Focus groups:** Guiding a small group of former patients through a common experience such as scheduling a test, admissions, or an ED visit, and asking open-ended questions about the experience. The system has used a process of patient and family partnership to test a "Know Me" form that assists the patient care team to understand needs and preferences, explore new ideas on how to handle patient delirium after surgery, and create a patient focused procedural consent form. Former patients who participate in these projects are passionate and empowered, helping uncover new innovations that would be missed without their input.

WE HAVE THE "WHY" BUT NEED THE "HOW"

Consciously or unconsciously, patients sometimes defy our best attempts at imposing a plan of care created on their behalf. Why? Because the plan is developed without them and therefore has an impoverished view. What the patient may want and expect from us can be misaligned with what we, as nurses, physicians, and clinicians—that is, experts—define as what is important for them.

In *Through the Patient's Eyes*, we learned what is important to patients in their care (Gerteis, Edgman-Levitan, Daley, and Delbanco, 1993). For hospital inpatients, the dimensions of care that matter are as follows:

- Respect for patient preferences, beliefs, and values
- Coordination of care
- Information and education
- Physical comfort
- Emotional support
- Involvement of family and friends
- Continuity and transition

Patients in ambulatory settings are concerned with these dimensions of care:

- Respect for patient preferences
- Access
- Information and education
- Emotional support
- Continuity and coordination

Do these requests seem surprising or unreasonable? Chances are, you are already providing "care that matters" to your patients and families to the best of your knowledge and skill and considering the system constraints. Yet as an industry, we're not reliably incorporating these requirements into the system of care, possibly because we do not have a process that fits our system, informs clinicians on processes, and includes quantitative measurement of engagement.

INTERACTIVE CARE MODEL (ICM)

The Interactive Care Model (ICM) (Drenkard, Swartwout, Deyo, and O'Neil, 2015), focuses on operationalizing patient engagement by providing a framework that translates the "'what' of patient engagement to the 'how'" (p. 503). Three key drivers inform the model:

- Shifting the mindset of clinicians from providers to partners

- Realizing that fully engaged consumers have a right to choose, and will choose, how they reach their optimal health

- Realizing that communication is changing and includes all types of technology

The model is divided into phases. These include the following:

- Assessing capacity for engagement-measuring patient activation, health literacy, and/or engagement on a regular basis with a validated tool.

- Exchanging information and communicating choices. Instead of offering a provider-driven plan, give options and use shared decision-making to assess the best choice.

- Having people and clinicians plan and explore mutually agreed upon goals, giving consideration to the person's support system and resources.

- Determining appropriate interventions based on the level of engagement and health literacy. The clinician helps the patient navigate through resources to find the most appropriate interventions, including use of peer groups, educational websites, and technological health applications.

- Conducting evaluations on a regular basis to assess changes in engagement or activation.

A VITAL SIGN: MEASURING AND CHANGING ACTIVATION LEVELS

The ICM implies that the level of patient engagement/activation is a vital sign. It is a piece of patient information that is as important as blood pressure or heart rate. However, the concept is elusive unless a clinician is able to measure it, make sense of the data obtained, and demonstrate how to change it to improve outcomes. That is one reason we have had difficulty advancing patient engagement. Scales exist or are in progress with various degrees of validation (Graffigna, Barello, Bonanomi, and Lozza, 2015). The Patient Activation Measure (PAM) (Hibbard, Stockard, Mahoney, and Tusler 2004) is one tool that has shown properties of reliability and validity (Murkoro, 2012). The PAM is a scale that measures activation in ways that make the concept practical and sensitive to change (Hibbard et al., 2004). The authors give an example that illustrates the need for measuring patient activation and using the results to guide care:

Imagine clinicians trying to treat a patient completely blind to the patient's record and list of clinical symptoms. Yet, when clinicians encourage patient engagement in their care, they do so blind to any information on the patient's capabilities for taking on a self-management role. What often results is a "one size fits all" patient education approach. If, however, clinicians had information on their patients' level of knowledge and skill to self-manage,

*they could target self-care education and support to individual patient needs and pre-
sumably be more effective in supporting patient's self-management. (Hibbard, Mahoney,
Stockard, and Tusler, p. 1999, 2005)*

The PAM was originally developed as a 22-item scale that measures patients' knowledge, skill,
and confidence in managing and taking control of their care (Hibbard et al., 2004). The scale
has been refined to a 13-item scale (Hibbard et al., 2005). The scale assesses activation through
questions designed to elicit responses that are then scored on a scale of 0 to 100 and place
patients into four levels of activation:

- **Level 1:** May not yet believe that the patient role is important

- **Level 2:** Lacks confidence and knowledge to take action

- **Level 3:** Is beginning to take action

- **Level 4:** Has adopted proactive behaviors but may have difficulty maintaining behaviors
  over time (Hibbard et al., 2005)

Additional information on the PAM can be found at http://www.insigniahealth.com/products/
pam-survey.

CASE STUDY: SARAH (ACTIVATION LEVEL 1)

Situation: Sarah has congestive heart failure and is discharged to home with all the standard information
about maintaining a low-sodium diet and quitting smoking, handouts on the importance of adherence
to medications, instructions on daily weights, and education on signs and symptoms of an exacerbation.
She takes all her medications as instructed but does not monitor weight or sodium intake. She receives a
message to call the heart failure discharge RN but she doesn't call. She returns to the emergency department and is admitted within 30 days of discharge for heart failure exacerbation. She receives the same
instructions upon discharge.

Discussion: We gather from the fact that she is readmitted that she might have problems adhering to her
healthcare regimen. If we had asked her, she might have said one of the following:

- "I don't like any of the foods on that list."

- "I don't do the shopping, and I rely on others to cook for me."

- "I don't understand why my weight going up a pound or two means I need to call the nurse."

- "I'm too tired to exercise."

- "The doctor knows what he is doing. He will ask me questions if they need more information."

- "I'm tired of people telling me I need to stop smoking and lose weight."

Discharging this patient with the standard educational packet and the standard follow-up call does not seem conducive to high reliability when the outcome is quality of life and reduced hospital readmissions. This patient's activation level, if known, might have been on the lower side. What kind of education and follow-up could have been tailored to this patient, knowing that she didn't understand her medications, didn't understand or know when to call for a subtle change, and didn't understand her role in her health-care? What kind of approach might be taken considering her experience with being judged due to her smoking and her weight?

Greene and Hibbard (2011) state that patients with lower activation levels need knowledge and success with small changes to build confidence. Motivational interviewing (MI) is a tool that can help. MI is a way of addressing patients who are ambivalent or resistant to changes (Rubak, Sandbaek, Lauritzen, and Christensen, 2005). MI focuses on discovering inner strengths of the client in order to resolve ambivalence about change. You can use MI for patient-centered change instead of giving patients a list of changes they need—but have no intention—to make (Berger and Villaume, 2013).

With MI, instead of the clinician prescribing a discharge plan, the clinician asks questions to come up with a mutually agreed upon goal. Characteristics of motivational interviewing include the following:

- Clarifying resistance (Rubak et al., 2005)
- Asking open-ended questions
- Showing empathy/understanding
- Informing and exploring realistic options
- Measuring the patient's desire to change using a scale
- Discussing the pros and cons of changes
- Remembering that the clinician is not there to "fix" but to inform and assist
- Using imagination (Berger and Villaume, 2013)

Conversations between the provider and the patient typically focus on making sense of the situation and examining beliefs and barriers to self-care, with an end goal of an action plan that is simple, is achievable, and can be monitored for success. Here are some examples of end goals:

- "I will keep a notebook and write down my weight on Monday and Friday."
- "I will make a list of some low-sodium foods to give to my son for when he goes to the store."
- "I will call this number (*XXX*) *XXX-XXXX* when my weight goes up by 3 pounds."

CASE STUDY: ALICE (ACTIVATION LEVEL 4)

Situation: Alice is in the hospital after a blood clot, has just discovered she is diabetic, and will be going home to resume taking care of her family, including a teenager and an elderly father. She is overwhelmed but understands that she needs to participate in her discharge plan and follow-up. She tries to exercise and eat well but is busy and sometimes forgets. She is very organized and does not have time in her life for complications.

Discussion: Again, the standard educational packet is not going to meet Alice's needs, especially while she is in the hospital and overwhelmed. She wants a practical and concrete plan that fits into her current life and situation so she can continue to feel in control.

Patients with high levels of activation need support with regard to their autonomy (Greene and Hibbard, 2011). Assisting Alice with an organized list of medications and their purpose and side effects, follow-up appointments, where to purchase blood glucose monitoring equipment and supplies, and signs and symptoms of adverse reactions to her medications is important to her. She might also benefit from electronic reminders to check her blood sugar and from Internet resources and support groups. What Alice does *not* need is information that is not tailored to her specific needs. She is motivated and wants a provider to work with her to come up with a practical plan.

A great resource for this type of patient is provided by the Robert Wood Johnson Foundation in the form of a discharge preparation checklist. This enables patients to check off the needed information, such as why they are taking certain medications, the side effects and management, and the number to call if they have problems. This type of checklist provides patients with a documented and practical plan for self-management. The checklist can be found at http://www.rwjf.org/content/dam/farm/toolkits/toolkits/2013/rwjf404048.

The components of the ICM coupled with a measurement tool for patient activation offer a concrete process that hard-wires patient engagement into the fabric of care. This model describes steps that quantify and personalize, placing emphasis on "seeing" the patient as a whole person. Table 12.2 summarizes levels of activation and suggested interventions as informed by the ICM.

TABLE. 12.2   ACTIVATION LEVEL CHARACTERISTICS AND INTERVENTIONS

Level of Activation	Belief	Expression	Interventions
1 (least)	Patients do not see that they have a role in their health status.	**Passive:** "My doctor will tell me what to do." **Passive:** "I feel safer just staying in the hospital." **Depressed:** "I can't do anything to change my situation."	Consider telehealth/telephone counseling options for ongoing support and education. Use motivational interviewing to break through ambivalence and fears about care.
2	Patients lack confidence in and knowledge of how to manage their health.	**Lack of confidence:** "I don't feel comfortable asking questions during rounds." **Lack of confidence:** "I don't even know what to ask."	Provide a checklist of questions before rounds. Place the checklist on the rounding documentation sheet.
3	Patients have a desire to manage their health.	**Seeking support:** "I really want to get out and walk every day after surgery but I don't want to walk by myself."	Provide information on peer support groups to facilitate motivation and decrease isolation.
4 (most)	Patients have adopted changes but may struggle with consistency. Expect to be an active participant in the plan of care.	**Seeking resources:** "I follow the low-sodium diet to a T when I cook for myself, but I have problems when I go out."	Provide electronic resources that can be used independently to provide guidance on ordering in restaurants.

CHALLENGES TO HIGHLY RELIABLE PATIENT ENGAGEMENT

Although high reliability is the ultimate objective, it is difficult to achieve without a commitment to a concrete goal. Several challenges exist and can become barriers if not addressed. These include the following:

- Clinician lack of knowledge about patient engagement and perceived lack of time
- Lack of leadership priority to support the initiative
- Lack of adequate support or resources to assist patients with low levels of activation or engagement
- Focus on other quality measures to advance patient engagement that don't include the patient

- Lack of a framework to support patient engagement with specific processes and actions
- Lack of measurement tools

Hopefully, this chapter has highlighted the need to combat these barriers to ensure that patient engagement is a priority that can be structured and measured and has a high impact.

SUMMARY

There is a two-part greeting in South Africa that translates to, "I am here to be seen" and "I see you." The greeting implies that to be a person is to be fully acknowledged as an individual and to be in an equally engaged state with the greeter. Isn't this what patients are saying to us? Aren't they saying, "See *me*, not solely my condition, my diagnosis-related group, my risk, my expected cost per hospital day, or my cost per member per month"? These things may be important data points for quality planning, but they are not important to the patient or to his or her family. The patient is here to be seen. You must see the patient as what he or she thinks, fears, needs, and prefers in his or her care and health.

Dignity Healthcare in California has one simple sign on its patient room doors: *Pause and Reflect.* Caregivers are urged to ask themselves the following questions:

- With whom am I entering into a relationship?
- What do I know and understand about this person?
- What can I do to engage the patient in safe and reliable care?

Being in the now and giving full attention to who's right there with you is called *mindfulness* (Vogus, Rothman, Sutcliffe, and Weick, 2014). Mindfulness supports the well-being of nurses and fellow care team members, patients, and family. Remaining mindful and relating to patients as partners has benefits for you as a nurse as well your patient. Engagement and reliable design have been shown to influence the expression of compassion and the experience of joy, meaning, and resilience. Ask yourself:

- Have you and your organization declared engagement and compassion as a property of your healthcare system?
- Have you and your organization committed to addressing abnormalities and defects in experience?
- Have you and your organization elevated gaps in patient respect and dignity to the same level of violation as other harm events?
- Have you and your organization redefined HRO to include the person and family receiving care?

Imagine a future in which the nurse/patient relationship is not replaced but is prefaced, individually and systemically, with "I see you"—nurse to patient, and patient to nurse. This is human-centered and reliable healthcare.

KEY POINTS

- Engagement and partnership in care begin with less emphasis on what we can do *for* patients and more emphasis on what we can do *with* patients.

- Reliability can be achieved in each patient encounter by designing standard work in the form of processes and measurement of patient engagement/activation.

- Lack of dignity and respect produces harm and needs to be reported, analyzed, and prevented.

- Human-centered care, through mindfulness, benefits both the nurse and the patient.

REFERENCES

Bate, P., & Glenn, R. (2006). Experience-based design: From redesigning the system around the patient to co-designing services with the patient. *Quality and Safety in Healthcare*, *15*(5), pp. 307–310.

Berger, B. A., & Villaume, W. A. (2013). *Motivational interviewing for health care professionals: A sensible approach*. Washington, DC: American Pharmacists Association Press.

The Beryl Institute. (n.d.). Defining patient experience. Retrieved from http://www.theberylinstitute.org/?page=definingpatientexp

Billingham, V. (1998). Through the patient's eyes. *Proceedings from Salzburg Global Seminar* (Session 356).

Center for Advancing Health (CFAH). (2010). *New definition of patient engagement: What is engagement and why is it important?* Washington, DC: CFAH.

Doyle, C., Lennox, L., and Bell, D. (2013). A systematic review of evidence on the links between patient experience and clinical safety and effectiveness. *BMJ Open*, *3*(e001570).

Drenkard, K. (2016). Are we really patient focused? Time to challenge ourselves. *Journal of Nursing Administration*, *46*(3 Suppl), pp. S1–S2.

Drenkard, K., Swartwout, E., Deyo, P., and O'Neil, M. B. (2015). Interactive care model: A framework for more fully engaging people in their healthcare. *Journal of Nursing Administration*, *45*(10), pp. 503–510.

Gerteis, M., Edgman-Levitan, S., Daley, J., and Delbanco, T. L. (Eds.). (1993). *Through the patient's eyes: Understanding and promoting patient-centered care*. San Francisco, CA: Jossey-Bass.

Goldenhar, L. M., Brady, P. W., Sutcliffe, K. M., and Muething, S. E. (2013). Huddling for high reliability and situational awareness. *British Medical Journal Quality and Safety*, *22*(11), pp. 899–906.

Graffigna, G., Barello, S., Bonanomi, A., and Lozza, E. (2015). Measuring patient engagement: Development and psychometric properties of the Patient Health Engagement (PHE) Scale. *Frontiers in Psychology*, *6*, p. 274.

Greene, J., and Hibbard, J. H. (2011). Why does patient activation matter? An examination of the relationships between patient activation and health-related outcomes. *Journal of General Internal Medicine*, *27*(5), pp. 520–526.

Haufe, S. (2014). Utilizing experience-based design to improve the patient experience. *Proceedings from Hospital Quality Institute Annual Conference*.

Hibbard, J. H., and Greene, J. (2013). What the evidence shows about patient activation: Better health outcomes and care experiences; fewer data on costs. *HealthAffairs*, *32*(2), pp. 207–214.

Hibbard, J. H., Greene, J., and Overton, V. (2013). Patients with lower activation associated with higher costs; delivery systems should know their patients' 'scores'. *HealthAffairs, 32*(2), pp. 216–222.

Hibbard, J. H., Mahoney, E. R., Stockard, J., and Tusler, M. (2005). Development and testing of a short form of the Patient Activation Measure. *Health Services Research, 40*(6 Pt 1), pp. 1918–1930.

Hibbard, J. H., Stockard, J., Mahoney, E. R., and Tusler, M. (2004). Development of the Patient Activation Measure (PAM): Conceptualizing and measuring activation in patients and consumers. *Health Services Research, 39*(4 Pt 1), pp. 1005–1026.

Institute of Medicine (IOM). (2001). *Crossing the quality chasm: A new healthcare system for the 21st century*. Washington, DC: The National Academies Press. Retrieved from http://www.nap.edu/openbook.php?record_id=10027

Knox, G. E., and Simpson, K. R. (2013). Teamwork: The fundamental building block of high reliability organizations and patient safety. In B. Youngberg (Ed.), *The patient safety handbook* (2nd ed.) (pp. 265–287). Chicago, IL: Jones & Bartlett Learning.

Merriam-Webster. (2016). *Merriam-Webster's Collegiate Dictionary*. Springfield, MA: Merriam-Webster Inc.

Morath, J. M. (1998). *The quality advantage: A strategic guide for health care leaders*. Chicago, IL: AHA Press.

Morath, J., and Turnball, J. (2010). *To do no harm: Ensuring patient safety in health care organizations*. San Francisco, CA: Jossey-Bass.

Murkoro, F. (2012). Summary of the evidence on performance of the Patient Activation Measure (PAM). Retrieved from http://selfmanagementsupport.health.org.uk/media_manager/public/179/SMS_resource-centre_publications/PatientActivation-1.pdf

Rubak, S., Sandbaek, A., Lauritzen, T., and Christensen, B. (2005). Motivational interviewing: a systematic review and meta-analysis. *The British Journal of General Practice, 55*(513), pp. 305–312.

Simmons, L. A., Wolever, R. Q., Bechard, E. M., and Snyderman, R. (2014). Patient engagement as a risk factor in personalized health care: A systematic review of the literature on chronic disease. *Genome Medicine, 6*(2), p. 16.

Smith, R., Hiatt, H., and Berwick, D. (1999). A shared statement of ethical principles for those who shape and give health care: A working draft from the Tavistock group. *Annals of Internal Medicine, 130*(2), pp. 143–147.

Sokol-Hessner, L., Folcarelli, P., and Sands, K. (2015). Insults to dignity: A neglected preventable harm. Presented at the 27th Annual National Forum on Quality Improvement in Health Care, Orlando, FL.

Taleb, N. N. (2007). *The black swan: The impact of the highly improbable*. New York, NY: Random House.

Vogus, T. J., Rothman, N. B., Sutcliffe, K. M., and Weick, K. E. (2014). The affective foundations of high-reliability organizing. *Journal of Organization Behavior, 35*(4), pp. 592–596.

Weick, K. E., and Sutcliffe, K. M. (2007). *Managing the unexpected: Resilient performance in an age of uncertainty* (2nd ed.). San Francisco, CA: Jossey-Bass.

PART 6

HRO CONCEPTS AND APPLICATION TO PRACTICE: RESILIENCE

CHAPTER 13

RESILIENCE:
A PATH TO HRO

Belinda Shaw, DNP, RN, NE-BC, CEN

Over the past decades, psychologists, psychiatrists, and sociologists have explored the concept of resilience. Early studies tended to be longitudinal and historical in nature and focused on individuals exposed to chronic oppressive environments (Garcia-Dia, DiNapoli, Garcia-Ona, Jakubowski, and O'Flaherty, 2013). Initial pioneering research centered on children who had been exposed to adverse family dynamics. Divergent explanations and theories regarding their resilience have been generated, with some common themes. Wolin and Wolin (1993) conducted 20 years of research on adult children of alcoholics and studied the factors that enabled them to rise above the adversity of their upbringing. Werner and Smith (1982) studied high-risk children in homes with poverty, abuse, and alcoholism in an attempt to determine the protective factors that facilitated a transition to healthy adulthood. Dr. Werner identified resilient children as possessing the following positive coping strategies:

- An active approach toward solving life's problems

- A tendency to perceive their experiences constructively

- An aptitude to gain others' positive attention

- An ability to use faith to maintain a positive vision of a meaningful life (Mallak, 1998)

> The strongest oak of the forest is not the one that is protected from the storm and is hidden from the sun. It is the one that stands in the open where it is compelled to struggle for its existence against the winds and rains and the scorching sun.
>
> —Napoleon Hill

Benard (1991) also studied the concept and asserted that resilient children share four common attributes:

- Social competence

- Problem-solving skills

- Autonomy

- A sense of purpose and future

The identification of post-traumatic stress disorder in the 1980s expanded the scope of resilience research to veterans and individuals who experience acute traumatic events. Bonnano (2004) studied the impact of these isolated and disruptive events on individuals and determined that resilience is the ability to maintain relatively stable levels of psychological and physical functioning as well as the ability to expand capacity for generative experiences and positive emotions. Bonnano (2004) found that strong social support, altruism, and discipline or focus were the protective factors for individuals to gain resilience (Garcia-Dia et al., 2013).

The application of resilience theory and study has since extended to the area of healthcare, including hospital organizations and healthcare workers. Emerging focus on nursing and resilience is prudent because of the stressful environment that exists on nursing units. Nurses frequently provide end-of-life care as well as skilled interventions and surveillance for a variety of critical illnesses. Unique safety hazards, including biological and chemical exposures, are part of the nursing work environment (Sexton, Teasley, Cox, and Carroll, 2007). Nursing teams adapt to rapid technological change and psychosocial concerns around healthy communication involving multidisciplinary team members including peers, physicians, and surgeons (Sexton et al., 2007). The conditions leading to a stressful work environment include shift work that frequently results in sleepiness, safety and performance issues, social disruption, and depression. Nurses are prone to musculoskeletal injuries, needle-stick injuries, chemical exposure to toxic medications and biohazards, and the mental health impact of incivility in the workplace (AFL-CIO Department for Professional Employees, 2014). Further evidence of the stressors in the nursing workplace has been described by Trinkoff et al. (2008), including the following:

- 75% of nurses experience workplace stress.

- 67% have been exposed to verbal aggression from a peer.

- 26% have been assaulted by a patient or family member.

- 40–49% experience burnout.

- 15% leave nursing because of moral distress.

Additional challenges for nurses include an aging workforce; shortages of nurses in specialty areas such as the emergency department, perioperative areas, and critical care; and an increase in the use of float pool and traveling or temporary nurses. Higher patient acuity, regulatory requirements, and ethical dilemmas add to job stressors on nursing units. Some work environments provide challenges around professional autonomy, imposed organizational change, occupational health and safety issues, and constant restructuring. The work environment may be perceived by some as hostile, abusive, or unrewarding (Jackson, Firtko, and Edenborough, 2007). These stressors may be manifested in illness, turnover, and high divorce rates among nurses (AFL-CIO Department for Professional Employees, 2014).

A recent significant event was the passing of the Affordable Care Act (ACA) of 2010, which promoted quality of patient care and financial incentives for hospitals to comply. As a result, and rightly so, an environment currently exists where quality and safety are paramount. Hospitals, healthcare providers, and nurses are now challenged by the ACA to provide the highest quality of patient care at the lowest possible cost, creating value. At the center of this value equation is nursing. Registered nurses (RNs) are the primary individuals who coordinate care in multiple healthcare environments, with responsibilities for patient education, technical expertise, surveillance, and prevention of patient harm. Nursing care is also integral to the patient experience, with a growing focus on patient and family satisfaction and reimbursement pressures to deliver top-level performance.

Additional forces have an impact on the work environment for nurses:

- **Economic forces:** These include declining reimbursement and bundled payments for care, causing hospitals to attempt to control expenses through pay practice changes. These changes may include limiting overtime, reducing shift differentials, increasing the use of unlicensed personnel, and adjusting nurse-patient ratios, inevitably resulting in a decrease in morale. With bundled payments, there is also pressure to decrease the hospital length of stay to increase income on the cost per case.

- **Social forces:** Multiple social forces affect the healthcare environment. Patients are now informed customers with access to publicly reported data. They have high expectations for quality care and customer service from healthcare providers and all others involved in the patient experience. Some members of the public also have expectations around sustaining life at all costs, causing moral distress for providers and nursing staff.

- **Technological forces:** These include the transition to electronic medical records and the fact that some nurses view the computer as a barrier to building relationships with patients. In addition to the perception of the computer as a barrier, the amount of time nurses allocate to documentation is onerous. The complexity of technology has also resulted in multiple alarms and alerts for caregivers to manage, leading to fatigue, tolerance, and overstimulation.

The stress of the job creates human and organizational challenges for the retention of nurses. Nursing administrators and managers must look for solutions not only to recruit nurses to their healthcare organizations, but more importantly, to become knowledgeable about how to support and retain nurses once they are employed (Hart, Brannan, and De Chesnay, 2014). As hospital systems focus on value, there is an effort to retain this valuable resource of nursing talent. Nursing turnover disrupts teams. This disruption may affect the quality of patient care, patient satisfaction, and employee satisfaction, and is financially costly. Nationally, nursing turnover is 16.5%, and the average cost to replace a vacancy is estimated to be between $36,000 to $88,000 depending on the nursing specialty (Li and Jones, 2013). Through awareness of the contributing factors and stressors for nurses, successful strategies in building resilience can assist in recruiting and retaining talent (Hart et al., 2014). As noted by Garcia-Dia et al., "Nurses bear witness to tragedy, suffering, and human distress as part of their daily working lives, and because of the stressors associated with assisting others to overcome adversity, resilience is identified as essential for nurses in their daily work" (2013, p. 267).

 Resilience in not necessarily dependent on nurses' age, experience, or education.

Contributing factors that decrease resilience for nursing include the following:

- **Challenging workplaces:** Workplaces that see constant change, that are demanding, and whose organizational goals are not congruent with nurses' professional or personal goals cause conflict within nurses when practicing.

- **Psychological emptiness:** This results from frustrations in the workplace and causes nurses to feel uncared for and to believe that their workplace does not value their opinions.

- **Diminished inner balance:** This occurs when nurses are unable to balance the demands of work with their outside lives.

- **Dissonance in the workplace:** This results in feelings of anxiety and ambiguity for new graduates (Hart et al., 2014).

There are many other healthcare professionals who deserve mention. First responders, including firefighters, paramedics, and emergency medical technicians (EMTs), face an equally challenging work environment. First responders work through high-stress scenarios and save lives in challenging social and environmental settings. They also serve witness to traumatic events that result in potential or actual loss of life. Cumulative traumatic events may lead to post-traumatic stress disorder (PTSD) for first responders, who have a higher prevalence for PTSD than the general population. This translates to a higher mortality rate, more accidental injuries, and early retirement for medical issues compared to the general population. In a longitudinal study of Chicago firefighters, it was determined that the likelihood of a current or retired member taking his or her own life was 25 times greater than the general population (Gunderson, Grill, Callahan, and Marks, 2014).

Physicians, particularly primary care physicians, are also at risk for job-related stress. Burnout is more prevalent among physicians than other professionals. Up to 60% of physicians convey that they have experienced burnout in their career, with up to 40% at any one given point in time. This negatively affects patient care during a time when the demand for primary care services is increasing. The aging population, the short supply of primary care providers, lower reimbursement, and increasing workload may increase the stress on physicians. Additional factors include an increasingly bureaucratic healthcare system at risk for depersonalization and physician self-care practices that tend to be sub-optimal (Fortney, Luchterhand, Zakletskaia, Zgierska, and Rakel, 2013).

THE DEFINITION OF RESILIENCE

Resilience has different meanings depending on the context in which it is used. According to the Merriam-Webster dictionary (2015), the Latin root of resilience is *resilens*, referring to the elastic quality of a substance. Individual resilience, first used as a term in 1824, is the ability to become strong, healthy, and successful after something bad happens. An additional meaning includes the ability to recover from or adjust easily to misfortune or change. In the context of organizations, resilience is the ability to withstand the impact of disruption and recuperate while resuming operations. In the field of physics and engineering, resilience is the capacity of a material to absorb energy, resist damage, and recover quickly (Merriam-Webster, 2015).

Definitions of resilience in the scientific literature are consistent. Jackson et al. (2007) explain the meaning of resilience as the ability of an individual to adjust to adversity, maintain equilibrium, retain some sense of control over his or her environment, and continue to move on in a positive manner. Adversity is central to this definition and is further described as a state of hardship or suffering associated with misfortune, trauma, distress, difficulty, or a tragic event. In the organizational context of nursing, workplace adversity may be viewed as any negative, stressful, traumatic, or difficult situation encountered in the workplace (Jackson et al., 2007).

RESILIENCE AS AN HRO PRINCIPLE

A high reliability health organization (HRO) has measurable near-perfect performance in quality and safety. High reliability is necessary in healthcare, where the consequences of error are high and the frequency is low (Riley, Davis, Miller, and McCullough, 2010). Organizations require resiliency to achieve high reliability.

A central tenet of resilient and reliable organizations is a collective sense of capability as well as a common sense of mission or future in their membership. When technical expertise is combined with a team's desire to contribute and its ability to be collaborative, the outcome is an elevated sense of team confidence. This confidence, in turn, enables the team to successfully make adjustments to unexpected adversity and emergent challenges (Bohn, 2010). A resilient organization will maintain a high level of performance despite mounting pressures, threats, and uncertainties.

There are several models of high reliability in the literature. The accepted principles of high reliability from The Joint Commission for the Accreditation of Hospital Organizations include the following:

- Preoccupation with failure
- Reluctance to simplify
- Sensitivity to operations
- Commitment to resilience
- Deference to expertise (Chassin and Loeb, 2013)

Boin and Van Eeten (2013) further define two types of organizational resilience:

- **Precursor resilience:** This describes the ability to accommodate change without catastrophic failure or a capacity to absorb shocks gracefully. High reliability concepts more closely align with precursor resilience.
- **Recovery resilience:** This is the ability to respond to a singular or unique event and bounce back to a state of normalcy. This may require different strategies, structures and practices.

Boin and Van Eeten (2013) determined the distinctive features that HROs share:

- High technical competence is pervasive throughout the organization.
- A clear awareness exists that certain core events must be prevented from occurring.
- Defined policies and procedures are aimed at avoiding harm.
- A formal structure of responsibilities, roles, and reporting relationships exists that may be transformed to a decentralized team structure in emergency conditions.
- Associates in the organization share the same values of care and caution, respect for procedures, individual responsibility, and the goal of safety.

Precursor resilience highlights the importance of decentralized decision-making, enabling associates to improvise in the moment. Resilient and reliable organizations are therefore nimble, increase the capacity for resourcefulness, highlight the importance of communication, and encourage creative solutions to respond to unique problems. Boin and Van Eeten's (2013) model may be contrary to typical HRO principles that are more structured, yet resilient organizations encourage and thrive on improvisation to avoid crisis management. Pidgeon (1997) concurs that decentralized decision-making during crisis assists with the flexibility and immediacy of response in reliable and resilient organizations.

A mention is warranted of the explosion of technology in healthcare. How do individuals and organizations achieve reliable performance when working with unreliable technology systems? Computer downtime and complex and fragile equipment frequently challenge healthcare providers to create workarounds. Technology that ensures patient safety is not always reliable.

According to Butler and Gray (2006), individuals and organizations achieve reliable performance in changing environments by changing how they think—how they gather information, how they perceive the world around them, and whether they are able to change their perspective to reflect the situation at hand. This may be accomplished through the following:

- Openness to novelty

- Alertness to distinction

- Sensitivity to different contexts

- Awareness of multiple perspectives

- Orientation in the present (Butler and Gray, 2006)

ESSENTIAL CHARACTERISTICS OF RESILIENCE

There are multiple characteristics of resilient individuals in the literature:

- **Self-efficacy:** This is associated with goal identification and perception of ability to execute tasks to attain a goal (Gillespie, Chaboyer, and Wallis, 2007). High efficacy associates have the following characteristics:

    - They have the ability needed.

    - They are capable of the effort required.

    - No outside events will deter them from performing at a high level.

    - A person with high self-efficacy will exert great effort toward goals and will be persistent in achieving a complex task through problem-solving behaviors (Mallak, 1998).

- **Hope:** Hope is the belief that goals may be created, pursued, and attained, resulting in a sense of empowerment. Hope has the potential to mitigate the effects of stress (Gillespie et al., 2007).

- **Coping:** This refers to the cognitive and behavioral efforts that may be exhibited in problem-solving or seeking social support to develop protective factors to stressors. Coping strategies may be positive or negative. A resilient person uses positive coping mechanisms (Gillespie et al., 2007; Mallak, 1998).

- **Rebounding:** This refers to the ability to bounce back after facing a life-altering event through acknowledgment of the event and moving toward a new normal (Garcia-Dia et al., 2013).

- **Determination:** This is a firm or fixed intention to achieve a desired end. Determined individuals possess the willpower and firmness of purpose to persevere and succeed (Taormina, 2015; Garcia-Dia et al., 2013).

- **Social support:** This means having at least one positive relationship with a significant person (Garcia-Dia et al., 2013).

- **Endurance:** This means possessing the mental and/or personal strength and fortitude that enable one to withstand difficult situations without giving up (Taormina, 2015).

- **Adaptability:** This is the capacity to be flexible and resourceful when faced with changing conditions (Taormina, 2015).

- **Recuperability:** This is the ability to recover physically and emotionally from harm, setbacks, or difficulties (Taormina, 2015).

- **Hardiness:** Hardiness comprises three dimensions:

    - Commitment to finding meaningful purpose in life

    - The belief that one can influence one's surroundings and the outcome of events

    - The belief that one can learn and grow from both positive and negative life experiences (Jackson et al., 2007)

In addition to these characteristics, resilient individuals possess an internal locus of control and positive self-esteem, pursue personal goals, adapt to change, and tend to have faith or a purpose in life. Resilient people also tend to have strong relationships, seek help when needed, look at stress as a way of becoming stronger, and use past experience to problem-solve current challenges. Humor, patience, tolerance, and optimism are personal traits of resilient people (Connor, 2006). Resilience can be developed and may help nurses remain in the profession rather than abandoning their career path when the complexities of providing healthcare seem overwhelming (Jackson et al., 2007).

THE CONCEPT OF RESILIENCE

Historically, the concept of resilience has been applied to the individual. There are a number of tools available to measure an individual's resilience. A recent topic of discussion and study, however, is organizational resilience. Relational resilience is a blending of individual and organizational resilience models. In this section, the concept of resilience will be explored in each context.

INDIVIDUAL RESILIENCE

Individuals are not born resilient. Resilience is forged through adversity, the environment, and life experiences. Resilience may be learned at any point across the life span and is an ongoing process of struggling with hardship and not giving up (Gillespie et al., 2007).

Resilience increases throughout life as a result of successfully coping with challenges. Through successful coping, an individual gains problem-solving skills and confidence. These inner strengths and capabilities are supplemented with external resources such as relationships with friends and family, meaningful work, and faith (Wagnild and Collins, 2009). The importance of relationships cannot be underestimated. Engagement in relationships enhances one's intellectual development, sense of worth, sense of competence, sense of empowerment, and most importantly, sense of connection. Resilience can be strengthened in all people through participation in growth-fostering relationships (Hartling, 2008).

Svetina (2014) has explored the concept of resilience as it relates to human development. Erikson's eight stages of human development provide a framework of internal conflict that is present during particular developmental periods. (See Table 13.1.) Each developmental "crisis" must be resolved to progress to the next stage of development.

TABLE 13.1   ERIKSON'S STAGES OF HUMAN DEVELOPMENT

Erikson's Developmental Stage	Corresponding Age of Developmental "Crisis"
Trust versus mistrust	Infant–18 months
Autonomy versus shame and doubt	18 months–3 years
Initiative versus guilt	3 years–5 years
Industry versus inferiority	5 years–13 years
Identity versus role confusion	13 years–21 years
Intimacy versus isolation	21 years–39 years
Generativity versus stagnation	39 years–65 years
Ego integrity versus despair	>65 years

(Source: Marcia and Josselson, 2013)

This theory suggests that resilience may be gained as an individual successfully progresses through the stages of development. This differs from traditional thinking about resilience building through external challenges or life events such as adversity, misfortune, or trauma as opposed to internal psychological conflicts (Svetina, 2014).

Scholarly work exploring resilience has generated tools to measure characteristics of individual resilience. (See Table 13.2.) The variety of tools and the components that are measured reflect the complexity of the concept. There is no gold standard resilience assessment survey (Windle, Bennett, and Noyes, 2011).

TABLE 13.2   INSTRUMENTS TO MEASURE INDIVIDUAL RESILIENCE

Instrument Name	Characteristics
Bartone Dispositional Resilience Scale Versions 1, 2, 3; 1989, 1991, 1995, 2007	Measures psychological hardiness: ■ Commitment ■ Control ■ Challenge
Biscoe and Harris Resiliency Attitudes Scale (RAS); 1998	Measures seven components of resilience: ■ Insight ■ Independence ■ Relationships ■ Initiative ■ Creativity ■ Humor ■ Morality
Block and Kremen ER 89; 1993	Components: ■ Ego control ■ Ego resilience

Connor and Davidson Resilience Scale (CD-RISC); 2003	Components:
	■ Personal competence
	■ Trust in own intuition
	■ Acceptance of change
	■ Personal control
	■ Spiritual influences
Donnon and Hammond Youth Resilience Scale; 2003, 2007	Components focus on protective factors:
	■ Personal competence
	■ Social competence
	■ Family coherence
	■ Social support
	■ Personal structure
Wagnild and Young Resilience Scale; 1993	Components:
	■ Equanimity
	■ Perseverance
	■ Self-reliance
	■ Meaningfulness
	■ Existential aloneness
Friborg Resilience Scale for Adults (RSA); 2003	Components associated with protective factors:
	■ Personal strength
	■ Social competence
	■ Structured style
	■ Family cohesion
	■ Social resources

continues

TABLE 13.2 INSTRUMENTS TO MEASURE INDIVIDUAL RESILIENCE (CONTINUED)

Instrument Name	Characteristics
Sinclair and Wallston Brief Resilient Coping Scale (BRSC); 2004	Components: ■ Personal coping resources ■ Pain coping behavior ■ Psychological well-being
Hurtes and Allen Resilience Attitudes and Skills Profile; 2001	Measures resiliency attitudes: ■ Independence ■ Creativity ■ Humor ■ Initiative ■ Relationships ■ Value orientation
Sun and Steward California Healthy Kids Survey; 2007	Assesses student perceptions of: ■ Their individual characteristics ■ Communication and cooperation ■ Self-esteem ■ Empathy ■ Problem-solving ■ Goals and aspirations ■ Family connection ■ School connection ■ Community connection ■ Autonomy experience ■ Pro-social peers ■ Meaningful participation in the community ■ Peer support

Four 5-Item Subscales of Adult Personal Resilience; 2013	Components:
	▪ Determination
	▪ Endurance
	▪ Adaptability
	▪ Recuperability

Gillespie et al. (2007); Taormina (2015); Svetina (2014); Windle et al. (2011)

Garmezy (1991) developed a triadic model of resilience that describes the interactions between protective and risk factors on three levels: the individual, the family, and the environment. Protective factors may be external, such as socioeconomic resources, family, and community. Additional protective factors are internal, such as personality, advanced motor skills, and self-help skills. Risks are described as stressful events that may be related to everyday issues, including death of a loved one, poverty, divorce, illness, and school or work stressors. Other stressful events include traumatic world events and exposure to violence and national disasters. Of key interest in the Garmezy model are environmental factors that may enhance resilience, such as work environments that have high levels of teamwork and that provide resources, structure, high expectations, stability, and opportunity.

ORGANIZATIONAL RESILIENCE

Resilient organizations have high reliability and maintain a high level of performance despite any mounting environmental pressures, threats, or uncertainties (Boin and Van Eeten, 2013). In the world of healthcare, high reliability means near-perfect performance for quality and safety. Resilient organizations can therefore be identified as having high-quality scores, which are available online through many public and private reporting firms.

According to Riley (2009), high reliability (and therefore resilient) organizations tend to have two characteristics:

- They have team-training programs.
- They engage in process and analysis design.

Team-Training Programs

One team-training program that Riley recommends is Team Strategies and Tools to Enhance Performance and Patient Safety (TeamSTEPPS), an interdisciplinary program created by the Agency for Healthcare Research and Quality (AHRQ). Multiple publications have documented improvement in pre- and post-test outcomes after TeamSTEPPS training as well as corresponding quality and safety outcomes (Castner, Foltz-Ramos, Schwartz, and Ceravolo, 2012; Brock et al., 2013; Thomas and Galla, 2013; Sheppard, Williams, and Klein, 2013; Ferguson, 2008; Mayer et al., 2011).

TeamSTEPPS identifies the barriers to effective teamwork as follows:

- Inconsistency in team membership
- Lack of time
- Lack of information sharing
- Hierarchical relationships
- Defensiveness
- Conventional thinking
- Complacency
- Varying communication styles
- Conflict
- Lack of coordination and follow-up
- Distractions
- Fatigue
- Workload
- Misinterpretation of cues
- Lack of role clarity (AHRQ, 2015)

The tools and strategies TeamSTEPPS uses include the following:

- Briefs
- Debriefs
- Huddles
- Cross monitoring
- Feedback
- Advocacy and assertion
- Collaboration

- Handoff

- The Two Challenge Rule

- Call-out

- Check-back (AHRQ, 2015)

The outcomes that may be achieved through the use of these tools include the following:

- A shared mental model

- Adaptability

- Team orientation

- Mutual trust

- Higher team performance

- Higher levels of patient safety (AHRQ, 2015)

There are three phases of implementation of TeamSTEPPS:

- **Site assessment:** This phase involves creating a change team of trainers, defining an opportunity to improve, and setting measurable goals.

- **Plan-train-implement:** This phase involves gaining organizational commitment, administrative support, and physician participation.

- **Sustaining gains:** Sustaining a TeamSTEPPS intervention involves practicing the skills, leadership emphasis on skills learned, providing feedback and coaching to team members, celebrating wins, celebrating successes, and updating and adjusting when needed (AHRQ, 2015).

A review of the literature indicates that there are a number of additional key variables in Team-STEPPS implementations, such as executive leadership oversight and participation, alignment of the program with organizational goals, early bedside staff involvement and trainer expertise, credibility and motivation of the trainers, and motivation and self-efficacy of the nursing staff. Patient safety, culture of safety, interprofessional communication, interprofessional education, and handoffs are frequently mentioned in TeamSTEPPS research. Concepts such as HROs, relationship-based care, and the American Association of Critical-Care Nurses (AACN) Healthy Work Environment also provide evidence to support teamwork as foundational to healthcare outcomes (Riley, 2009; Koloroutis, 2004; AACN, 2005).

Process and Analysis Design

The second characteristic of highly reliable (resilient) organizations is process design. Process design starts with process mapping, an exercise that identifies bottlenecks, workarounds, unnecessary redundancies, and potential points of error. Involving the team who performs the work as well as the patient in the design process is key to understanding inefficiencies and waste. Additionally, having a team commitment to the standardization of stable processes with low variation is the key to reliability. It has been proven that 5% of medical errors are caused by incompetence, while 95% of errors are made by conscientious individuals who are outcome-focused working in poorly designed systems without uniformity (Riley, 2009).

Mallak (1998) describes two types of organizations:

- **Mechanistic organizations:** These are like a machine—efficient, programmed with low levels of uncertainty in a closed system.

- **Organic organizations:** These are like an organism—complex responses, flexible, and with higher levels of uncertainty in an open system design.

Mallak (1998) contends that organizational structure should fit the type of organization. That is, structures with tight decision-making control and scarce information would not work in an organic organization. Healthcare systems are certainly organic in nature, necessitating process design and teamwork to heighten certainty, reliability, and resilience.

Resilient organizations have the following characteristics:

- They perceive all experiences constructively, even those that may be difficult.

- They demonstrate positive adaptive behaviors, viewing change as an opportunity.

- They ensure adequate external resources to maximize the potential for positive adaptive responses. Additional resources may be in the form of advice, information, finances, emotional support, and practical help.

- They empower individuals to expand decision-making boundaries.

- They practice *bricolage*—the practice of creating order out of chaos. This may be accomplished through survival training courses, which simulate finding solutions on the fly in the practice environment. Practice enhances an individual's comfort level when taking risks.

- They develop tolerance for uncertainty. They have the ability to make a decision when all of the needed information is not available.

- They build virtual role systems—a work environment where the team can continue in the absence of one or more members.

- They use positive reinforcement, such as feedback, public recognition, reward systems, and encouragement.

- They provide constructive feedback when individuals fail so that they may walk away from the experience with a positive mental framework and learn from the experience (Mallak, 1998).

Hopkin (2014) has researched the principles and practices of resilient organizations. He asserts that managing risk is the key to resilience. Through an extensive analysis of eight organizations, he determined that the key to achieving resilience in an organization is to focus on behavior and culture.

Hopkin (2014) contends that to achieve resilience, five criteria must be met:

- **The ability to anticipate problems:** This requires high involvement and constant vigilance from all members of the team. It is important to avoid complacency or overconfidence. All members of the team should be encouraged to raise concerns and ask challenging questions.

- **The diversification of resources:** Diversification allows for a flexible response to adverse circumstances and opportunities. This may be achieved by establishing risk parameters that are acceptable, limiting dependencies and expanding partners to limit single points of failure, building flexibility into the business, and practicing scenario planning and response exercises.

- **Strong relationships and networks:** Members of the organization should have a shared purpose and shared values, which lead to trust. A no-blame culture balanced with accountability, open communication, and focus on the customer are the cornerstones of these relationships.

- **The ability to launch a rapid response in times of crisis to normalize operations quickly:** To achieve this, organizations must identify cross-functional teams and processes, empower those teams, and rehearse risk scenarios.

- **The ability to learn from experience and make improvements accordingly:** Associates should be knowledgeable about risk management, structured learning, near-miss reporting, and peer review. A desire to improve is an important underpinning of this principle.

Similar themes of highly reliable and resilient organizations were studied by Taylor, Clay-Williams, Hogden, Braithwaite, and Groene (2015). The seven underlying themes are as follows:

- A positive organizational culture. This is demonstrated through respect, trust, a focus on excellence, recognition, and a non-threatening environment.

- A responsive senior management team that is supportive, involved, and accessible.

- Effective performance monitoring that includes accurate goal-setting measurements, adequate data systems to monitor improvement, a continuous improvement culture, and accountability.

- The ability to attract, retain, and develop talented and proficient professionals. The workforce must also be aligned with the organization's mission, participate in competency training, and be knowledgeable about the organization's policies and procedures.

- Effective, committed leaders.

- Practice must be driven by evidence and expertise. The front-line staff must also have autonomy, flexibility, and empowerment to be creative and innovative.

- Effective, multidisciplinary teamwork, collaboration, and a coordinated effort with the patient in the center of the team.

The connection between high reliability and organizational resilience was also made by Boin and Van Eeten (2013). In this thorough analysis, essential elements for organizational resilience were defined as follows:

- High technical competence throughout the organization

- A clear awareness of risk avoidance

- Policies and procedures that help to minimize risk

- A culture of reliability

- A formal reporting structure

- Authorization to transform to a decentralized, team-based approach to problem-solving when emergencies arise

RELATIONAL RESILIENCE

Relational resilience is important for individuals and organizations. Relational resilience implies that resilience may be strengthened through relationships that bolster an individual's intellectual development, sense of worth, empowerment, competence, and connection.

Hartling (2008) contends that the concept of resilience should migrate from the idea of individual intrinsic toughness to one of a human capacity that may be developed and strengthened through relationships. The proposed definition of resilience in this adapted view involves the ability to connect, reconnect, and resist disconnection in response to hardships, adversities, trauma, and alienating social and cultural practices. Relational resilience is based on engagement in relationships in which the individuals feel known, valued, and recognized. Knowing that one makes a difference to another provides the boost of emotional energy that strengthens one's ability to be resilient. The sense of connection that results from relationships provides the groundwork for mutual empathy, responsiveness to others, mutual empowerment, and authenticity (Hartling, 2008).

Jordan (2004) also made the case for moving beyond the concept of resilience as an individual trait. Jordan (2004) suggested five ways to enhance capacity for relational resilience:

- Migration from individual control to an archetype of supported vulnerability
- Movement from a unidirectional need for support to mutual empathetic involvement
- Separation of self-esteem from relational confidence
- Leveling hierarchy and encouragement of mutual growth and constructive conflict resolution
- Movement from self-motivated meaning to more expansive relational awareness

Through the lens of relational resilience, higher team functioning or teamwork may be affected through development of a culture of supported vulnerability, flexibility, empowered conflict resolution, mutuality, confidence, and awareness (Jordan, 2004). Mutual support, one of the concepts presented in TeamSTEPPS training, has crosswalks to relational resilience. (See Table 13.3.) The mutual support tools, task assistance, feedback, advocacy and assertion, Two Challenge Rule, CUS, and DESC Script all enhance relationships.

TABLE 13.3   TEAMSTEPPS MUTUAL SUPPORT TOOLS AND INFLUENCE ON RELATIONAL RESILIENCE

TeamSTEPPS Mutual Support Tool	Influence on Relational Resilience
Task assistance	Helping others with tasks.
	Fostering a climate where it is expected that assistance will be actively sought and offered.
Feedback	Shared information that is timely, respectful, specific, directed toward improvement, and considerate.
Advocacy and assertion	Asserting corrective action when viewpoints differ in a firm and respectful manner.
Two-Challenge Rule	Leveling hierarchy and empowering all team members to stop the line when there is a patient-safety issue.
CUS	Assertive statement.
	I'm concerned, I'm uncomfortable, this is a safety issue!
DESC Script	Constructive approach for managing and resolving conflict.

RESILIENCE-BUILDING STRATEGIES

Many organizations have stressed individual resilience, aimed at retaining their valuable healthcare professionals. It is intuitive that engaged and resilient staff are central to the goal of attaining organizational resilience. This section explores strategies aimed at building individual and organizational resilience.

PERSONAL STRATEGIES

Individual resilience strategies are consistent regardless of one's roles or responsibilities in the healthcare system. Hart et al. (2014) proposed the following individual strategies to build resilience:

- Engaging in extracurricular activities such as exercise, social networks, and volunteerism.

- Practicing cognitive reframing—the exercise of revisioning or re-creating the work environment into a more effective workplace.

- Developing emotional toughness and detachment. This allows nurses and clinicians to perform painful, unpleasant patient procedures that are necessary for patient healing.

- Cultivating connections with family, friends, and colleagues.

- Maintaining work-life balance.

- Using critical reflection for problem-solving and adapting to the realities of professional practice. This frequently takes the form of reflective journaling and may be especially helpful for new professionals entering the workforce.

- Reaffirming professional commitment and finding meaning and congruency between one's work life and one's personal beliefs and value system.

- Maintaining a positive attitude through humor, laughter, visualizations, and positive affirmations.

- Seeking and establishing a relationship with a trusted mentor to provide professional and personal guidance.

Jackson et al. (2007) have an abbreviated but similar strategy to build individual resilience through the following protective factors:

- Building positive, nurturing networks and professional relationships inside and outside the work area, including mentorship.

- Maintaining positivity, positive emotions, and laughter.

- Developing emotional insight.

- Achieving work-life balance and spirituality.

- Becoming more reflective as a means of developing insight and understanding into experiences and knowledge that can be used in subsequent situations.

Parse's Human Becoming School of Thought (HBST) teaches strategies of reflective learning and practice (Jackson et al., 2007). Kupperschmidt, Keintz, Ward, and Reinholz (2010) used Parse's theory to conceptualize a five-factor model for becoming a skilled communicator. Skilled communication is one of the tenets of a healthy work environment (HWE). Historically, communication has been interpreted as being the responsibility of a manager. Kupperschmidt et al. (2010), however, argue that all members of the healthcare team share the responsibility for healthy communication. Enhancing communication is a personal resilience strategy that also benefits the team.

The five-factor model involves the following:

- **Becoming aware of self-deception:** This awareness enables all members of the team to focus on their contributions and accountability for the development of the HWE. This includes individual team members being willing to acknowledge and change problematic past behavior and become more open and trusting and less defensive.

- **Becoming more reflective in practice:** Reflection is the process of stepping back from an experience to evaluate its meaning and to guide future behavior. Self-questioning is integral to becoming reflective.

- **Becoming real, genuine, and authentic in relationships:** An authentic individual understands his or her purpose, strengths, weaknesses, and values. Authentic people tend to have enduring relationships, practice self-discipline, and live their personal and professional values.

- **Practicing mindfulness:** To be mindful is to be present and focused on a current experience without interference from past experience. Mindfulness means choosing to respond positively, being present-centered, acknowledging all thoughts and feelings, and being aware of verbal and nonverbal communication.

- **Being candid:** This means speaking with candor, free from bias, and with truth. This may only happen in environments where there is trust.

Mutual support in relationships is another recommendation that is a personal strategy with team benefits. Mutual support involves concern for and assistance to other members of the healthcare team. In teams with high levels of mutual support, someone always "has your back."

There is an individual responsibility on the healthcare team to demonstrate mutual support in the following ways:

- By assisting other team members during high workload

- By requesting assistance from team members when feeling overwhelmed and providing assistance when asked or when sensing that another team member is overwhelmed

- By acknowledging and communicating potentially dangerous situations to team members

- By providing feedback in a way that promotes positive interactions and future change

- By advocating for patients, even when one's opinion conflicts with that of a senior member of the unit

- By challenging team members when concerns about patient safety are recognized

- By resolving conflicts, even when those conflicts have become personal (TeamSTEPPS Curriculum, 2.0, 2013)

Mutual support is also central to relational resilience. Creating caring relationships is the responsibility of the individuals who are part of the team.

ORGANIZATIONAL STRATEGIES

Managerial opportunities to increase the resilience of healthcare teams and organizations are numerous. The individual strategies of enhanced communication and mutual support may also translate as organizational strategies. Indeed, the AACN describes a healthy work environment as one that includes skilled communication, true collaboration, effective decision-making, appropriate staffing, and meaningful recognition (AACN, 2005). There is an assessment tool on the AACN website that organizations may use to assess the components of an HWE in their individual or collective teams.

The nursing profession has created an additional resilience strategy in the American Nurse Credentialing Center (ANCC, 2015) Magnet Recognition Program®. Magnet® recognized organizations possess components that create positive nursing environments in which to practice. The components include the following:

- **Transformational leadership:** There is advocacy and support for nursing at the organizational level. This ensures the voice of nursing is heard, the input is valued, and practice is supported. The chief nursing officer (CNO) is an executive stakeholder in the organization.

- **Structural empowerment:** There is shared governance for decision-making regarding nursing practice.

- **Exemplary professional practice:** Organizational outcomes are grounded in safety, quality, and interdisciplinary teamwork.

- **New knowledge, innovations, and improvement:** This includes evidence-based practices.

- **Empirical outcomes:** This is the report card that reflects clinical, workforce, patient, and organizational outcomes.

It makes sense that Magnet nursing environments are resilient nursing environments. This intuition is corroborated by Hart et al. (2014). Magnet nursing environments promote additional strategies, such as the following:

- Implementing new graduate nurse residency programs

- Establishing mentorship programs for new graduate and newly hired nurses

- Establishing a mechanism for formal and informal debriefing sessions for nurses involved in traumatic or stressful patient and family situations

- Hosting personal resilience workshops for nurses

- Implementing employee assistance programs

- Providing professional development programs, such as the programs that cover the following:

    - Interdisciplinary effective communication

    - Coping strategies

    - Effective team building/teamwork (TeamSTEPPS)

    - Emotional intelligence

    - Conflict management and resolution

    - Stress reduction

    - Implementing and enforcing a zero-tolerance policy for disruptive behaviors

    - Promoting personal health incentives

    - Offering smoking-cessation classes

    - Offering workout/gym facilities

    - Offering free health screenings

Other organizational resilience strategies include the following:

- **An integrated human resources (HR) department:** HR generalists should be known faces to the employees in an organization. Developing partnerships and relationships with teams by attending team meetings ensures that employees see HR as a department that is a resource for them, not solely a resource for management. This partnership is preferable to the perception by employees that they see HR representatives only when there is a problem.

- **Employee assistance counseling:** This is an essential benefit for employees to tap into for help in their personal or professional lives.

- **Employee crisis fund availability:** The option to donate paid time off or contribute to a team member financially through an employee assistance fund is an additional organizational measure for resilience.

- **Time off and scheduling policies:** Extended illness, funeral leave, and other paid time off policies are beneficial, as is adherence to the Family Medical Leave Act (FMLA). Many organizational healthcare units have also implemented self-scheduling practices to assist employees with work-life balance.

Riley's (2009) analysis of HRO—and by extension resilient organizations—concluded that team training such as TeamSTEPPS and process redesign are essential. TeamSTEPPS has been discussed at length, while further discussion on process redesign is warranted. Six Sigma and lean process design originated in industry and has more recently been applied to healthcare. Through the application of these process-redesign strategies, the many complex processes in healthcare can be streamlined and create environments where patient care is enhanced and practices are simplified for the professionals who deliver care. Supply placement to minimize nursing steps, patient admission and throughput, the discharge process, and overall patient-care coordination are examples of how the work environment can be improved for patients and professionals. The standardization of workflow decreases ambiguity and increases reliability.

A few last words on organizational resilience strategies focus on the role of the manager. According to Taormina (2013), when employees are given information about a problem, they will better understand and be more likely to accept the changes that are imposed to deal with the problem. Therefore, to strengthen people's endurance for life's vicissitudes in general, it would be beneficial to increase their understanding of the world and the way that it works. Organizational support, which refers to the positive treatment of employees by their managers, can increase the emotional commitment of the workforce and decrease turnover. This leads to a more enthusiastic workforce, which, in turn, benefits the entire organization.

PRACTICAL APPLICATIONS

A number of resilience training programs have emerged over the past decade. The following serve as exemplars that have similar themes in their curricula. While not an exhaustive list of available programs, the examples serve varied target audiences, including all multidisciplinary team members and pre-hospital providers.

EXAMPLE 1: DUKE UNIVERSITY AND MINNESOTA HOSPITAL ASSOCIATION

A partnership between Duke and Minnesota Hospital Association resulted in Webinar Implementation for the Science of Enhancing Resiliency (WISER) training. The webinar focuses on caregivers but is also open to leaders, executives, and physicians. The program provides in-time feedback to participants as well as allowing for a structure and protected time to practice using the tools introduced in the training.

The webinar is a series of eight 60-minute sessions that focuses on self-awareness, mindfulness, purpose, self-care, and relationships. Mindfulness involves two exercises: three good things and the practice of observation without evaluating. The three good things exercise was initially developed by Marty Seligman in the field of positive psychology. It involves keeping a gratitude journal, in which the healthcare professional should write during the last 2 hours of the day, when recall of events is enhanced. It has been proven that recalling three positive things each evening will enhance individuals' ability to recognize positive moments in their day (Mid-Michigan Health, 2015).

WISER training addresses purpose through resilience writing and journaling, discussion around blame and forgiveness, and the recognition and avoidance of negative loops of thought and communication. Self-care training involves fatigue management, nutrition, and spending time in nature. Relationship training centers on showing gratitude, support, and validation and on social support (Minnesota Hospital Association, n.d.).

Duke has developed a patient-safety center with the following education and training:

- Patient-safety leadership training and certification course
- Physician leadership in patient safety and quality
- TeamSTEPPS train the trainer (16 hours)
- Bite-sized resilience: three good things
- TeamSTEPPS essentials (4 hours)
- Enhancing Caregiver Resilience: Burnout and Quality Improvement (3 days)
- Enhancing Caregiver Resilience Essentials (1 day) (Duke University Health System, n.d.)

As this program matures, it will be interesting to gauge any changes in staff retention and other organizational outcomes.

EXAMPLE 2: MAYO CLINIC

Mayo Clinic also has a very developed resilience training program through its website (Mayo Clinic, 2015). The content of the training describes strategies to build skills to better endure hardship. Strategy approaches include cultivating positive relationships, making every day meaningful, developing successful coping skills, remaining hopeful, performing self-care, planning in order to be proactive, and seeking professional advice assistance when needed (Mayo Clinic, 2015). Individual tactics include the following:

- **Getting connected:** This involves establishing positive relationships for support and acceptance and making connections through volunteering or joining faith/spiritual communities.

- **Making every day meaningful:** Do something each day that gives you a sense of purpose or accomplishment, and set goals for the future.

- **Learning from experience:** Use coping strategies that have worked for you in the past.

- **Remaining hopeful:** You can't change the past. Look to the future to accept and anticipate change.

- **Taking care of yourself:** Participate in hobbies and activities you enjoy. Sleep, maintain a healthy diet, be physically active, and engage in stress-management activities such as yoga, meditation, guided imagery, deep breathing, and prayer.

- **Being proactive:** Don't ignore your problems. Figure out what needs to be done, make a plan, and take action.

- **Seeking professional advice:** Professionals may include employee assistance programs or private practitioners (Mayo Clinic, n.d.).

This is currently a web initiative. It will be interesting to track progress over time for staff retention and organizational outcomes. Comparing the outcomes of a web-only program with in-person, interactive strategies over time will be valuable.

EXAMPLE 3: FIRST RESPONDERS

The first responder resilience training program is a collaboration among the Colorado Department of Public Health Office of Emergency Preparedness and Response; Centura Health Prehospital Emergency Services; Philip Callahan, PhD; and Michael Marks, PhD. The origins of the training program were in the Southern Arizona Veteran's Administration Health Care

System and the University of Arizona as an effort to re-integrate returning war veterans into the academic setting. The program spread to Colorado after the Aurora theater shooting in July 2012. Signs of PTSD were identified in first responders after this event, and the Colorado Department of Public Health reached out to Dr. Callahan and Dr. Marks to assist with training efforts (Gunderson et al., 2014).

The First Response Resilience curriculum addresses 12 resilience skills:

- Goal setting
- Nutrition
- Exercise
- Sleep
- Relaxation
- Activating events, beliefs, and consequences (ABCs)
- Perspective
- Self-defeating thoughts
- Empathy
- Wins and losses
- Reaching out
- Social support

Many of these skills are addressed in the 1-day training. Others are assigned to be discussed in small groups during the month following training. Each classroom skill is discussed in less than 1 hour, with extensive interaction and reflection in small groups. Studies with pre- and post-assessment tools by Callahan and Marks are encouraging (Gunderson et al., 2014).

SUMMARY

The application of resilience theory and study expanded to the healthcare sector after the 1980s, following recognition that nursing and healthcare providers are vulnerable to the stressful environment in which they practice. Healthcare professionals, including nurses, physicians, and first responders, are susceptible to many factors, including shift work; injury; verbal aggression from patients, families, and co-workers; assault; moral distress; workforce shortages; rapid technological changes; performance pressures; pay practice changes; complex and unreliable technology; overstimulation; and fatigue. The stressors in the work environment translate to high levels of burnout.

Multiple strategies are presented to develop individual and organizational resilience. Exemplars are provided to demonstrate how strategies have been packaged by Duke and the Minnesota Hospital Association, Mayo Clinic, as well as collaboration between the Colorado Department of Public Health Office of Emergency Preparedness and Response, Centura Health Prehospital Emergency Services, Philip Callahan, and Michael Marks.

KEY POINTS

- Individual resilience is the ability to become strong or recover after facing adversity.

- Resilience is a quality that may be developed throughout life.

- Organizational resilience is the ability to withstand disruption and recuperate while resuming operations.

- High reliability organizations are resilient organizations.

- Relational resilience implies that individual and organizational resilience may be enhanced through strengthening relationships.

- There are multiple strategies to increase and monitor individual and organizational resilience.

REFERENCES

Agency for Healthcare Research and Quality. (2015). TeamSTEPPS: Strategies and Tools to Enhance Performance and Patient Safety. Retrieved from http://teamstepps.ahrq.gov/

American Association of Critical-Care Nurses (AACN). (2005). Standards for establishing and sustaining healthy work environments. Retrieved from http://www.aacn.org/wd/hwe/docs/hwestandards.pdf

American Federation of Labor Department for Professional Employees. (2014). Nursing: A profile of the profession. Retrieved from http://dpeaflcio.org/wp-content/uploads/Nursing-2014.pdf

American Nurses Credentialing Center. (2015). Magnet Recognition Program® overview. Retrieved from http://nursecredentialing.org/Documents/Magnet/Magoverview-92011.pdf

Benard, B. (1991). Fostering resilience in kids: Protective factors in the family, school, and community. Retrieved from http://crahd.phi.org/papers/fostering.pdf

Bohn, J. G. (2010). Development and exploratory validation of an organizational efficacy scale. *Human Resource Development Quarterly*, *21*(3), pp. 227–251.

Boin, A., and Van Eeten, M. J. G. (2013). The resilient organization. *Public Management Review*, *15*(3), pp. 429–445.

Bonnano, G. A. (2004). Loss, trauma and human resilience: Have we underestimated the human capacity to thrive after extremely aversive events? *The American Psychologist*, *59*(1), pp. 20–28.

Brock, D., Abu-Rish, E., Chiu, C. R., Hammer, D., Wilson, S., Vorvick, L., … Zierler, B. (2013). Interprofessional education in team communication: Working together to improve patient safety. *BMJ Quality and Safety*, *22*(5), pp. 414–423.

Butler, B. S., and Gray, P. H. (2006). Reliability, mindfulness and information systems. *MIS Quarterly*, *30*(2), pp. 211–224.

Castner, J., Foltz-Ramos, K., Schwartz, D. G., and Ceravolo, D. J. (2012). A leadership challenge: Staff nurse perceptions after an organizational TeamSTEPPS initiative. *The Journal of Nursing Administration*, *42*(10), pp. 467–472.

Chassin, M. R., and Loeb, J. M. (2013). High reliability health care: Getting there from here. *The Milbank Quarterly*, *91*(3), pp. 459–490.

Connor, K. M. (2006). Assessment of resilience in the aftermath of trauma. *Journal of Clinical Psychiatry*, *67*(Suppl. 2), pp. 46–49.

Duke University Health System. (n.d.). Duke Patient Safety Center. Retrieved from http://www.dukepatientsafetycenter.com

Ferguson, S. L. (2008). TeamSTEPPS: Integrating teamwork principles into adult health/medical-surgical practice. *Medsurg Nursing*, *17*(2), pp. 122–125.

Fortney, L., Luchterhand, C., Zakletskaia, L., Zgierska, A., and Rakel, D. (2013). Abbreviated mindfulness intervention for job satisfaction, quality of life, and compassion in primary care clinicians: A pilot study. *Annals of Family Medicine*, *11*(5), pp. 412–420.

Garcia-Dia, M. J., DiNapoli, J. M., Garcia-Ona, L., Jakubowski, R., and O'Flaherty, D. (2013). Concept analysis: Resilience. *Archives of Psychiatric Nursing*, *27*(6), pp. 264–270.

Garmezy, N. (1991). Resiliency and vulnerability to adverse developmental outcomes associated with poverty. *American Behavioral Scientist*, *34*(4), pp. 416–430.

Gillespie, B. M., Chaboyer, W., and Wallis, M. (2007). Development of a theoretically derived model of resilience through concept analysis. *Contemporary Nurse*, *25*(1–2), pp. 124–135.

Gunderson, J., Grill, M., Callahan, P., and Marks, M. (2014). Responder resilience. *Journal of Emergency Medical Services*, *39*(3), pp. 57–61.

Hart, P. L., Brannan, J. D., and De Chesnay, M. (2014). Resilience in nurses: An integrative review. *Journal of Nursing Management*, *22*(6), pp. 720–734.

Hartling, L. M. (2008). Strengthening resilience in a risky world: It's all about relationships. *Women & Therapy*, *31*(2–4), pp. 51–70.

Hill, N. (n.d.). Points to ponder on resilience. Retrieved from http://resiliencefirst.com/resilience_quotes.html

Hopkin, P. (2014). Achieving enhanced organisational resilience by improved management of risk: Summary of research into the principles of resilience and the practices of resilient organizations. *Journal of Business Continuity & Emergency Planning*, *8*(3), pp. 252–262.

Jackson, D., Firtko, A., and Edenborough, M. (2007). Personal resilience as a strategy for surviving and thriving in the face of workplace adversity: A literature review. *Journal of Advanced Nursing*, *60*(1), pp. 1–9.

Jordan, J. V. (2004). Relational resilience. In J. V. Jordan, M. Walker, and L. M. Hartling (Eds.), *The complexity of connection: Writings from the Stone Center's Jean Baker Miller Training Institute* (pp. 28–46). New York, NY: Guilford Press.

Koloroutis, M. (2004). *Relationship-based care: A model for transforming practice*. Minneapolis, MN: Creative Health Care Management.

Kupperschmidt, B., Kientz, E., Ward, J., and Reinholz, B. (2010). A healthy work environment: It begins with you. *Online Journal of Issues in Nursing*, *15*(1), pp. 1–4.

Li, Y., and Jones, C. B. (2013). A literature review of nursing turnover costs. *Journal of Nursing Management*, *21*(3), pp. 405–418.

Mallak, L. (1998). Putting organizational resilience to work. *Industrial Management*, *40*(6), pp. 8–13.

Marcia, J., and Josselson, R. (2013). Eriksonian personality research and its implications for psychotherapy. *Journal of Personality*, *81*(6), pp. 617–629.

Mayer, C. M., Cluff, L., Lin, W. T., Willis, T. S., Stafford, R. E., Williams, C., … Amoozegar, J. (2011). Evaluating efforts to optimize TeamSTEPPS implementation in surgical and pediatric intensive care units. *The Joint Commission Journal on Quality and Patient Safety*, *37*(8), pp. 365–374.

Mayo Clinic. (n.d.). Tests and procedures: Resilience training. Retrieved from http://www.mayoclinic.org/tests-procedures/resilience/art-20046311?pg=2

Mayo Clinic. (2015). Resilience: Build skills to endure hardship. Retrieved from http://www.mayoclinic.org/tests-procedures/resilience-training/in-depth/resilience/art-20046311

Merriam-Webster. (2015). Resilience. Retrieved from http://www.merriam-webster.com/dictionary/resilience

Mid-Michigan Health. (2015). 3 good things. Retrieved from http://www.midmichigan.org/3goodthings

Minnesota Hospital Association. (n.d.). Resilience training. Retrieved from http://www.health.state.mn.us/patientsafety/preventionofviolence/mharesiliencytrng.pdf

Pidgeon, N. (1997). The limits to safety? Culture, politics, learning and man-made disasters. *Journal of Contingencies and Crisis Management*, *5*(1), pp. 1–14.

Riley, W. (2009). High reliability and implications for nursing leaders. *Journal of Nursing Management*, *17*(2), pp. 238–246.

Riley, W., Davis, S. E., Miller, K. K., and McCullough, M. (2010). A model for developing high-reliability teams. *Journal of Nursing Management, 18*(5), pp. 556–563.

Sexton, K. A., Teasley, S. L., Cox, K. S., and Carroll, C. A. (2007). United States operating room nurses: Work environment perceptions. *Journal of Perioperative Practice, 17*(3), pp. 116–117.

Sheppard, F., Williams, M., and Klein, V. R. (2013). TeamSTEPPS and patient safety in healthcare. *Journal of Healthcare Risk Management, 32*(3), pp. 5–10.

Svetina, M. (2014). Resilience in the context of Erikson's theory of human development. *Current Psychology, 33*(3), pp. 393–404.

Taormina, R. J. (2015). Adult personal resilience: A new theory, new measure, and practical implications. *Psychological Thought, 8*(1), pp. 35–46.

Taylor, N., Clay-Williams, R., Hogden, E., Braithwaite, J., and Groene, O. (2015). High performing hospitals: A qualitative systematic review of associated factors and practical strategies for improvement. *BMC Health Services Research, 15*, pp. 1–22.

TeamSTEPPS Curriculum 2.0. (2013). Retrieved from http://teamstepps.ahrq.gov/

Thomas, L., and Galla, C. (2013). Building a culture of safety through team training and engagement. *Postgraduate Medical Journal, 89*(1053), pp. 394–401.

Trinkoff, A. M., Geiger-Brown, J. M., Caruso, C. C., Lipscomb, J. A., Johantgen, M., Nelson, A. L., … Selby, V. L. (2008). Personal safety for nurses. In R. G. Hughes (Ed.), *Patient safety and quality: An evidence-based handbook for nurses* (pp. 473–508). Rockville, MD: Agency for Healthcare Research and Quality.

Wagnild, G. M., and Collins, J. A. (2009). Assessing resilience. *Journal of Psychosocial Nursing and Mental Health Services, 47*(12), pp. 28–33.

Werner, E. E., and Smith, R. S. (1982). *Vulnerable but not invincible: A longitudinal study of resilient children and youth*. New York, NY: McGraw-Hill.

Windle, G., Bennett, K. M., and Noyes, J. (2011). A methodological review of resilience measurement scales. *Health and Quality of Life Outcomes, 9*(8), pp. 1–18.

Wolin, S. J., and Wolin, S. (1993). *The resilient self: How survivors of troubled families rise above adversity*. New York, NY: Villard Books.

CHAPTER 14

BUILDING HIGH RELIABILITY THROUGH SIMULATION

Kelly D. Wallin, MS, RN, CHSE

Frances C. Kelly, MSN, RNC-OB, NEA-BC, CPHQ

Kerry A. Sembera, MSN, RN, CCRN

In the healthcare setting, simulation has traditionally been employed as an educational strategy, enabling healthcare providers to practice procedures and develop competence before caring for real patients. Simulation immerses the individual in a realistic experience in which he or she can practice or test skills, reflect on gaps or strengths, and better understand performance, thereby exemplifying the wisdom of Confucius in this chapter's opening quote.

Until recently, simulation has been predominantly used in pre-practice settings, such as schools of nursing, medicine, and allied health, to prepare students for post-graduation practice. This chapter describes the emerging use of simulation in hospitals and other healthcare organizations as an advanced quality-improvement and patient-safety tool. We suggest that this tool—when used according to current best practices in healthcare simulation—is uniquely well-suited to underpin and promote each of the five principles essential to high reliability organizations (HROs) in ways that traditional quality-improvement tools have been limited.

> Tell me, and I will forget. Show me, and I may remember. Involve me, and I will understand.
>
> —*Confucius*

This chapter:

- Provides an overview of healthcare simulation, including current definitions, modalities, methods, and implications for best practice

- Identifies the benefits of employing simulation as an advanced quality improvement (AQI) and patient-safety tool

- Integrates the principles of HRO and simulation within a key driver diagram, providing a framework aimed at reducing preventable harm and improving the quality of care in an organization

- Describes examples of how this framework has been used, highlighting various concepts central to high reliability within various clinical settings

OVERVIEW OF HEALTHCARE SIMULATION

The use of simulation in healthcare settings is a rapidly growing field. Experts are increasingly defining the systems, methods, guidelines, and standards necessary for healthcare simulation to be officially recognized as its own professional community of practice (Palaganas, Maxworthy, Epps, and Mancini, 2014). Because readers of this handbook likely possess a variety of backgrounds, some may not be as familiar with the healthcare simulation currently emerging in hospitals as a quality and patient-safety tool. To provide a common foundation in simulation for all, this section provides an overview of essential elements and practices in simulation.

Healthcare simulation is defined by the Society for Simulation in Healthcare (SSH) as follows (SSH, n.d.):

> *A technique that uses a situation or environment created to allow persons to experience a representation of a real healthcare event for the purpose of practice, learning, evaluation, testing, or to gain an understanding of systems or human actions; the application of a simulator to training, assessment, research, or systems integration toward patient safety.*

At its most basic, a simulation activity consists of the following "molecule" of elements:

- **The scenario:** A realistic situation in which participants are immersed.

- **The simulator:** A physical space, equipment, mannequins, and/or humans used within the situation to replicate real life.

- **The experience:** "Near-life" immersion in the situation, as experienced by the participants. This is then reflected upon in a facilitated debriefing either during or after the event.

The degree to which the simulated experience approaches reality is known as *fidelity*.

The following section provides a more in-depth review of the elements, or anatomy, of a simulation.

THE SCENARIO

More than just a case study in which participants practice a clinical procedure, the scenario is a multidimensional plan that provides all the contextual cues needed to immerse participants in a realistic clinical situation. In designing scenarios, simulationists consider not only the expected (and unexpected) clinical progression of the case based on learning objectives, but also such things as the following:

- Pre-simulation information needed by participants, such as clinical knowledge/skills, orientation to simulation, and/or simulated patient information

- Staging—that is, preparing the setting and simulator to look realistic, with appropriate equipment, moulage (techniques to simulate injury or symptoms), and other props needed either initially or later as participants manage their situation

- Scripts for embedded/simulated persons to augment the fidelity of the scenario

- Programming mannequin software to interact appropriately with participants

- Planning for audio-visual recording and playback if used for debriefing or research

- Participant roles and responsibilities related to scenario objectives

- Process for and the key points to be addressed during debriefing

THE SIMULATOR

More than just a mannequin, the simulator can take various forms, depending on the goals of the simulation. Some examples include the following:

- **Anatomical simulator:** These include full-body mannequins that interact with the learner in varying degrees (for example, pulses, breath sounds, or vocalization), depending on the level of fidelity required. Partial-body task trainers, such as a torso for placement of chest tubes or an airway trainer for intubation practice, may also be used.

- **Simulated persons (SPs)/embedded actors:** An SP or embedded actor is a person trained in particular actions and responses essential to the goals of the simulation. This person is embedded in the scenario and influences the flow of the scenario. He or she may also provide feedback during debriefing.

- **Equipment/technology:** This could include haptic trainers (devices that interact with the user's own body motions to produce tactile or other sensory feedback) or virtual reality applications (computer-based applications that interact with users to immerse them in a virtual environment).

- **Physical space/environment:** This is a mocked-up facility or space used to simulate patient rooms, units, hospitals, or an ambulance.

- **In situ simulation:** Rather than using mocked-up spaces, this type of simulation is conducted in the real patient care environment with participants who are "on duty" in their actual work setting.

- **Hybrid:** This describes a combination of modalities, such as combining a simulated person with a mannequin or partial-body task trainer.

THE EXPERIENCE

More than just play-acting or role-playing, an effectively designed and conducted simulation experience allows participants to suspend disbelief, immersing themselves in realistic sights, sounds, smells, feelings, emotions, stressors, and human dynamics—all of which are consistent with the situation being simulated and the goals of the simulation.

Additionally, the facilitated debriefing immerses participants in a structured reflection on their performance to access deeper layers of meaning behind how things happened as they did. This includes risk-free discussion of *sacred cows,* or well-known norms regarded as immune from open discussion or questioning, and of human/system weaknesses and errors (Rudolph, Simon, Dufresne, and Raemer, 2006).

Providing "psychological safety" (Dieckmann, Gaba, and Rall, 2007) for participants in the simulation is essential to achieving the full benefits of both the scenario and the debriefing. This cannot be overemphasized. Ensuring that simulation participants perceive that they are psychologically safe to speak up about what they know and how they believe things should or could be done is an absolutely essential element in any simulation. It is even more important when simulation is being employed as a strategy for improving reliability and the culture of safety in an organization (Edmondson, 2014). Failure to ensure a safe environment during the simulation and debriefing experience will hamper efforts to promote thoughtful reflection and transparency. Worse, it could harm a weak or fledgling organizational safety culture.

The term *high-fidelity simulation* is often used to imply the use of high-tech mannequins. However, it should be noted that even a low-tech simulator can be used to produce a high-fidelity simulation, depending on the goals of the simulation. An effective healthcare simulation activity requires attention to all three of the noted elements—the scenario, the simulator, and the experience—not just what simulator you use.

METHODS

A wide variety of teaching, learning, assessment, or research methods are considered when developing and conducting effective healthcare simulations. The methods used should match the objectives and aims of the simulation as well as the simulator and modality chosen. For example, if the goal of the simulation is to assess or validate competence, the degree of fidelity (realism) experienced by the learner as well as standardized scenarios and debriefing and evaluation tools are much more important than if the goal is for learners or participants to practice interdisciplinary teamwork. In the latter case, it is much more important that the team of learners or participants is representative of all the appropriate disciplines, and that the debriefing is facilitated effectively to address each discipline's role and point of view. Finally, if the goal of the simulation is to learn or practice communication skills, it may be more important to use simulated persons as the simulator rather than mannequins to ensure an effective and realistic communication experience.

The technology of the simulator should never drive the simulation. Rather, the goals of the simulation should drive whatever technology is used.

Debriefing is widely known to be the most important element in any simulation. This is because, as many simulationists believe, the learning *really* occurs in the debriefing rather than in the scenario itself. Debriefing methods vary. Which method you should use depends on the objectives of the simulation and logistical limitations, such as time available and the facilitation skills of the debriefer. Some frequently used debriefing methods are described in Table 14.1.

TABLE 14.1   DEBRIEFING METHODS

Method	Description	Practice Implications

Plus/Delta	Generic framework adapted from flight crew debriefings.
	
	After the scenario, debriefers guide learners/participants to reflect on two elements:
	
	  ■ What went well and why
	
	  ■ What needs improvement and why
		This is a fairly simple approach that is useful when time is short and/or the debriefer has not been trained in other methods.

Advocacy-Inquiry (Rudolph et al., 2006)	A framework guiding learners or participants to reflect not only on observed performance in the scenario but also on each participant's unobservable thoughts and frame of mind that may have led to the observed behaviors.
	
	Debriefers guide learners/participants to reflect on performance with an inquiry consisting of three parts:
	
	  ■ Identify a particular action or behavior observed in the scenario
	
	  ■ Advocate/state his or her own (the debriefer's) take on what he or she observed (bad, good, or indifferent)
	
	  ■ Ask in a genuinely curious and supportive manner for the participant's take on what happened and why
		Although this method requires more training for debriefers and takes more time, it offers a pathway to gaining a deeper understanding about why things happened as they did in simulation.
		
		This is a very useful technique for supporting a culture of safety during debriefing as well as uncovering less obvious factors that contribute to errors or near misses.

Rapid Cycle Deliberate Practice (Hunt et al., 2014)	An emerging method of debriefing that occurs during the scenario instead of afterward. The scenario is stopped (at either pre-selected points or when an opportunity for improvement is noted), the debriefer gives directed feedback on performance, and the scenario starts over again or resumes until the next debrief point.	This approach prioritizes opportunities for learners to immediately identify errors and then try again during the scenario rather than wait for a lengthy debriefing later.

During the debriefing, participants may gain additional learning from watching their video-recorded performance in the scenario. However, use of videorecording is not necessary, depending on the goals of the simulation and the overall method used.

BENEFITS AND OUTCOMES OF SIMULATION

One of the greatest benefits of simulation as a learning methodology is that it enables the participant to apply knowledge, skills, or behaviors in a realistic (and often stressful) situation to gain proficiency without causing risk to patients or other providers. For many, the first real opportunity they have to practice working as a healthcare team in a crisis situation in a complex hospital system is when they encounter these situations while caring for real patients. In fact, in the traditional apprenticeship model of transitioning to practice after completion of basic professional preparation, the post-graduate clinician in any discipline becomes very familiar with the "watch one, do one, teach one" model. Thankfully, simulation offers an alternative that promotes a safer and more reliable healthcare delivery system. Errors made in simulation become errors prevented in actual patient care.

Benefits of simulation that are particularly relevant to organizations striving to improve patient safety and reduce preventable harm through increasing reliability include the following:

- Unlimited exposure to rare and high-risk clinical events
- Safe atmosphere for training in procedures and clinical scenarios that are risky to both clinicians and patients
- Unlimited practice of technical skills as well as nontechnical skills such as teamwork and communication
- Immediate feedback and learning, with or without video-assisted debriefing
- The opportunity to teach and learn about skills or outcomes that are difficult to teach or assess using traditional methods of education and clinical practice

Teamwork and communication are nontechnical skills that have historically been omitted from professional education curricula, perhaps because they are difficult to teach or to improve using conventional means. Yet, they have been identified as critically important to underpin a culture of safety and improve patient outcomes. Not surprisingly, the literature is replete with studies identifying that the lack of teamwork and failures in communication among our modern-day interprofessional teams remain high on the list of root causes of errors and preventable harm in healthcare. In its hallmark 1999 publication, "To Err Is Human: Building a Safer Health System," the Institute of Medicine (IOM) reported that 70% of mistakes in healthcare were the result of human error, and that this human error was due not to lack of medical knowledge but rather to failures in communication and teamwork (IOM, 1999).

Much attention has been given to the fact that nurses, physicians, and other healthcare professionals train in silos. Yet, today's complex healthcare system depends much more on effective teamwork than autonomy, much like the pit crews in professional automobile racing (Gawande, 2011). A hospital is like "the pit." In order to function effectively, efficiently, and safely, we who work there must cultivate "pit crew" skill sets we probably did not learn or practice in school.

Characteristics of our modern healthcare system that call for a different approach include the following:

- Healthcare organizations are complex systems. No longer can any one individual possess all the information and skills needed to care for patients safely and effectively.

- Clinicians are specialized, yet must work together to achieve common goals for patients.

- Healthcare requires effective coordination, communication, and standardized practice.

- To function as a coordinated team, these skills must not only be taught but also practiced...and practiced...and practiced, much like the pit crew that accomplishes everything needed to keep its car in the race in an 8-second pit stop.

According to Gawande (2011), what we lack in healthcare are opportunities to practice teamwork. Therefore, healthcare is increasingly adopting crew resource management (CRM) principles. These principles guide the efficient coordination of individuals within teams. They're what propelled the aviation and aerospace industries into HROs. Simulation is one of the only ways that healthcare team members can practice CRM skills, learning about and improving the unique technical and nontechnical skills required to effectively coordinate care and communicate across disciplines, especially in clinical emergencies.

It is gratifying to see an increasing number of reports in the literature describing improved provider performance, improved patient outcomes, and reduced preventable harm to patients and errors in healthcare, resulting—at least in part—from simulation training. Examples of the positive impact of simulation include the following:

- Improved operating room performance of surgical residents (Seymour et al., 2002)

- Improved Apgar scores, decreased incidence of hypoxia encephalopathy, and 70% reduction in brachial plexus injuries with shoulder dystocia for newborns after delivery (Draycott et al., 2008)

- Improved survival from 33% to 50% of pediatric inpatients after cardiac arrest (Andreatta, Saxton, Thompson, and Annich, 2011)

- Decreased medical error rates from 30.9% to 4.4% (Morey et al., 2002)

- Decreased rates of central line–associated bloodstream infection (CLABSI) from 4.9/1000 to 3.2/1000 with an annual cost savings of $3.9 million (Scholtz, Monachino, Nishisaki, Nadkarni, and Lengetti, 2013)

Healthcare simulation, in its basic form as an educational tool, offers a wide variety of modalities and methods for training individuals and teams in technical as well as nontechnical skills. However, simulation can also be employed as a quality-improvement and patient-safety tool, targeting specific quality and safety outcomes and contributing to the reduction of error and risk in an organization. The next section outlines a framework for how simulation may be used as a patient-safety and quality-improvement tool, incorporating each of the five HRO principles.

USING SIMULATION TO DRIVE FOR HIGH RELIABILITY

At its core, healthcare simulation is an educational methodology. However, it can be used for much more than teaching. It can also be used as a tool for organizational learning and change management, skill sets that are critical for HROs.

According to Chassin and Loeb (2013), there is little guidance in the published literature on a framework or pathway for hospitals (or any other industry, for that matter) to use to elevate a low reliability organization into a highly reliable one. However, those seeking to develop such a pathway are giving increasing attention to three domains important for organizations to address when making the changes necessary to advance toward high reliability: leadership, safety culture, and robust process-improvement tools (Chassin and Loeb, 2013). Employing simulation as a robust process-improvement tool targeting each of the five HRO principles is a unique methodology that supports change in all three of these domains. This section describes a framework for using healthcare simulation as a process/quality improvement tool aimed at advancing each of the five concepts of HROs.

KEY DRIVER DIAGRAMS

Key driver diagrams are often used within quality improvement initiatives to demonstrate a pathway for achieving a desired outcome (Institute for Healthcare Improvement, n.d.). The driver diagram is used as a planning and analysis tool at the beginning of a project and provides a theory of change that can facilitate the organization of work and communication throughout the project.

As depicted in Figure 14.1, driver diagrams are structured flowcharts that help teams see the relationships among the goal (aim), the factors (drivers) felt to be most influential to meeting the goal, and the action plan (interventions). When faced with a quality or patient-safety concern, quality improvement teams try to answer the question, "What change can we make that will result in the desired improvement?" Use of the driver diagram requires teams to identify their theories about what key factors are really driving or influencing the results. When these drivers have been identified, teams can determine how to address each driver by identifying areas for improvement, specific interventions, or change concepts to achieve the goal (aim).

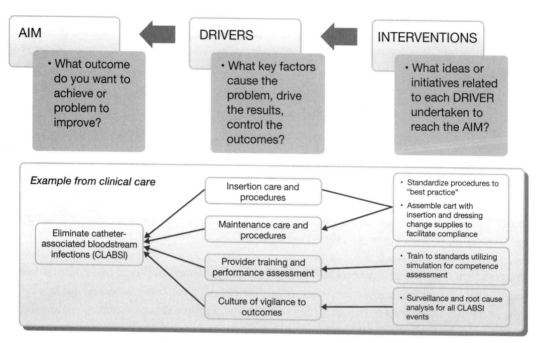

Figure 14.1   Example of key driver diagram.

What if you could apply the key driver diagram framework to outline a pathway for building high reliability in a healthcare organization by aligning a toolkit of simulation interventions with each of the HRO principles? Within such a framework, evidence-based quality and process improvement strategies may be integrated with innovative applications of simulation to target the primary drivers of high reliability. Figure 14.2 illustrates a framework in which at least three types of simulation methods are employed within a quality improvement model to assist an organization to promote reliability. These are as follows:

- Simulation-based clinical system testing
- Simulation-based solution testing
- Simulation-based just-in-time training and clinical rehearsal

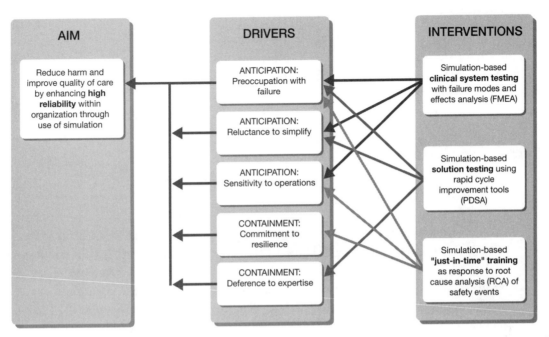

Figure 14.2   Key driver diagram for using simulation as a patient-safety and quality tool to build high reliability.

The following section describes each of these interventions. This discussion includes examples of how simulation may be used in any organization to improve reliability, which will improve the quality and safety of care.

SIMULATION-BASED METHODOLOGIES SUPPORTING HRO

The integration of high-fidelity clinical simulation with established quality and patient-safety methods represents an innovative way to more robustly develop strategies and processes for improving reliability. The remaining portion of this chapter describes recipes for employing simulation within your own organization's quality and patient-safety toolbox to improve quality, safety, and reliability.

Simulation-Based Clinical System Testing (SbCST) with Failure Modes and Effects Analysis (FMEA)

What Is It?

This refers to the use of *in situ* clinical simulation to test current or new patient-care environments, systems, processes, or equipment to proactively identify actual system failures or latent (unrecognized) safety threats. The focus is *not* to educate providers but rather to evaluate complex systems in which healthcare providers interact with the physical environment (facility, equipment, processes). It is often used in conjunction with FMEA to prioritize the risk of each identified threat based on the potential severity and probability that these threats may actually occur in real patient care. An example of this method is the staging of high-fidelity clinical simulations to test patient and provider safety in a newly built unit before move-in.

How Can It Help an Organization Build High Reliability?

This approach addresses the following tenets of high reliability:

- **Preoccupation with failure:** Catastrophic patient harm often occurs as a result of an unanticipated sequence of active failures and latent conditions that are difficult to foresee (Davis, Riley, Gurses, Miller, and Hansen, 2008; Reason, 1997). FMEA is an established and widely used means of proactively seeking out both latent and active weaknesses and failures in healthcare systems to analyze causes, assess risk, and address resolutions (The Joint Commission, 2005). Combining high-fidelity clinical simulation with the FMEA technique moves it out of the conference room and right to the bedside, resulting in a much more robust patient-safety tool.

- **Reluctance to simplify:** Taking the time to thoroughly test complex clinical systems (processes + facilities + equipment + people) with a realistic simulation of typical or high-risk/-impact clinical care situations can aid in recognition of active or latent threats to the safety of patients or clinicians. This enables teams to develop solutions to mitigate the identified risks when it is easier to correct rather than failing to recognize it until after patient harm occurs.

- **Sensitivity to operations:** Engaging front-line clinical providers performing in "near real" clinical situations to assist in identifying safety concerns or deviations from expected performance harnesses the power of those closest to even the smallest operational details at the point of care to detect concerns. Simulation participants are then encouraged in debriefings to share potential concern, no matter how small, as well as suggested solutions, so that early indicators of system threats can be identified and addressed effectively.

How Do You Do It?

Here's how this process works:

1. Engage all stakeholders early to clarify priorities, scope, and their level of involvement in the project. Include formal leaders (including architects and facilities leaders), who will have both the authority to support the project and the accountability to take action on findings.

2. Conduct a needs assessment to identify the specific systems to be tested and the priority concerns. If the intent is to test a new space, this should be initiated well in advance of the anticipated opening date to ensure operational readiness to conduct an effective simulation. Keep in mind that simulation can be used to inform decisions and identify latent safety threats throughout the design and construction phases of building a new hospital environment, not just after construction and before opening.

3. Develop simulation scenarios incorporating appropriate fidelity to test for the identified concerns. (Refer to the section "Overview of Healthcare Simulation" for standard components.)

4. Identify and clarify roles of qualified clinical and nonclinical observers for the day of the simulation. In SbCSTs, including experts from nonclinical disciplines such as regulatory readiness, environmental/facility services, security, and information technology provides valuable insight based on their areas of expertise, further enhancing dialogue and the understanding of system weaknesses.

5. Develop tools for collecting and documenting findings. Scripted debriefing questions aimed at uncovering latent threats to patient safety or weaknesses in the system are often developed to gather specific information from participants. Trained facilitators play a critical role in observing participants' communications, interactions, and body language during the debriefing.

6. Conduct the simulation. Then document all findings, categorizing them as follows:

   - **Resource issues:** This includes issues related to personnel, medication, and equipment—whether missing, malfunctioning, or unusable due to the provider's unfamiliarity with the device.

   - **Process issues:** This includes issues related to workflows, policies, or procedures that do not work as anticipated in the clinical setting.

   - **Facility or space setup concerns:** This includes issues that impair effective, efficient, and safe patient care or teamwork.

   - **Clinical performance gaps:** This includes issues related to cognitive and technical skills of clinical personnel that may be a focus for inservice, orientation, or future simulation-based training.

7. Engage appropriate stakeholders to prioritize the risk of each finding using an appropriate FMEA risk-prioritization tool. Then finalize the report of all findings. Distribute the final report to those responsible and accountable for taking action to mitigate the identified patient-safety risk.

FMEA tools are covered elsewhere in this book. In addition, you can visit http://www.ihi.org and http://www.jointcommission.org for examples of FMEA tools.

CASE EXAMPLE

The Problem

How did we know we were ready to safely care for hospitalized patients in our new hospital for women and newborns before we opened for care? After 5-plus years of designing, building, and developing written processes and systems for workflow, we wanted a realistic test of the many complex interactions involved in putting new patient care teams in a new building with a new patient population and new workflow processes. Finding weaknesses through trial and error with real patients seemed an unacceptable alternative, especially as we seek higher reliability.

Our Project Aim

Test clinical systems in the new setting after construction was completed but before opening for patient care using *in-situ* simulation to identify, prioritize, and address potential safety threats.

Measures

- Number of latent safety threats (LSTs) identified
- Self-reported ratings on confidence, self-efficacy, and preparedness for opening from participants and leaders, before and after simulation
- Post-simulation survey ratings from participants on effectiveness and safety of simulation

Methods

Six months before the opening date for the inpatient side of the hospital, the simulation center team met with key administrative and clinical leaders to assess their priorities for testing and to ensure their commitment to supporting resources for the project. Key questions driving the needs assessment were as follows:

- What is new or different compared to the way we do things currently?
- What are the top-priority patient-care units and clinical processes to test?

Based on their prioritization of top concerns for testing, we designed two different formats for our simulation series:

- **Virtual unit:** The new neonatal ICU (NICU) was a unit of private rooms rather than an open ward, as used with previous NICUs. Given this significant change, it would be important to test systems for a nurse inside a patient's room to communicate with the rest of the unit, particularly in an emergency.

Our simulation, therefore, consisted of a virtual unit—11 simulated patients being cared for in the unit simultaneously over the course of 1 hour followed by a 2-hour debriefing. These simulations occurred over 3 days.

- **Worst day in the life:** Priority concerns from women's services leaders included testing units that were new to our hospital (for example, labor and delivery) as well as responsiveness to clinical emergencies for a laboring mother moving through the different patient-care locations. To test those systems, we developed a simulation format in which the same patient moved from one care location to another within the hospital, experiencing a series of activities, procedures, and critical events. The simulation consisted of 3 days of simulation and three simulated patients, each day taking a different patient through four scenarios and debriefings.

Outcomes

As a result of these system tests, we discovered over 100 LSTs, all of which were resolved or had contingency planning in progress before the hospital opened. Some examples were as follows:

- **Resource issue:** Planned quantities on unit of urgently needed meds like magnesium sulfate and surfactant were insufficient for true clinical emergencies. Corrected before opening.
- **Facility issue:** Computer workstations mounted on articulating arms for convenient nurse charting interfered with the ability of code-team personnel to access the patient during an emergency. Arms were removed from all NICU rooms, and workstations were repositioned before opening.
- **Systems issue:** Some essential team members responding to an emergency were unable to access (badge in to) unit. All departments were re-evaluated for access, and security clearances were corrected before opening.
- **Clinical performance:** Some staff were unaware of the new procedure for transporting infants on bubble CPAP. Education was incorporated into the final pre-opening staff orientation.

Outcomes related to the confidence and preparedness before and after the simulation were interesting. Immersed simulation participants (usually front-line clinical staff) were less confident that they were prepared to safely care for patients in the new facility before the simulation but much more confident afterward. On the other hand, leaders and observers were much more confident before the simulation but less confident afterward. Although we don't know why this happened, it is possible the leaders became more aware of potential issues they had never imagined by observing the simulation. Either way, the simulation proved to be a catalyst for both groups to address any remaining or previously unrecognized loose ends to ensure a successful and safe opening!

Simulation-Based Solution Testing with Rapid Cycle Improvement

What Is It?

This refers to the use of high-fidelity clinical simulation in repeated cycles to test changes or potential solutions for process weaknesses before implementation in a real patient-care setting. Simulation is conducted within the widely accepted rapid-cycle improvement model (Plan-Do-Study-Act, or PDSA) to solicit ideas for improving and then retest until satisfied with the results. This type of simulation can be conducted in a center or *in situ*, depending on the scope of the project. An example of this method would be testing a new central line maintenance bundle before implementation to determine whether it works within your culture, people, and environment.

How Can It Help an Organization Build High Reliability?

This approach addresses the following tenets of high reliability:

- **Preoccupation with failure:** This approach demonstrates a preoccupation with failure by validating that a new or revised process actually works in a clinical environment before conducting training and implementing it in real patient care. This can help leaders identify and address unrecognized weaknesses, failures, and latent safety threats in the process in a proactive fashion rather than waiting to see how it works in a real clinical setting after implementation.

- **Reluctance to simplify:** Quality problems are often approached with a simple, one-size-fits-all, "best-practice" solution. By using the "Sim-as-PDSA" methodology, alternative approaches to a complicated process, algorithm, or workflow can be thoroughly tested, tweaked, and retested in a simulated clinical environment before arriving at the final solution to be implemented.

- **Deference to expertise:** Solutions are generally developed after an adverse event or near miss encountered by front-line providers who may or may not be involved in follow-up as the solutions are being developed. This methodology engages individuals who routinely navigate the complexities of front-line care along with leadership experts to plan, simulate, evaluate, revise, and simulate again to get to the best solution.

How Do You Do It?

You design the simulation activity as a curriculum based on the principles of the rapid-cycle improvement model:

1. **Plan:** Assemble the appropriate stakeholders. Then identify the problem, aims for improvement, proposed solutions, and measures of success for improvement. Finally, develop the plan for simulating the proposed solutions (refer to the section "Overview

of Healthcare Simulation"), including scheduling appropriate clinical participants and qualified observers.

2. **Do:** Conduct the simulation.

3. **Study:** Debrief participants and observers to identify both what worked well and any concerns.

4. **Act:** Determine what changes are to be made to plan for next scenario.

5. **Repeat:** Repeat the PDSA approach on the same or different day, incorporating the suggested changes into the scenarios.

CASE EXAMPLE

The Problem

Due to the increasing complexity and acuity of obstetrical patients, severe maternal morbidity is on the rise. One of the leading causes of maternal morbidity and mortality is post-partum hemorrhage (PPH). Effective management of PPH requires the immediate and coordinated response of an interprofessional team and timely escalation to mass transfusion protocols (MTP) for a variety of interventions to occur within a very short time frame. Our organization wanted to ensure that new protocols and algorithms developed in conference rooms and offices were actually tested and refined in a near-real (simulated) clinical environment before finalizing and initiating hospital-wide training.

Our Project Aim

Test proposed PPH management algorithms to identify changes needed and refine procedures before service-wide training and implementation.

Measures

- Number of changes identified in existing protocols/algorithms before house-wide training
- Post-simulation survey ratings from participants on effectiveness and safety of simulation

Methods

Support was received from operational leadership for an interprofessional team of up to 25 front-line staff members and leadership observers from 10 different departments to participate in one full day of simulations. The day consisted of three high-fidelity obstetric hemorrhage simulations that were conducted in the actual clinical setting *(in-situ)*. Each simulation was followed by a facilitated debriefing in nearby conference rooms. Participants and observers were asked to evaluate (study) the degree to which the proposed algorithms worked effectively in near-real life and give suggestions for improvements. Suggestions were then prioritized and incorporated into subsequent simulations for evaluation, congruent with PDSA methodology. At the end of the day, clinical leaders synthesized all findings, then made decisions on changes to be made to the originally proposed algorithms.

Outcomes

Along with a much-improved understanding by all departments of how their individual workflows affected the overall team and the patient, three key changes in the protocol were identified and implemented:

- A mass transfusion protocol (MTP) button was added to the automated smart panel in each room, which would automatically activate the departments required to respond in the event of mass transfusion needs.
- Code and MTP nursing roles and zones in the protocol were modified to more efficiently support interventions needed.
- A new role for a dedicated recorder was added to better keep up with blood loss and notifications to the team.

Participants favorably rated the effectiveness of the simulation in improving their approach to management of PPH. In the 2 months following the simulation, staff throughout the hospital were trained on PPH and the refined procedures for management. After their training, 85% of staff and physicians participated in a series of simulation-based scenarios to practice their role in the management of PPH.

Simulation-Based Just-in-Time/Place (JITP) Training and Clinical Rehearsals as an Adjunct to RCA

What Is It?

Simulation-based just-in-time/place (JITP) training involves the use of simulation as an embedded practice that is no longer an extra but rather is integrated into work expectations for all clinicians to improve their performance and patient-care outcomes through frequent training and rehearsal opportunities. Simulation-based JITP training occurs in very close timing and/ or location to when and where the actual clinical encounter being simulated may take place. This strategy enhances the ability to meet rapidly emerging or changing patient-care or provider needs, either before or after patient-safety events occur. When used in conjunction with a simulation-based clinical rehearsal, focus is on using simulation to rehearse rare, unusual, or complex situations before they happen, or before a provider must perform an unusual, high-risk, or complex procedure. An example might be rehearsing the coordination of surgical teams involved in the separation of conjoined twins.

How Can It Help Organizations Build High Reliability?

This approach addresses the following tenets of high reliability:

- **Preoccupation with failure:** Healthcare providers must be constantly vigilant to changes in healthcare that affect the provision of patient care—new therapies, changing technology, and unique patient conditions. Complacency is a threat to patient safety. By using simulation-based JITP with clinical rehearsal before high-risk or low-frequency procedures or situations, providers can improve performance and outcomes.

- **Sensitivity to operations:** Clinical rehearsals, especially when incorporated into day-to-day operations at the unit level, can improve situational awareness and provider recognition of unsafe conditions or practices. The just-in-time format enables a unit to individualize the timing and content of the rehearsal to meet the specific provider or patient need and can lead to improved performance and outcomes when part of routine preparation for care. By targeting CRM skills as part of just-in-time simulation, the specific members of the team on duty that day can practice teamwork skills in high-risk situations.

- **Commitment to resilience:** Simulation-based JITP can be used in conjunction with root cause analysis (RCA) to transform a reactive culture into a forward-looking one that solves problems before they occur or escalate. By incorporating the routine use of clinical rehearsals aimed at the primary causal factors for the safety event into everyday practice, simulation can help transition lessons learned into early recognition and prevention.

How Do You Do It?

Here's how this process works:

1. Engage all levels of stakeholders to assess their level of commitment to the project. Include formal leaders who will have the authority to support the project and encourage participation at the unit level.

2. Identify unit priorities or quality goals that need to be practiced. If using simulation as an intervention following an RCA, several key priorities might have already been identified, which provides a good starting point for just-in-time simulation.

3. Find the right space for unit simulations. A location highly accessible, on the unit, and/or close to everyday patient care is ideal. If space is not available, consider incorporating mobile equipment to bring the simulation to the providers.

4. Identify simulation experts from like clinical disciplines that can both perform the simulation and debrief afterward.

5. Develop tools for collecting and documenting findings. Given the time pressures associated with *in situ* simulation, the debriefing in this setting is by necessity brief and concise. Scripted debriefing questions aimed at uncovering knowledge and performance deficits as well as system issues are used to try to gather specific information from the providers participating in the scenarios. By using a scripted and standardized debriefing format, critical components are covered in a relatively short time frame.

6. Conduct the simulation. Then document all findings, categorizing them as follows:

   - **Cognitive objective(s):** What was the learning objective for the simulation? Was it met? For example, did the group recognize impending respiratory failure and respond appropriately?

   - **Behavioral objective(s):** How well did the team perform together and follow CRM principles? For example, were team roles clearly identified and followed? Given the time restraints of the just-in-time training, often only one or two CRM principles are discussed.

   - **Technical objective(s):** What task or skill was needed to successfully accomplish the simulation objective? An example would be proper bag/mask ventilation in the respiratory failure scenario.

   - **Systems issues:** Was a personnel, medication, equipment, or process issue identified in the simulation? As an example, during the simulation, there may have been missing or malfunctioning equipment, or a provider error with a device.

7. Follow up with appropriate stakeholders to communicate any system threats identified as a result of the simulation so that action can be taken to mitigate the identified patient-safety risk.

CASE EXAMPLE

The Problem

An RCA in a high-risk area demonstrated a need for increased training and practice in early recognition of deteriorating patients, management of critical events, and team skills training. This area also had a growing population of high-risk patients as well as an increased incidence of codes compared to other acute care areas.

Our Project Aim

Our aim was to provide high-fidelity, just-in-time simulations on this high-risk unit at regular intervals (twice a week to start) to improve patient safety and team skills as evidenced by an increase in the number of rapid response team (RRT) referrals and a decrease in incidence of codes by 25% over the next year.

Measures

- Days between codes
- Number of RRT calls
- Scores on safety attitudes questionnaire before project began and 1 year after

Methods

With full institutional support, including medical and nursing leaders on the unit, we converted an underused treatment room into a dedicated, full-time simulation room. We then installed high-fidelity simulation equipment and supplies. We collaborated with the simulation center for support with equipment, curriculum, study design, and database development. Using simulation-trained educators and debriefers, we developed just-in-time scenarios, objectives, and outcomes, as well as a database to log all activity and objectives. Next, we oriented all staff to simulation, the mannequin, and the simulation room. As we started, we quickly realized the scenarios would need to be revised to capture more just-in-time cases. Most scenarios were developed just before the event to account for all the patient's current factors, including vital signs, labs, etc., instead of the already-developed scenarios. A scripted debriefing style was used to streamline the process and allow for easier tracking for quality-improvement purposes.

Outcomes

- After the first year of twice-weekly scenarios, the incidence of RRTs increased by 60%.
- SAQ scores improved with regard to physician-nurse teamwork, collaboration, and work environment like being part of a large family.
- Most recently, the unit has gone more than 18 months without a cardiopulmonary arrest!

COMMON QUESTIONS

Following are two common questions regarding simulation:

- **I want to use one of these simulation methods to improve quality and patient safety in my organization. How do I get started?**

  - Healthcare simulation is increasingly a professional practice community, with its own art and science. It is a powerful tool that enables us to achieve previously elusive goals. However, if not practiced in accordance with current best practices and standards, it can also cause harm—particularly to a culture of safety. If you want to incorporate simulation into your quality-safety toolbox and you are not trained in current standards and practices for healthcare simulation educators, it is essential that you partner with a trained simulationist before initiating any of these projects. Alternatively, you can get formalized training from an accredited institution on how to implement healthcare simulation.

■ **How do I obtain institutional/leadership support to start a healthcare simulation program aimed at improving patient safety?**

■ The literature is growing with reports of the positive impact of simulation-based efforts on quality of care and patient safety. Review these findings (many are cited in this chapter's reference list) and compare them with your own organization's top patient safety and quality concerns. Does your organization have similar concerns? If so, begin building the case for how simulation can provide a new and much-needed tool for addressing those concerns in your organization. Don't hesitate to network with leaders from other simulation programs or other patient-safety departments who use simulation. The Society for Simulation in Healthcare (SSH) is a great resource with a robust website (http://www.ssih.org). Becoming a member of this organization provides access to even more resources and networking groups. Your goal is to communicate to your leaders the value of adding simulation to their patient-safety program, and it will be essential to find one or more leaders with appropriate authority and influence to become champions for healthcare simulation in your organization.

SUMMARY

Using healthcare simulation as an advanced quality improvement tool is an innovative and effective method for improving patient safety. Immersing clinical providers in high-fidelity scenarios with debriefing allows a unique method for examining and mitigating the latent safety threats inherent in healthcare systems that result in errors and harm to patients. A framework outlining three types of simulation that specifically target HRO principles has been offered in this chapter, along with "recipes" and case examples for readers' reference in translating to their own clinical setting.

KEY POINTS

■ Healthcare simulation is increasingly being used as an innovative quality-improvement and patient-safety tool within hospital settings. Using simulation in conjunction with traditional quality-improvement strategies such as FMEA and PDSA results in a more powerful tool for improving high reliability in an organization.

■ Effective simulations are designed and facilitated by trained simulationists and consist of the following key elements:

■ **Scenario:** A realistic situation in which participants are immersed

■ **Simulator:** A physical space, equipment, mannequins, and/or humans used within the scenario to replicate real life

- **Experience:** The multi-sensory experience of participants in the scenario followed by reflective learning during a post-scenario debriefing

- Ineffective teamwork and communication have been reported to be the leading contributor to medical errors and patient harm. Teamwork and communication are difficult skills to practice and improve through conventional means of education. Simulation is a unique and powerful tool for learning about, practicing, and improving communication and teamwork, especially in critical and complex clinical situations.

- Effectively designed simulation-based interventions directly support the following HRO concepts:

  - **Preoccupation with failure:** Scenarios immerse participants in error-prone situations and expose previously unrecognized factors that contribute to failure. Post-scenario debriefings encourage individual and organizational learning about how to prevent errors. The net effect is greater anticipation (and subsequent removal) of precursors to potential failure.

  - **Reluctance to simplify:** Hospitals are complex interactive systems. Using clinical simulation to examine all the moving parts, verify assumptions, and correct course and practice until perfect enhances understanding and avoidance of errors.

  - **Sensitivity to operations:** Engaging front-line personnel in clinical simulations—sometimes even in their own actual clinical settings—enables you to identify what is really happening (as opposed to what you *think* is happening) on the front lines of healthcare.

  - **Commitment to resilience:** After an analysis of errors, simulation can be incorporated into action plans to practice and refine skills and processes designed to prevent future errors. In addition, ongoing simulation-based clinical rehearsals or just-in-time simulation training can spread lessons learned and increase everyone's vigilance and responsiveness to precursors for error.

  - **Deference to expertise:** Simulation methodology depends on the engaged participation of subject matter experts at every phase of development and implementation to achieve the degree of realism needed to attain its goals—and subject matter expertise is relative to what is being simulated. A key principle in simulation is that everyone participates, everyone speaks up, and everyone's contribution is equally valued in the interest of learning and eliminating preventable harm to patients. Simulation is truly a team sport.

ACKNOWLEDGMENTS

The authors would like to acknowledge our physician partners, especially Dr. Jennifer Arnold, medical director of the Texas Children's Simulation Center, for their contributions to our work in developing the use of simulation as a tool for promoting HROs.

REFERENCES

Andreatta, P., Saxton, E., Thompson, M., and Annich, G. (2011). Simulation-based mock codes significantly correlate with improved pediatric patient cardiopulmonary arrest survival rates. *Pediatric Critical Care Medicine, 12*(1), pp. 33–38.

Chassin, M. R., and Loeb, J. M. (2013). High-reliability health care: Getting there from here. *The Joint Commission.* Retrieved from http://www.jointcommission.org/assets/1/6/Chassin_and_Loeb_0913_final.pdf

Davis, S., Riley, W., Gurses, A. P., Miller, K., and Hansen, H. (2008). Failure modes and effects analysis based on in situ simulations: A methodology to improve understanding of risks and failures. In K. Henriksen, J. B. Battles, M. A. Keyes, and M. L. Grady (Eds.), *Advances in patient safety: New directions and alternative approaches* (Vol. 3). Rockville, MD: Agency for Healthcare Research and Quality.

Dieckmann, P., Gaba, D., and Rall, M. (2007). Deepening the theoretical foundations of patient simulation as a social practice. *Simulation in Healthcare, 2*(3), pp. 183–193.

Draycott, T. J., Crofts, J. F., Ash, J. P., Wilson, L. V., Yard, E., Sibanda, T., and Whitelaw, A. (2008). Improving neonatal outcome through practical shoulder dystocia training. *Obstetrics and Gynecology, 112*(1), pp. 14–20.

Edmondson, A. (2014). *Teaming: How organizations learn, innovate, and compete in the knowledge economy.* San Francisco, CA: Jossey-Bass.

Gawande, A. (2011). Cowboys and pit crews. *The New Yorker.* Retrieved from http://www.newyorker.com/news/news-desk/cowboys-and-pit-crews

Hunt, E. A., Duval-Arnould, J. M., Nelson-McMillan, K. L., Bradshaw, J. H., Diener-West, M., Perretta, J. S., and Shilkofski, N. A. (2014). Pediatric resident resuscitation skills improve after "rapid cycle deliberate practice" training. *Resuscitation, 85*(7), pp. 945–951.

Institute for Healthcare Improvement. (n.d.). Rapid response teams. Retrieved from http://www.ihi.org/topics/rapidresponseteams

Institute of Medicine (IOM). (1999). To err is human: Building a safer health system. Washington, DC: The National Academies Press.

The Joint Commission. (2005). *Failure mode and effects analysis in healthcare: Proactive risk reduction* (3rd ed.). Chicago, IL: Joint Commission Resources.

Morey, J. C., Simon, R., Jay, G. D., Wears, R. L., Salisbury, M., Dukes, K. A., and Berns, S. (2002). Error reduction and performance improvement in the emergency department through formal teamwork training: Evaluation results of the MedTeams project. *Health Services Research, 37*(6), pp. 1553–1581.

Palaganas, J. C., Maxworthy, J. C., Epps, C. A., and Mancini, M. E., Eds. (2014). *Defining excellence in simulation programs.* Philadelphia, PA: Lippincott Williams & Wilkins.

Reason, J. T. (1997). *Managing the risks of organizational accidents.* Farnham, UK: Ashgate Publishing.

Rudolph, J. W., Simon, R., Dufresne, R. L., and Raemer, D. B. (2006). There's no such thing as a "non-judgmental" debriefing: A theory and method for debriefing with good judgment. *Simulation in Healthcare, 1*(1), pp. 49–55.

Scholtz, A. K., Monachino, A. M., Nishisaki, A., Nadkarni, V. M., and Lengetti, E. (2013). Central venous catheter dress rehearsals: Translating simulation training into patient care and outcomes. *Simulation in Healthcare, 8*(5), pp. 341–349.

Seymour, N. E., Gallagher, A. G., Roman, S. A., O'Brien, M. K., Bansal, V. K., Andersen, D. K., and Satava, R. M. (2002). Virtual reality training improves operating room performance: Results of a randomized, double-blinded study. *Annals of Surgery, 236*(4), pp. 458–463.

Society for Simulation in Healthcare (SSH). (n.d.). Full accreditation. Retrieved from http://www.ssih.org/Accreditation/Full-Accreditation

CHAPTER 15

HIGH RELIABILITY IS BUILT WITH RESILIENCE

Julie Benz, DNP, RN, CNS-BC, CCRN

Most readers of this book are searching for ideas and suggestions to improve their healthcare organization's quality services. Unless you are a student on the quest of knowledge for academic reasons alone, you are likely interested in viable examples and best practice models that may be useful within your system and practice.

All healthcare organizations have active quality departments that perform many process-improvement projects and regulatory readiness functions. Organizations are overwhelmed with regulatory measures that dictate care delivery models and use reimbursement incentives to gather an audience within every healthcare facility. These departments may vary in size and focus. Some consist of one employee or have dozens of regulatory experts, depending on the data-collection and analysis needs of the populations served. It is popular to have researchers, nurse scientists, and trained certified abstractors within the quality departments.

In addition to minimal regulatory requirements, specialty accreditations are often desired, purchased, and achieved. These have blossomed in number within the last decade. Some popular examples of specialty accreditations include The Joint Commission (TJC) Certification of Comprehensive Stroke Centers, TJC Healthcare Facilities Accreditation Program, as well as Trauma Level I accreditations by the

> It is not the strongest of the species that survive, nor the most intelligent, but the one most responsive to change.
>
> —Charles Darwin

American College of Surgeons and State Departments of Health or Chest Pain Center by the Society of Cardiovascular Patient Care.

Achieving excellence in care delivery, safety, patient satisfaction, and outcomes seems to reach beyond regulatory minimal standards and accreditations, however. The desire for high-quality, measurable, and tangible excellence is prevalent among the leadership of most healthcare facilities and systems of care. This causes quality experts to search for excellence examples outside the healthcare industry. The industrial and manufacturing industries have offered many approaches to excellence. Change management, lean process improvements, and Six Sigma programs were introduced and translated for healthcare delivery services. These tools received robust support for guiding complex problem-solving with highly effective and reproducible solutions (Chassin and Loeb, 2011).

National organizations—public and private—such as the Institute for Healthcare Improvement (IHI), the Robert Wood Johnson Foundation, and the Agency for Healthcare Research and Quality (AHRQ)—support research, randomized controlled studies, and meta-analysis to produce white papers, or landmark reports, designed to galvanize efforts for high-quality care. These reports expose clusters of excellence in care delivery in healthcare systems or facilities with variable performance. Adaptation of industrial methods of quality performances contributed to growth and process improvement models. Still, the goal of ongoing, consistent performance at the level of superior excellence remained elusive and out of reach for healthcare delivery systems.

The desire for consistent performance at peak safety levels appeared to exist only in organizations that simply must avoid extreme hazards or in industries that could not accept any level of error for public safety. These organizations have become a super-set of best practice performers, referred to as high reliability organizations (HROs). Examples to emulate were found at nuclear power plants, among commercial airlines, and on the flight decks of aircraft carriers (Chassin and Loeb, 2011).

HRO PRINCIPLES

HROs are defined as high risk, dynamic and hazardous, and nearly error-free (Weick and Sutcliffe, 2007). As mentioned, best examples come from the commercial airline industry, nuclear energy plants, and defense systems such as aircraft carriers. Healthcare systems and facilities benefit from an understanding of the culture within these organizations and may emulate the methods used to remain error-free. Industry leaders have dissected, analyzed, replicated, and planned their efforts based on the culture of HROs.

As discussed, HROs ascribe to the following principles:

- Preoccupation with failure

- Reluctance to simplify

- Sensitivity to operations

- Deference to expertise

- Commitment to resilience

PREOCCUPATION WITH FAILURE AND RELUCTANCE TO SIMPLIFY

HROs display a preoccupation with failure. As a result, the identification of errors is paramount to HROs. Most errors are systems errors. Errors occur when sound processes are eroded by those who skip steps, impede workflow, or speed up tedious, technical processes. Workarounds are often a result of a desire to simplify. A *workaround* is a behavior that temporarily overcomes a barrier or bypasses a problem in the system (Debono et al., 2013). When an organization accepts the creation of workaround techniques, a culture of "normalization of deviance" exists (Safer Healthcare, 2015). A gradual shift in standards becomes acceptable, and the norm becomes the nonstandard, or workaround, behavior.

The Challenger space shuttle is an example. The O rings on the Challenger were designed to function only at temperatures greater than 56 degrees. The shuttle had been launched successfully during progressively lower temperatures; therefore, out-of-range testing had become the "new norm." The morning of the Challenger launch, the temperature on the launch pad was 29 degrees. The O ring was compromised, resulting in the Challenger explosion. This occurred, in part, because it had become acceptable to work around the manufacturer's guidelines for the O rings (History, n.d.).

Breaking points such as these may be caused by the following:

- Illogical workflow patterns

- Leadership pressure to meet ever-compressed timelines

- Rewards for productivity that may be achieved by skipped steps

- Inner-team competitiveness

- Workflow variance created by team members

Teams at breaking points may frequently employ workarounds that temporarily lead to safety but hide problems in the system. This leads to a less safe environment in the long run (Debono et al., 2013).

HROs strive for event-free processes and look for warning signs of variance or possible trouble. Very small warning signs are seen as red flags. These are used for insight into the entire system. Near misses or events that *almost* happen are red flags and are examined to prevent future system failures. Actual failure is not needed to identify a problem if the smallest hint of variance is subject to recognition and resolution before the failure causes an adverse event.

An example of this concept in healthcare is found in medication delivery. Medications are often stored by product—for example, all the furosemide (Lasix) may be stored in a designated area. But medication is offered in various strengths, volumes, and routes. If variable dose strengths are together in storage, the possibility of someone retrieving the wrong dose strength is very real. However, it is possible to use built-in systems that clearly identify dose, strengths, volumes, and routes. Proactive institutions review this regularly and design dispensing to limit error. Other solutions might be the establishment of silent zones around medication-dispensing machines to enhance concentration, barcoded medications, barcoded medication orders, and barcoded name bands. Workaround processes are eliminated, and time is allowed for multiple stop checks during medication delivery to reduce process decay. Routine observation of medication dispensing helps to identify near misses. Efforts made to ensure the accuracy of medication delivery are considered energy well spent to prevent adverse medication events from reaching a patient and causing harm.

Anticipation of variance becomes the norm at HRO facilities. Catching failures early involves a preoccupation with failure (Weick and Sutcliffe, 2007). This should be discussed across departments connected to the function under scrutiny. If variance is anticipated, unexpected events are less disruptive, and the focus may shift to containment of the error or potential variance.

Even if events are planned and practiced, more risk may exist than realized. The expectation of "what should happen" might limit observation of variance, causing people to find only what they expect to find. Routines do not allow for novel events, and people could lose flexibility in activities. Strict plans or algorithms will dictate expectations. An example found in hospitals is multiple casualty training. Emergency department and emergency medical service providers often engage in drills to practice the sudden arrival of high-volume, high-acuity patients. Participants master triage so that patients can be categorized into predetermined groups for treatment and care. In discussion after real events with high-volume, high-acuity admissions, most staff report that they were extremely focused on their role and did not see or experience the bigger picture. Their task became the most important event, and their focus was extreme. So, in effect, although the drills included needed activities, they failed to capture the thought process in the manner of an actual event.

Human factors play into the reliability of processes. Crew resource management (CRM) began with pilots and the National Aeronautics and Space Administration in 1979 (Safer Healthcare, 2015). Workshops were held to review every airline crisis from the last decade. Pilots, on simulators, retrained for those disasters, which included crisis decision-making skills. The focus was on the safety, efficiency, and morale of those forming work teams. Pre-flight briefings and post-flight debriefings plus measurements of crew performance were successful in reducing in-flight crisis. In 2000, the Institute of Medicine (IOM) reviewed CRM techniques and publications on The Joint Commission (TJC) website (Pronovost et al., 2009) and validated the need for team training. Knowing that human performance depends on health, attitude, knowledge, emotions, cognitive ability, circadian rhythms, and other personality traits increases the challenge of teamwork. Teams may be stronger than individuals for error-free processes. Improved process design and technology assistance are crucial in safety-focused environments. The health of the healthcare team, working in cohesive patterns, may allow the mention of error potential and the admission of human error.

SENSITIVITY TO OPERATIONS AND DEFERENCE TO EXPERTISE

HROs solicit input from all levels of the organization. Information about working situations and processes is highly valued. No employee's thoughts about safety issues are considered irrelevant. If suggestions for improvements are sought out from the employees who do the job, the entire team is successful.

A multitude of healthcare examples abound. One success story is found in patient registration. In the modern emergency department, patients with time-sensitive health issues must move quickly through admission and into treatment. Patients experiencing stroke, heart attack, or severe trauma should quickly be seen by physicians and receive diagnostic or treatment interventions. The first hour of these diagnoses is often called the *golden hour*, and clinical management of this period can predict outcomes and mortality rates. As cardiologists often say, "time is muscle." However, historically, the average admission, including the collection of all demographic data, took between 10 and 15 minutes. A wise admissions clerk designed the top line of the admission screen to receive two sources of patient identification and to issue a registration number. The patient could then begin to receive care. The registration number was later matched with past medical records and facilities visits. This was not a "John Doe" number, which had to be converted to obtain old medical records. By the time the patient had the CT scan, arrived in the catheterization lab, or had diagnostic blood testing, the old medical record was linked and available for safer planning of patient care.

The HRO culture of communication would embrace this suggestion, from any level of employee. There is no rank or pretense about speaking up to improve the product, safety, or the system. Frequent team meetings to share thoughts and allow for suggestions abound. Even messages that originate from the bottom up to challenge traditions are given an opportunity to be expressed, to be heard, and possibly be operationalized.

In the early 2010s, news shows captured footage of factory workers stopping assembly lines if the product appeared questionable. The idea that each team was as strong as its weakest link was strengthened and celebrated. Around the same time, tech companies in Silicon Valley had developed think tanks and oasis lounges and had dedicated time to groups of workers to collaborate in free thought and creative manners. The value of thoughts arising in every corner of the workplace was beginning to take hold and mature.

HROs are seen as creative and innovative. No idea is too small to consider, weigh the risk-benefit ratio, and pilot. This is not to spur capricious decision-making but to encourage some risk-taking with simple solutions to common problems. An example from a patient care delivery system is problem-solving regarding home medication use during a patient's stay in hospital. Fixed income patients are at risk of suffering following hospitalizations due to costs. The pharmacy item markup is industry standard but causes strife. Typically, elderly males take one prescription medication per decade of life. So a 74-year-old male, retired, living on Social Security and savings, may use seven prescription medications prior to hospitalization. These may be expensive. If the patient is permitted to bring these medications to the hospital for self-administration, hundreds of dollars could be saved per admission. A clinical pharmacist could inspect the medication, reconcile the prescription with the primary care provider, and supervise the patient application. Dosing errors or techniques can be noted. The patient need not endure a second bottle of expensive eye drops for glaucoma or eczema lotion.

COMMITMENT TO RESILIENCE

Reports of humans tolerating horrific natural events such as hurricanes and floods fill the news. People avidly follow stories about tsunamis and sinking cruise ships half a world away. Man-made tragedies also garner a strong reaction. When such events occur, people often experience initial pain, shock, and trauma, but move quickly to bounce back, recover, and continue with their lives. Shouts such as "Boston Strong!" rang across the Internet shortly after the Boston Marathon bombings in 2013. Often, news reports emphasize these post-event shows of strength rather than the horrific loss of life and limb.

Recovery after unpredicted personal tragedy confirms that it is human nature to recover, move forward, and be brave, as demonstrated by Olympic swimmer Amy Van Dyken after a traumatic spinal cord injury. Her commitment to walk again was a virtue attributed to an Olympic gold medal athlete. Once her focus turned to resilience, references were abundant in the news, Internet, social media, and personal discussions. Recovery and resilience are acknowledged as human traits.

Organizations have demonstrated resilience as well. Some examples include the direct fiscal lifesavers offered to the American automotive industry. Initially, the monies, known as "bailouts" (suggesting a very negative connotation), were not seen as useful, with so much funding on the line. The return to economic success and repayment of these hefty loans demonstrated resilience on the part of automotive firms, which worked hard to rebuild their organizations, products, and reputations. Currently, the same companies are facing safety violations and recalled sold items. The outcome of these events is not yet known. Will resilience prevail? The automotive industry is certainly not error-free.

Deliberately capturing resilience as a trait is the challenge for the healthcare industry. Resilience is a desirable trait, worthy of replication, although possibly elusive.

STRESSORS

According to Weick and Sutcliffe (2007), resilience consists of three components:

- The ability to absorb stress and continue to function

- The ability to bounce back from untoward events

- The capacity to learn from episodes of resilience

Stressors may appear in a variety of forms—for example, internal adversity from poor leadership decisions, stakeholder/board member pressures, inadequate supplies or equipment, lack of technical sophistication, and many more. (Anyone who has worked in a healthcare facility can list many more internal stressors!) External stressors come from regulations, competition from other facilities, third-party payment systems, available workforce, etc. (See Table 15.1.)

In addition to internal and external stressors, there are also predictable and unpredictable stressors. Examples of predictable stressors include budget deadlines and constraints, turnover of leadership positions, profit loss, and payer limitations. Modern healthcare organizations use strategies to predict stresses and define responses to mitigate outcomes. Each of these stressors has its own planned, predictable response. For example, stressors such as payer limitations may be managed ahead of time by negotiating insurance contracts.

TABLE 15.1 STRESSORS IN HEALTHCARE

	Internal Stressors	External Stressors
Predictable	Poor leadership decisions	Federal regulations
	Stakeholder pressures	Facility competition
	Board of directors pressures	Third-party payment systems
	Inadequate equipment/supplies	Salary adjustments
	Budget deadlines	
Unpredictable	Technical sophistication changes	Workforce availability
	Variation in census	Publication of events
	Hospital-acquired complications	Community support
	Variation in payer mix	Local legislation
	Payer contract variation	
	Leadership turnover rates	

 Less predictable but necessary changes were brought about by the new challenges in healthcare due to the Affordable Care Act. Healthcare institutions have needed to create solutions not previously imagined. Reimbursement is now based on quality outcomes and patient satisfaction. All care providers play a part in the success or failure of this new reimbursement program. Every employee is part of the solution. Still, planning and decision-making occur at the top levels of administration. Most hospitals have struggled to find unique solutions and have spent much administrative energy on achieving higher standards of care.

As mentioned, some stressors are less predictable. Examples include hospital-acquired infections (HAIs) and pressure ulcers. Historically, people viewed hospitals as places where they went to die. More recently, however, people's views of hospitals have evolved. Now, hospitals are seen as places of healing. Today, patients do not enter a hospital with the expectation of becoming more ill or feeling worse. The hospital, as a facility, is responsible for ensuring a complication-free recovery for patients, *without* an HAI or pressure ulcer. Unfortunately, whether this outcome is achieved is not necessarily within the control of the facility. For example, a patient with extremely unstable vital signs might not tolerate movement from side to side. These physiologic responses, coupled with low perfusion or circulation to the skin, could set the stage for skin breakdowns or pressure ulcerations. Yet the hospital remains responsible for the complications developed during the hospitalization.

Solutions and responses developed by hospitals have shown their resilience to address HAIs and pressure ulcers. Some solutions include the following:

- The development of new bed surfaces
- Positional alarms, which notify staff when time limits for a position are met
- Increased assessments
- Improved nutritional support
- Laboratory testing of albumin and pre-albumin to quantify the nutritional state
- Audits of skin complications
- Skin specialist consultations
- Quality data reporting for analysis and process improvement

All this attention, time, money, and focus have not eliminated the pressure ulcer issue. Still, the focus of patient care has shifted, and the outcomes are more free of complications than in the past. It is not an error-free process, and care is far from perfect, but evidence of reduced complications is present.

RESPONSES TO UNTOWARD EVENTS

Resilience implies that after being faced by a stressor, the person or organization will recover or return to the previous state or level of performance. Often, however, a return to the previous state is not desired. Some events result in revolutionary change.

An example of this is the response to the violent attacks on the United States on September 11, 2001. The resilience shown by the nation permeated many aspects of society. Multiple layers of safety checks against terrorism emerged through various national and international organizations. Some of these safety measures are reported to have prevented further terrorism. Other responses included a surge in patriotism and an increased respect for the military. The impact was profound, and no one returned to the previous state.

Healthcare examples of resilience that surge to a new level may be found in patient safety at the point-of-care delivery (Riley, 2009). Two methods have been used to increase patient safety at the level of care delivery: developing interdisciplinary teams and improving process design. As an example, consider patient falls. To help eliminate them, organizations no longer limit the accountability for patient falls to nurses. Now, accountability for patient falls is shared by inter-disciplinary teams of care providers, including physicians, radiology, lab phlebotomists, physical therapists, and pharmacists. As a result, everyone is invested in the elimination of patient falls.

Process design changes have also been brought to bear on the issue of patient falls. These include the following:

- Assessment and risk stratification for fall risk on admission
- The addition of safety alarms to beds and chairs, which broadcast an audible sound when weight is removed from the surface
- Frequent toileting rounds to minimize the urgent need to empty bladders or bowels
- Keeping patient rooms free of clutter
- Hourly safety rounds to assess comfort, position, and other interventions

In addition to these process changes, most institutions require some documentation of when pa-tients are seen by care providers. Many facilities have clocks or numbers near the door, with the last time someone entered to provide care. Name tags can be used to electronically track door entry and patient contacts. Audible alarms can be set for when rounding for a patient is noted to have been infrequent. Technology continues to offer more assistance for the monitoring of patient position, patient needs, and contact with care providers. Data is collected and shared, usually on a monthly or quarterly basis.

All the data from this technology can overwhelm front-line managers. The use of electronics and the data created by them must be supported and valued at the highest levels of administration.

The importance of patient safety is now reflected in the larger values of healthcare facilities, and teams take any variance seriously. Many facilities now identify falls with injury as major events, allowing resources to determine the weakness of the care delivery or of the barriers created to prevent that fall. A team may meet to debrief or recap the fall situation, and all possible controls on the variables are reinforced and reviewed.

In an effort to respond to untoward events, many organizations practice error mitigation. HRO organizations often use resiliency to return to a steady state. This is common on aircraft carriers. If an issue is found on the landing deck, the only goal is to return to a safe landing or take-off deck. The same happens in healthcare facilities.

Correctly identifying a patient is critical. If a patient is misidentified, tragedy could result. No one wants to give medication to or draw blood for diagnostic testing from the wrong patient. Caregivers can take some simple steps to ensure patients are identified correctly:

- Rather than asking the patient, "Are you Mary Smith?" bedside caregivers should change the question to, "Could you please state your name for identification?" This eliminates the chance that a patient could respond to the wrong name.

- Ask the patient to state his or her birth date. This prevents, for example, a patient named Anthony who answers to Tony from responding to the name Tommy.

Using technology can also help. Most facilities use barcoded name bracelets, medication packaging, and medication administration records.

This seemingly would result in error-free drug administration, yet some caregivers may skip steps to save time or reduce redundancy. When asked, one nurse reported she felt "silly" asking for the patient's name on the fourth medication delivery of the day. Some caregivers affix the patient's hospital bracelet—which features the patient's name, date of birth, medical record number, physician, and allergies—to the bed rather than the patient, which could result in an error. Skipped steps and condensed processes open the opportunity for system failures. When technology, training, policies, and expectations are ignored, the result is a tenuous and unsafe patient-care situation.

ERROR MITIGATION

It's important to recognize that errors may exist. The HRO response is to correct the error before an adverse outcome affects safety. This seemingly implies the recognition of errors prior to occurrence. Opportunities for pre-event recognition occur with risk identification tools for falls, orientation and training on barcoded medication delivery, hard stops in computer technology (that is, the program will not proceed without certain data elements or the documentation of certain process steps), and the identification of allergies on admission to the facility.

After an error has occurred, palliation becomes a priority. First, you must identify and define the exact nature of the problem (Safer Healthcare, 2015). All employees should be aware of the steps needed to identify problems. Those involved in the event should share the story of their experience to accurately identify the exact moment the error transitioned from potential to real. Teams must also recognize the obstacles faced in problem identification.

For best results, organizations should do the following:

- Eliminate fear of retribution from leadership.

- Recognize negative implications of performance.

- Recognize the urgent need for reconstruction of the process prior to the error.

- Acknowledge the possibility of bias and watch for evidence of personal or professional bias in error mitigation.

HROs verify conclusions and determine event etiologies (Safer Healthcare, 2015). They look for cues and solicit input from those directly involved in events. Taking the incident back in time and creating a review to the realistic level of occurrence will be the fastest data-collection method and eliminate interpretation and assumptions. The method requires the inclusion of all present at the original event and works effectively if done quickly after the occurrence.

An HRO healthcare facility must offer error-free care over a long period of time. The care may not be perfect, but errors with complications should be avoided.

BUILDING RESILIENCE THROUGH TEAM TRAINING: CARDIAC ARREST EVENTS

Creating an HRO and demonstrating resilience involves taking small steps over time. This allows the value and culture of safety to permeate all layers of the work teams in healthcare. Examples can be found in all healthcare delivery departments. The in-depth example used here will be the development, use, and review of healthcare emergencies—in this case, the cardiac arrest of a patient, which is a high-risk, low-volume experience.

Response to cardiac arrest must be swift and accurate. Where some clinical disasters are always handled by the same team members—for example, complications during a surgical case would involve the surgeon, anesthesiologist, and perioperative team members in the room—a cardiac arrest event may occur in a variety of patient care areas, arise at different times of day, and have specific roles filled by a number of different care professionals. This emergency commonly results in death if interventions are not applied in a precise sequence that reflects up-to-date, current knowledge. The outcome of a cardiac arrest event depends on the ability of the physicians, staff, and other providers to focus on the situation and respond with near perfect execution.

PLANNING FOR CARDIAC ARREST EVENTS

Preparing for cardiac arrest situations involves long-term planning. The facility must plan to have the necessary equipment and medications immediately available throughout the facility. This is no small task. The usual method is to collate the equipment and medication on a crash cart, with several identical carts placed throughout the facility. To secure these supplies, it is typical to have a cart that locks—that is, the cart has a removable locking system to protect the integrity of its contents. The lock is broken or opened for immediate use during a cardiac arrest event. Most carts have a defibrillator device on the top of the cart. Other equipment is secured to the outside of the cart, such as a back board, IV poles, and electrode patches for heart monitoring.

Because the cart is locked to secure the contents, most staff are not familiar with the contents of the cart and cannot locate needed items rapidly. Staff often report that their lack of familiarity with the cart creates stress and interferes with smooth processes during cardiac arrests. To address this, drawers should be labeled with contents, and a menu of cart contents should be displayed on the outside of the cart. Finally, checklists should be provided to show that the contents have been assessed daily. Figure 15.1 shows an example.

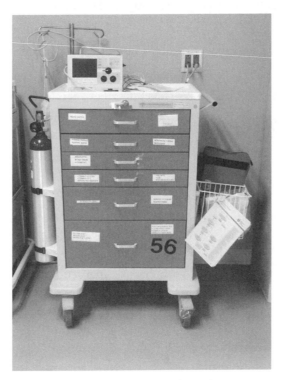

Figure 15.1   Labeled crash cart.

Team members should have assigned roles for the event (Field et al., 2010). These are likely to include the following:

- **Medical director:** This person is responsible for the overall orders and interventions selected.

- **Lead RN:** This person is responsible for the activities, documentation, closed-loop communications, and supervision of all care. This often involves assessing chest compression rate and depth.

- **Respiratory therapist:** This person is responsible for achieving and maintaining the airway, assisting in intubation, and securing the endotracheal tube.

- **At least one to two other RNs:** These team members will handle medication delivery, defibrillation, and the assessment of vital signs and central pulse (usually obtained at the femoral artery).

Other team members may include the following:

- **Clinical pharmacist:** This person is responsible for medication preparation, labeling, and handoff to the med delivery RN.

- **Chaplain or spiritual care provider:** This person is responsible for caring for the patient's family.

- **Other staff from the area:** These team members will handle the procurement of supplies.

- **Observers, students, and orientees:** These people will have learning roles.

TRAINING FOR CARDIAC ARREST EVENTS

The training and preparation for any cardiac arrest situation is usually done through the American Heart Association, using the 2010 evidence-based standards for care (Field et al., 2010). The course is designed for physicians, nurses, respiratory therapists, and other healthcare providers (clinical pharmacists, operating room technicians, emergency medical providers, etc.). This course, called Advanced Cardiac Life Support (ACLS), contains text with details and content, a pre-test, a rhythm strip test of cardiac rhythms identification, and demonstrations at several skill stations. Classes are initially 2-day events with re-certification every 2 years. Other lifesaving certifications include pediatric events, neonatal events, obstetrics, trauma-specific events, heart surgery–specific, and so on. For this example, we will focus on ACLS standards and clinical event training.

The key aspect of any ACLS application is the recognition of clinical symptoms. Because these events may take place outside the emergency department or critical care unit, all staff must recognize and offer initial lifesaving support. The recognition and initial steps in resuscitation are collated into a program called Basic Life Support (BLS), also based on American Heart Association standards (Berg et al., 2010). There are many versions of these steps—Life Saver, Basic Rescue, and so on. All follow the same premise: the identification of a catastrophic set of symptoms including loss of pulse, loss of consciousness, absent or ineffective breathing efforts, or choking.

RESPONDING TO CARDIAC ARREST EVENTS

The BLS responder role includes an assessment for the aforementioned symptoms, activation of the emergency response system, and commencement of chest compressions. As simple as it is to list those few steps, completing them successfully is complex. This author's facility, located in Lakewood, Colorado, has developed a system that acknowledges the importance of the first five minutes of BLS. The American Heart Association (n.d.) purports the fast and accurate use of BLS weighs heavily on the outcome of any ACLS efforts:

- **Minute 1:** The responder has 1 minute to identify the absence of a pulse or breathing. If absent, 2 minutes of chest compressions are begun while the responder calls for help. The call for help may be a shout to others during chest compressions or use of a wall button for code blue (the name used for cardiac arrest at this facility). An overhead page is sent immediately to notify ACLS responders.

- **Minute 2:** Nearby responders have 1 minute to bring the crash cart and connect the automatic external defibrillator (AED). (AED use is taught in BLS.) Chest compressions continue.

- **Minutes 3–4:** The AED requires the placement of large pads on the bare-skinned chest for monitoring rhythm and delivering defibrillation shocks. The computer in the AED interprets the heart rhythm. If needed, it gives a shock to the chest. It then reanalyzes the heart rhythm. The AED will advise if chest compressions should continue. The back board is placed under the patient for improved chest compression circulation.

- **Minute 5:** ACLS responders are at the bedside, continue chest compressions, and begin more sophisticated interventions, medications, etc.

A cardiac arrest event can last from 1 minute to hours, depending on the patient response to therapy and the original catastrophic event. Following cardiac arrest events is a debriefing (Berenholtz et al., 2009) or discussion period. This facility calls them *post-code pauses* (PCPs). During the PCP, team members spend 10 seconds in quiet thought about the patient and about their experience. This occurs whether the patient responds well or does not survive. (Surviving patients often need critical care attention, in which case the PCP can be moved outside the patient room.) Next is a discussion of technical skills. Or, the discussion may start with the responder's experiences. The order is not as important as the identification of things that went well and of things responders could have done differently. On occasion, participants will bring their own feelings into focus; that type of discussion is allowed within the time parameters of the PCP.

POST-CODE PAUSE

The modern emergency department (ED) is the quintessential master of resiliency. The physicians, nursing staff, support staff, and emergency medical services staff move rapidly from one patient to the next. The team endures unimaginable human circumstances but is quickly prepared for and awaiting the next admission, the next patient, and possibly the next tragic encounter. Having roots in combat wars, EDs function with military precision. Care is distributed to those with greatest need (triage systems). Situations are rapidly assessed and prioritized. The military concept of debriefing is well-known to these practitioners and is used in cases of mass casualties, horrific outcomes, and pediatric experiences.

St. Anthony Hospital is a busy, urban, private Level I trauma center just west of Denver. Nestled close to the mountains, it is commonly involved in the rescue of locals and tourists. The first civilian air rescue team, Flight for Life, calls St. Anthony its home base. When asked to pilot a debriefing system after cardiac resuscitation, the St. Anthony ED developed a gentle, more desirable format of the post-code pause (PCP). Critical incident teams existed for robust tragedies (public shootings, weather disasters, etc.); the PCP was designed to assist with significant emotional events, which occur with some regularity for the ED team. The PCP is designed specifically to address technical, procedural, and emotional reactions to emergency situations.

The pilot development team was led by a unit-based educator, Heather Liska, RN, CEN; a hospital chaplain, Elizabeth Phelan; and the unit-based council. Staff surveys were completed before the first PCP, at 6 months, and at 1 year. The following is a brief listing of results of the survey at the 6-month point:

- **What is your perception of support of leaders and peers during code blue?** 25% improvement

- **Do you perceive compassion fatigue and homage is paid to the patient?** 40% improvement

- **Do you still talk about code blue events 24 hours later?** 56% in agreement

- **Do you feel pressure to return to work immediately after a code blue?** No change in response from first survey

Figure 15.2 shows the PCP format. This activity has gained recognition from the American Nurses Association, Emergency Nurses Association, and Colorado Nightingale Nursing Awards for Excellence. It is unique in ED care and worthy of replication to build a more resilient team. As one staff nurse said of this program, "We reboot our machines and it is time for us to reboot ourselves."

Date:_____ Age of Patient:_____Type of Alert:_____

**Names of all staff members involved in post-resuscitation pause

_____   _____   _____

_____   _____   _____

**After the Event, everyone pauses for 10 seconds of silence to either remember the life of the person or celebrate the success of the Code Blue

What did the team do well?

What intervention(s) do you wish had or had not been offered?

How is your satisfaction with the equipment and medications available?

Where can we grow and improve?

How did we support the family (if they are present)?

How are you doing after the code?

What do you need to be able to be successful for returning to work right now?

Additional comments or concerns:

Figure 15.2 Sample PCP record.

Best success will be achieved if consistent criteria are used in the consideration of a PCP experience, such as having one immediately after a code blue. Strong unit-based champions for the project have increased its acceptance and kept the process on care providers' radar. Our chaplains are at every code blue event and have become a consistent and strong support system. The PCP has evolved in the ED from a post-code pause to a post-event pause, as some non-code events prompt an equally emotional response from staff. The PCP is now applied throughout acute care services, critical care areas, and perioperative services.

PCP builds resilience in the most prized asset of every hospital: care providers, from physicians to nurses to clinical pharmacists to chaplains to support services. The process takes just 10 minutes but enhances staff emotional resources, reduces ED post-traumatic stress among staff, and allows staff to express their private respect for life's most fragile moments. If it can work effectively in a busy urban emergency department, it can work wonders for other caregivers.

CARDIAC ARREST MOCK DRILLS

To prepare for cardiac arrest events, team members can participate in mock drills. The mock drill should involve all the same complex steps as the real event. An extra step of briefing the staff often precedes the mock cardiac arrest drill (Bandari et al., 2012). During this briefing, staff involved in the drill receive information about the drill. Role expectations and crisis steps are reviewed. Staff are informed of the time and place of the drill. All on-duty staff are asked to participate, as they would if the drill were a real event. The mock cardiac arrest team has the same membership as a real event. When the drill begins, notification is also done in the same manner as a real event. A wall button may notify operators to overhead page "Code blue in room 444" as well as trigger a beeper group of predetermined responders.

The event itself is scripted with a high-fidelity mannequin, preprogrammed for the clinical scenario. If the event involves a regular resuscitation mannequin, a rhythm simulator should be employed. The goal is to have the team respond to the clinical presentation of the mannequin and not involve the educational staff with questions and prompts. To conserve resources, the events are between 5 and 10 minutes in length. The clinical events follow the more complex algorithms for ACLS (Field et al., 2010) and include starting IV access lines, medication delivery, airway maneuvers, and vital-sign assessments.

The greatest gain of this (or any) mock drill is found in the debriefing phase. Structured toward the positive, debriefings capture the strengths of the teamwork (Bandari et al., 2012). If the technology is available, it is best to video the event. Then allow the team to watch the action and verbally report their impressions and findings.

If developing mock drills is too cumbersome, build resilience through the debriefing of highly complex, high-risk, low-to-moderate volume real-life events.

IDENTIFYING RESILIENCE

The concept of resilience in healthcare delivery is important for any healthcare organization that wants to become highly reliable. Although the concepts are tangible, will you know resilience when you see it? Are you able to help others identify resilience? Everyone works each day hoping to offer the best level of service possible and not create harm. Reducing errors and being mindful of potential errors is important. But are we demonstrating resilience?

Organizations interested in employing the concept of resilience can perform a resilience gap analysis. Ponder each question in Table 15.2. You may find the team needs some redirection based on the indicators and choose to build the team before completing the gap analysis.

TABLE 15.2   RESILIENCE QUALITIES TO CONSIDER DURING GAP ANALYSIS

Indicator	Present	Absent	Follow-up	Outcome Date
Are red-flag events or near misses reported?				
Is reporting of red-flag events rewarded?				
Is reporting of red-flag events punished?				
Have suggestions for workflow come from the workforce level?				
Do team meetings allow time for open discussion of everyday processes?				
Is the workflow regularly observed and evaluated by others?				
Does this process allow variation or is variation open to safety issues?				
Have there been action-based mock drills?				
Are pre-process briefings used regularly?				
Are post-event debriefings used regularly?				
Is crew resource management training used with supervisors, and are the results monitored by leadership?				
Are stressful events (with or without outcome errors) reviewed?				

continues

TABLE 15.2   RESILIENCE QUALITIES TO CONSIDER DURING GAP ANALYSIS   (CONTINUED)

Indicator	Present	Absent	Follow-up	Outcome Date
Are predictable workforce stressors identified and mitigated?				
After error mitigation, is the goal to return to a steady state?				
Are the values of safety supported on every level of the workforce?				
Is data about safety, productivity, or processes well-known and understood at all levels of the workforce?				

The gap analysis will involve a review of the entire facility, not just one event. It would behoove leadership to invest in planning and development of skill sets to enhance resilience. Response to change is a feature of every business, and having resilient characteristics will become essential. Not all changes affect healthcare delivery positively. Most will want their hospital, organization, department, or service to move fluidly through change. HROs can offer their attributes to healthcare for adoption and employment. It is up to healthcare organizations to reduce vulnerabilities by enhancing resilience.

SUMMARY

Excellence in healthcare delivery, patient safety, satisfaction with care delivery systems, and positive outcomes are common findings in HROs and valued by all care delivery systems. To accomplish these goals, healthcare facilities benefit from mimicking key properties: preoccupation with failure, reluctance to simplify, sensitivity to operations, deference to expertise, and commitment to resilience.

The development of resilience can involve a deliberate set of processes, which includes emphasis on recovery after an event, development of planned reactions to events, early identification of stressors causing events, encouragement of the development of new solutions, and measuring the return to previous performance steady states (usually with data from process improvement activities). Future avoidance of system errors requires mitigation of errors. Often-used techniques for mitigation of errors include team training, mock event practice sessions, post-event debrief session(s), and the development of improved processes from the knowledge gained from past experiences.

Resilience is a valued and common attribute of organizations, groups, and countries. Because all events cannot be controlled, people move forward after untoward events through a regathering of spirit, focus, and responses. These same activities, applied to healthcare facilities, lead care delivery teams toward resilience and HRO positive outcomes.

KEY POINTS

- Resilience is an important key component of HRO processes. These processes include preoccupation with failure, reluctance to simplify, sensitivity to operations, deference to expertise, and commitment to resilience.

- Resilience can be developed using the following processes:

  - Attention to recovery after an untoward event or outcome

  - Development of planned reactions to events that value system error redevelopment

  - Identification of stressors (both predictable and unpredictable)

  - Creative encouragement of the development of new solutions by staff involved at focal event level

  - Measuring many processes that impact outcome and using data to evaluate progress

  - Setting goal(s) upon return to steady states of performance

  - Developing team training

  - Using mock events in practice sessions

  - Using post-event debriefing

  - Emphasizing improvement gained from knowledge of previous experiences

REFERENCES

American Heart Association. (n.d.). About CPR and first aid. Retrieved from http://cpr.heart.org/AHAECC/CPRAndECC/AboutCPRFirstAid/UCM_473210_About-CPR-FirstAid.jsp

Bandari, J., Schumacher, K., Simon, M., Cameron, D., Goeschel, C. A., Holzmueller, C. G., ... Berenholtz, S. M. (2012). Surfacing safety hazards using standardized operating room briefings and debriefings at a large regional medical center. *Joint Commission Journal on Quality and Patient Safety, 38*(4), pp. 154–160.

Berenholtz, S. M., Schumacher, K., Hayanga, A. J., Simon, M., Goeschel, C., Pronovost, P. J., ... Welsh, R. J. (2009). Implementing standardized operating room briefings and debriefings at a large regional medical center. *Joint Commission Journal on Quality and Patient Safety, 35*(8), pp. 391–397.

Berg, R. A., Hemphill, R., Abella, B. S., Aufderheide, T. P., Cave, D. M., Hazinski, M. F., ... Swor, R. A. (2010). Part 5: Adult basic life support 2010 American Heart Association guidelines for cardiopulmonary resuscitation and emergency cardiovascular care. *Circulation, 122*(18 suppl. 3), pp. S685–S705.

Chassin, M. R., and Loeb, J. M. (2011). The ongoing quality improvement journey: Next stop, high reliability. *Health Affairs, 30*(4), pp. 559–568.

Debono, D. S., Greenfield, D., Travaglia, J. F., Long, J. C., Black, D., Johnson, J., and Braithwaite, J. (2013). Nurses' workarounds in acute healthcare settings: A scoping review. *BMC Health Services Research, 13*(175).

Field, J. M., Hazinski, M. F., Sayre, M. R., Chameides, L., Schexnayder, S. M., Hemphill, R., … Vanden Hoek, T. L. (2010). 2010 American Heart Association guidelines for cardiopulmonary resuscitation and emergency cardiovascular care science, part 1: Executive summary. *Circulation, 122*(18 suppl. 3), pp. S640–S656.

History. (n.d.). Challenger disaster. Retrieved from http://www.history.com/topics/challenger-disaster

Pronovost, P. J., Goeschel, C. A., Olsen, K. L., Pham, J. C., Miller, M. R., Berenholtz, S. M., … Loeb, J. M. (2009). Reducing health care hazards: Lessons from the commercial aviation safety team. *Health Affairs, 28*(3), pp. w479–w489.

Riley, W. (2009). High reliability and implications for nursing leaders. *Journal of Nursing Management, 17*(2), pp. 238–246.

Safer Healthcare. (2015). Effecting positive cultural change…crew resource management. Retrieved from http://www.saferhealthcare.com/crew-resource-management/crew-resource-management-healthcare/

Weick, K. E., and Sutcliffe, K. M. (2007). *Managing the unexpected: Resilient performance in an age of uncertainty* (2nd ed.). San Francisco, CA: Jossey-Bass.

CHAPTER 16

SUSTAINING A CULTURE OF SAFETY: STRATEGIES TO MAINTAIN THE GAINS

Cynthia A. Oster, PhD, MBA, APRN, ACNS-BC, ANP

"To Err Is Human," the landmark report by the Institute of Medicine (IOM) (1999), calls on all healthcare organizations to create a culture of safety. A safety culture is unlikely to be fully realized without organizational commitment. The "Keeping Patients Safe" report (IOM, 2003) reaffirms the importance of creating and sustaining a culture of safety. A culture of safety permeates an organization and is expressed in the beliefs, attitudes, and values of employees. In addition, it is present in an organization's structures, practices, policies, and procedures. Sustaining a culture of safety "begins with the human aspects but must reach beyond the underlying systems and processes, which enable resilience and error prevention in today's complex healthcare environment" (Blouin and McDonagh, 2011, p. 450).

Resilience describes organizations that achieve very high levels of safety despite high risk, difficult tasks, and constantly increasing pressures (Woods, 2006). These high reliability organizations (HROs) have extremely strong and resilient cultures of safety that pervade the organization. According to Woods (2006), resilient organizations are proactive and adaptive. They do not wait for an adverse event to occur to make corrections. Resilient organizations focus on

> Lasting change starts from the inside out— by first changing individuals... By changing individuals, we can really change organizations.
>
> —*J. Stewart Black and Hal B. Gregersen*

anticipating changes in risk and plan for adaptation. Critical to patient safety is engineering resilience into workflows and patient care processes, enabling healthcare organizations to move toward high reliability. Sustaining a culture of safety requires organizational resilience—commitment to vigilance for potential errors and the detection, analysis, and redressing of errors when they occur.

The purpose of this chapter is to describe how resilient organizations can sustain a culture of safety by creating an organizational culture of personal and professional accountability. This chapter begins by discussing organizational vulnerabilities, related performance, and adherence to regulations and policies across the care continuum as a rationale for sustaining a culture of safety. The chapter provides a framework for change needed to sustain a culture of safety and concludes with strategies to maintain the gains within a culture of safety.

FRAMEWORK FOR ORGANIZATIONAL CHANGE

Healthcare delivery is complex, and complexity affects the quality and safety of care given to patients (IOM, 2010). Complexity is often cited as the reason for significant unpredictability and variation in clinical outcomes within a healthcare organization (IOM, 1999; IOM, 2001; IOM, 2003). According to Wachter and Shojania (2004), most errors are made by good people working in a dysfunctional system. That means making care safer depends on strengthening the system to prevent or catch errors made by fallible people. The complexities of our healthcare systems provide a combination of individual events that can create a disastrous outcome, thus creating a perfect storm.

 Perfect storm is an expression that describes an event where a rare combination of circumstances drastically aggravates a situation (Fields, 2006). The term is also used to describe an actual phenomenon that happens to occur in such a confluence, resulting in an event of unusual magnitude.

Improving and sustaining a culture of safety requires organizational commitment and an understanding of the fundamental dynamics of leading strategic change. Creating and sustaining a culture of safety requires every healthcare organization to change, and change is very difficult. Black and Gregersen (2008) identify the core problem: Changing individuals and the mental maps inside their heads must happen before you can change the organization. (Mental maps guide daily behavior.) Successful strategic change requires changing individual mental maps and behaviors first, because they *are* the organization. Changing individual behaviors creates an organizational culture of personal and professional accountability that can sustain a culture of safety.

Regulatory bodies specify quality indicator expectations. Practitioners perceive care as "excellent," whereas regulatory agencies expect "perfect" care. Culture affects performance. To keep patients safe, an HRO must be willing and ready to change.

To change an organization, you must break through your own brain barriers and help those around you do the same—one step at a time. Black and Gregersen (2008) identify three barriers that stand in the way of changing an organization:

- Failure to see
- Failure to move
- Failure to finish

Sustaining change requires the organization to understand the nature of each of these barriers and make the needed adjustments to break through each barrier. Overcoming these three barriers provides a conceptual framework for changing an organization and sustaining a culture of safety. This section offers tools and strategies for overcoming each of the three barriers as an approach to sustaining a culture of safety.

FAILURE TO SEE → WHAT DO WE SEE?

Sustaining a culture of safety requires an organization to see the need for a culture of safety. Simply put, "we fail to see because we are blinded by the light of what we already see" (Black and Gregersen, 2008, p. 24). Even when opportunities or threats stare the organization in the face, the organization fails to see the need to change. Organizations fail to break through this barrier not because they do not know it is there but because they underestimate its strength. Organizations underestimate its strength by failing to take the time or make the effort to fully understand the nature of the barrier.

Failure to see stems from the blinding light of past successful mental maps (Black and Gregerson, 2008). Mental maps determine how people see the world of work, guiding their daily steps and behaviors. Organizations place themselves at the center of the universe with everything else revolving around them. Thus, our view tends to be distorted, inflating what we know and deflating what we do not know. The organization believes that what it knows is everything and what it does not know is nothing. Consequently, the organization sees the future the way things have been seen in the past—in other words, "this is the way we do it here." The longer these successful maps have been in place and been effective, the more difficult it is to see beyond the working mental maps and identify the need for change—even when opportunities or threats stare people in the face.

A culture of safety requires the organization to move from "failure to see" to "what do we see?" Transparency and system and individual accountability characterize seeing organizations. Shifting from a culture of blame to one of transparency enables organizations to recognize that often, the system has created a series of small failures that unfortunately places the individual at the end of a series of mistakes. James Reason's Swiss cheese model of medical errors depicts this scenario (Reason, 1990). Healthcare has traditionally treated errors as failings on the part of individual providers, reflecting inadequate skill or knowledge. The holes in the Swiss cheese represent a failure. Each hole or failure, by itself, doesn't cause the catastrophic result. But when a combination of failures occurs—when the holes line up—the cumulative effect can. The systems approach takes the view that most errors reflect predictable human failings in the context of poorly designed systems.

Rather than focusing corrective action on punishment or remediation, the systems approach seeks to identify situations or factors likely to give rise to human error. This approach also seeks to change the underlying systems of care to reduce the reoccurrence of errors or minimize their impact on patients. Transparency helps an organization identify all the layers of an error so the organization can see and apply appropriate solutions. The seeing organization focuses on plugging the holes in the Swiss cheese. It is a transparent organization with system and individual accountability that works to prevent the failure to occur in the first place. Things like redundant systems and the use of checklists plug the holes in the Swiss cheese!

 Use of Just Culture, discussed elsewhere in this text, helps the organization to determine both system and/or individual accountability. This process moves an organization from "failure to see" to "what do we see?"

The organizational challenge is to break through the barrier of "failure to see." If an organization fails to see threats or opportunities, it will not make needed changes. To break through this barrier, people must see that the environment has changed and that the old "right thing" is now wrong. A variety of tools can be used to help organizations see that the environment has changed:

- **Clinical audit and feedback:** Audits, which can be either prospective or retrospective in nature, are a crucial component to improving quality and safety. They also provide baseline adherence to guidelines of care (Patel, 2010). Observation of actual or real-time clinical practice can be part of the auditing process. An audit, coupled with feedback, generally leads to small but potentially important improvements in professional practice (Ivers et al., 2012). (See Figure 16.1.)

Elements of Documentation	1	2		3	4	5	6			
	Admit RN Akin Man (Applies to Element 1)	Braden Risk Assessment q24th or per unit standard		Skin Assessed qShift	Manage Moisture on Skin qShift	Optimize Nutrition and Hydration qShift	Minimize Pressure		Were elements 2–6 met?	What correction measure was done?
	Skin Man Completed upon arrival to the unit?						Turning Documentation per Guidelines throughout shiftmize Pressure	Mattress/Bed Documentation qShift		
Patient Name and PA Number	Yes/No	Yes/No	Score	Yes/No	Yes/No/NA	Yes/No	Yes/No/NA	Yes/No/NA	Yes/No	
Totals	(NA)									

Guidance for completing Audit Tool:

■ Skin Man completion should be done on admission and/or transfer into your unit. If skin is intact, a physician signature is not required.

■ Manage Moisture on Skin: If the patient is not incontinent and does not have moisture concerns, audit response may be NA (not applicable).

■ Optimize Nutrition & Hydration: Is there documentation regarding eating, TPN, tube feedings, supplements, etc.?

Figure 16.1 Example of a documentation audit tool.

■ **Open discussion of events:** Interviews with those involved can give clarity to various issues and complexities surrounding a situation.

■ **Peer review:** Peer review empowers staff to identify clinical practice learning needs, improve quality and safety of care for patients, and build trust, which helps create transparency (Boehm and Bonnel, 2010; Garner, 2015).

■ **Adverse event analysis:** Adverse events are injuries resulting from medical care (Wachter, 2012). Analysis of these events can create system changes that reduce the likelihood of the adverse event occurring again.

■ **Cause and effect:** The Ishikawa cause and effect diagram, also called a fishbone diagram, is commonly used to illustrate how various causes and sub-causes create a particular effect on an outcome. This strategy can help organize the causes contributing to a complex problem (Warren, 2008).

■ **RAPID decision making:** This process involves the right people in the decision-making process, which means more impact. This tool trades ambiguity for transparency (Huggett and Moran, 2007).

■ **Lean tools:** Process mapping helps reveal the flow of events from a customer perspective. Simple lean tools and techniques such as Gemba walk, visual control, daily huddles, standard work, value stream mapping, error proofing, and A3 thinking can be used to improve quality and safety (Imai, 2012; Kimsey, 2010; Simon and Canacari, 2012).

People will not change unless they see the need for change. Data is a powerful tool to help an organization see the need for change. One tool that is very helpful to clarify "what do we see?" or where to focus is the adverse event analysis tool. The tool in Figure 16.2 has the following categories, which a manager reviews against the event:

■ Policy

■ Staffing

■ Equipment

■ Other external factors

■ Communication

■ Unit or organizational impact

■ Conclusion

■ Improvement plan

Patient Name		Occurrence ID	
Patient PA#		Date of Occurrence	
Clinical Leader		Date Assigned	
Unit		Date Analysis Due	
Severity			
Summary			

Instructions:

1. The clinical leader facilitates the analysis by answering the questions below and returns to the Patient Safety Manager within one business day. DUE
2. Upon completion of the analysis, use the Just Culture algorithm to determine if event involves individual accountability, systems error, or both Please complete the following:
   a. For Individual Accountability — The clinical leader determines action then completes individual monitoring log. Submit to Patient Safety Manager upon completion.
   b. For Systems Errors — The clinical leader initiates the PDCA worksheet. The Patient Safety Manager will provide guidance, as necessary.
      i. Analyze the information captured under "Explanations" to identify the appropriate actions to prevent this event from happening in the future.
      ii. Record these actions on the PDCA worksheet.
3. The PDCA worksheet becomes the proposed plan of action and should be returned to Patient Safety Manager within 3 business days. DUE
4. The clinical leader presents the plan at the next scheduled Patient Safety Council meeting (fourth Wednesday 8-10 am) for review and approval. DUE

Question	Response		Explanations
1. Were policies, procedures and/or protocols followed?	Yes	No	
	If "No" explain →		
2. List the relevant policies, procedures, and/or protocols that governed actions before, during, and after the event.			
3. Was the expected level of care met?	Yes	No	
	If "No" explain →		
4. Were the policies, procedures, protocols in place, andcare delivered at the time of the event adequate to have prevented the event from happening?	Yes	No	
	If "No" explain →		
5. Related to policies, procedures, protocols, and/orexpected level of care, did staff have appropriate:			
☐ Training/education?	Yes	No	
☐ Competency?	Yes	No	
☐ Orientation?	Yes	No	
	If "No" explain →		
6. Did the capability and number of staff match the acuity and number of patients?	Yes	No	
	If "No" explain →		
7. Were non-facility staff involved in the event?	Yes	No	
	If "Yes" explain →		
8. Did equipment performance contribute to this event?	Yes	No	
	If "Yes" explain →		
9. What other external/ environmental factors contributed to this event?			
10. What role did communication play in this event? For example, shift-to-shift handoffs, MD-to-RN communication, MD-to-MD communication,			
11. Could this event happen in another department?	Yes	No	
	If "Yes" explain →		
12. Additional comments:			
13. Conclusion based on analysis:			
14. Improvement plan:	☐ Individual Accountability (Provide follow-up monitoring document to Patient Safety) ☐ Systems Error (Complete PDCA document)		

Figure 16.2   Sample adverse event analysis form.

This tool uses the basic concepts of human factors science in safety event review to assist in getting to the main causes of the issue—in essence, a root cause analysis (RCA) at the unit/manager level (The Joint Commission [TJC], 2013). It is then reviewed at a committee level for group action.

FAILURE TO MOVE → HOW DO WE MOVE?

Sustaining a culture of safety requires an organization to move. "Failure to move" occurs even when smart organizations see the need to change or move to a culture of safety. Organizations fail to break through this barrier not because they do not know it is there but because new mental maps or processes are required to move to a culture of safety. It occurs because people are not motivated to go from doing the wrong thing well to doing the right thing poorly (Black and Gregersen, 2008). Breaking through "failure to move" requires the people within an organization to comprehend that the old right thing is now wrong and that the new right thing is now right and what they need to do.

Organizations will fail to move if the new right thing is not clearly identified (Black and Gregersen, 2008). "How do we move?" requires clear vision or direction to a specific goal or target. People will hesitate to move when the question "where are we going?" is clearly answered. The clearer the new vision, the more immobilized people can become. They often strengthen their resolve to continue to do the old right thing very well, refusing to do the new right thing poorly. The new mental map must answer the question "where are we going?" and identify the new right thing. Leaders must make the organization believe that the new mental map will route and guide everyone through the quagmire of doing the new right thing poorly to doing it very well.

Organizational change initiatives often fail because people fail to move even when they clearly see the need to move. "Failure to move" occurs because people do not believe in the destination, much less the route to get there, their ability to walk it, or that the journey will be rewarding. As a result, employees continue to be very competent at the old way of doing things and resist change for fear of appearing incompetent at doing the new thing right. For an organization to really get moving, employees must clearly see in their own minds where they are going, have the required resources to make the trip, and believe the desired destination is worth the journey.

A culture of safety requires an organization to move from a perspective of "failure to move" to a viewpoint of "how do we move?" To break through this barrier, people must travel a trail that will take them from doing the new right thing poorly to doing it well. It requires a clear target, the right capabilities and tools in place, and rewards for employees to believe that they can do the new right thing well. An assortment of tools can be used to help organizations navigate a trail that will take them from doing the new right thing poorly to doing it well. Organizations can move using the following tools:

- **Process improvement cycles:** Plan, Do, Study, Act (PDSA) is a systematic series of steps for gaining knowledge for the continual improvement of a process. Each step is repeated over and over as part of a never-ending cycle of continual improvement (The W. Edwards Deming Institute, 2015).

- **Evidence-based practice models:** These models tell us how to move good evidence into clinical practice to optimize patient outcomes. Various models have been developed and are often very different from each other. Each model has advantages and disadvantages that may make one more useful in an organization than another. Select one that works for your organization to systematically implement and continually evaluate the effectiveness of change over time (Oster, 2011).

- **RAPID decision-making sessions:** A group of individuals who review the issues and determine solutions in a short session assist in building momentum for a desired improvement (Huggett and Moran, 2007).

- **Lean tools:** These tools help eliminate waste, standardize work where appropriate, and use visual management boards to show progress in real time to help move a project forward (Kimsey, 2010; Simon and Canacari, 2012). (See Figure 16.3.)

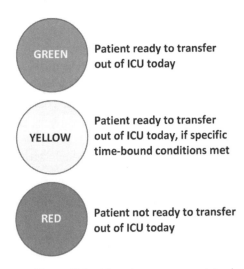

GREEN — Patient ready to transfer out of ICU today

YELLOW — Patient ready to transfer out of ICU today, if specific time-bound conditions met

RED — Patient not ready to transfer out of ICU today

Figure 16.3 Visual management tool.

FAILURE TO FINISH → ARE WE FINISHED?

Sustaining a culture of safety requires an organization to finish. Even when employees see the need and begin to move, they often fail to finish by not going far or fast enough for the change to ultimately succeed. The full impact of a culture of safety cannot be realized until the majority of individuals in an organization change. Quite simply, strategies to create and sustain a culture of safety will not make a difference until the majority of people think and act differently. A cultural shift to safety is an organizational change, involving hundreds if not thousands of individuals. It is impossible to implement overnight. It can take months or even years for the desired changes to ripple through an organization.

"Failure to finish" occurs because people get tired and lost during the time it takes to change. "People get tired because organizational transformation is fundamentally not about transforming the organization; it is about transforming the people who work in it" (Black and Gregersen, 2008, p. 86). Overcoming "failure to finish" requires large numbers of employees to shift their philosophical perspective from "seeing is believing" to "believing is seeing" (Black and Gregersen, 2008). Moving from a position of "failure to finish" to "are we finished?" requires employees to think and behave differently. This in turn requires trust in the organization. Employees who trust the organization willingly follow the desired route to the target destination. Those who do not trust the organization will deviate from the desired route.

The journey to organizational transformation is long and tiresome. People get worn out along the journey. They do not remember where they started, know where they are now, or know where they are going. Uncertainty sets in. The mental map detailing the desired route is not clear. Consequently, employees feel lost, lack the desire to press ahead, and fail to finish.

A culture of safety requires an organization to pass from a place of "failure to finish" to the position of "are we finished?" "Failure to finish" happens because employees get tired and lost, and therefore do not go fast or far enough. Finishing requires champions to reinforce and encourage fellow employees when the change occurs and to applaud early successes. It requires monitoring progress and communicating individual and collective improvement. Organizations can finish using the following tools:

- **Champions:** Identify local or unit-based individuals with a passion for the project (Pronovost et al., 2013).

- **Reward accountability:** Focusing on the positive tends to yield healthy competition and more buy-in (Roberts, Madsen, Desai, and Van Stralen, 2005).

- **Just-in-time training:** This is usually done peer to peer to create awareness in the moment and can be a powerful teaching tool.

- **Just Culture:** Understanding system and individual accountability creates fair practice for behavior changes (Reason, 1997).

- **Rank order of error reduction strategies:** We continually ask ourselves to move up the rank order of error reduction strategies whenever possible (Carroll, 2009).

■ **Lean safe design principles:** Lean safe design principles help us make the work visible. How can we have the work tell us what to do? How can we create checks beyond our humanness? How can we standardize the work using evidence-based knowledge to improve our care to our patients? Knowing this should yield positive outcomes for our patients and streamline value-based care (Womack and Jones, 2003). (See Figure 16.4.)

How good we need to be drives the finish line. While all of us would agree we want perfection, you have to choose priorities. Priorities that have the most potential for negative impact on patients might be the ones you target for a higher compliance and/or improvement rate. The level of priority helps to determine the type of measure to use. If an organization strives for near perfection, then performance means 3.4 defects per million opportunities, or 99.9999% adherence as defined by Six Sigma (Kubiak and Benbow, 2009; Six Sigma, n.d.). If process improvement is the objective, a target of 96% is acceptable (Pronovost et al., 2013). A regulatory priority may require 90 to 100% adherence depending on the standard you are working to improve. Identify your goal and select the most robust improvement measurement strategy to achieve your goal.

Porter Adventist Hospital Admission Criteria to the ICU
Defined by the Society of Critical Care Medicine and approved by PAH MEC

Critically ill, unstable patients that need intensive treatment and monitoring that cannot be provided outside of the ICU:

1. Mechanical ventilation
2. Non-invasive (BiPAP) ventilation (which by definition is an unstable ventilator mode) for patients with acute respiratory failure (CHF, pneumonia, COPD). *Specific exceptions: patients on BIPAP for OSA, and chronic respiratory failure on BiPAP at home.*
3. Vasoactive drips:
    a. Any anti-hypertensive drip including nipride, nicardipine
    b. Any pressor including dopamine, levophed, vasopressin, neosynephrine
    c. Any medication, per policy 165.368: IV Medications: Guidelines for Use, that can only be given in a critical care area of the hospital
4. Medication drips with potential CNS side effects:
    a. Benzodiazepines
    b. Narcotics (exception is comfort care)
5. Medications or drug overdose with high risk hemodynamic, neurological (GCS < 9) or respiratory compromise
6. Sepsis with organ dysfunction
7. Intensive monitoring:
    a. DKA due to insulin drip, frequent blood glucose monitoring, or pH < 7.20 with unstable vital signs
    b. Atrial fibrillation with uncontrolled ventricular response, with unstable vitals/symptomatic
    c. Post cardiac arrest, CPR, or cardioversion (if cardioversion done for hemodynamic instability)
    d. Altered MS, any cause, with high risk for respiratory failure, GCS 8 or less, acute unstable CVA, seizure/status epilepticus, intracerebral hemorrhage
8. Hemodynamic instability:
    a. Shock with hypovolemia, acute blood loss anemia, sepsis, cardiogenic
9. Metabolic derangements with high risk for complications including but not limited to:
    a. Sodium derangements (< 110 or > 170)
    b. Potassium derangements (< 2 or > 7 with EKG changes or cardiac instability)
    c. Alterations in glucose (refractory hypoglycemia or > 800) or calcium (> 15)
10. Post-operative patients requiring extensive nursing care or at high risk for complications listed above
11. Any patient deemed by the Attending physician to be at high risk of becoming critically ill in the next 12 hours

Figure 16.4 Lean principle of making the work visible via poster display.

STRATEGIES TO MAINTAIN THE GAINS

A culture of safety within an organization shows a commitment to consistently safe operations, encourages error and near-miss reporting, promotes interprofessional collaboration, and commits resources to address top safety concerns (Agency for Healthcare Research and Quality [AHRQ], 2014). Sustaining a culture of safety is needed if an organization is to be resilient, maintain gains, and sustain the success of an HRO (Hershey, 2015). Maintaining and sustaining gains requires organizational commitment to vigilance for potential errors and the detection, analysis, and redressing of errors when they occur. The following sections discuss organizational strategies to maintain gains in patient safety. These strategies encompass leadership, infrastructure and resource investment, data analysis and feedback, transparency, and professionalism and accountability.

LEADERSHIP

The commitment of leadership to safety is crucial to sustaining and maintaining gains in a culture of patient safety within an organization. "Words alone are an ineffective leadership tool" (IOM, 2003, p. 288). The commitment to a culture of safety is needed from all organizational leaders from the boardroom to the bedside, including management. Safety must be a priority from the very top of the organization to the newest member of the team to the person delivering services at the bedside.

The importance of governance to quality and safety must not be overlooked. Sustaining a culture of safety requires board engagement in quality and safety. For almost a decade, both the Institute for Healthcare Improvement (IHI) and the National Quality Forum (NQF) have sought to engage board leadership and called for hospital board members to focus on quality and safety (IHI, 2008; NQF, 2004). However, Jha and Epstein (2010) report that fewer than half of the boards surveyed in their study rated quality of care as one of their top two priorities, and only some reported receiving any training in quality. Boards should understand how serious the quality and safety issue is in healthcare, be educated on high reliability principles, and highly prioritize safety (Heenan, Khan, and Binkley, 2010; Joshi and Hines, 2006). Endorsement of a safety governance structure by the board of directors and leadership may be the single most important element needed to sustain a culture of safety (Hilliard et al., 2012).

Senior leadership commitment must be expressed by actions observable to employees. It is a challenge for leaders to move from a bureaucratic-autonomous structure to a transformational-interdependent structure that integrates reliable and consistent processes and procedures throughout the organization (Kerfoot, 2006). Observable leadership actions may include:

- Undergoing formal training to gain an understanding of safety culture and safety concepts (Hilliard et al., 2012)

- Ensuring that safety is addressed as a priority in the strategic plans of the organization (Shabot, Monroe, Inurria, Garbade, and France, 2013)

- Having facility-wide patient-safety policies and procedures that clearly articulate responsibility and accountability of employee performance affecting patient safety (IOM, 2003)

- Including safety as a priority meeting-agenda item (Shabot et al., 2013)

- Ensuring blame-free and non-punitive management responses to staff members reporting errors (Tschannen and Lee, 2012)

- Providing fair analyses of causes after near misses and critical incidents to create an environment of open communication regarding error reporting (Benn et al., 2009)

- Supporting, recognizing, and rewarding those achieving safety improvement goals (International Atomic Energy Agency [IAEA], 2006)

Research suggests that executive leadership directly affects safety climate and employees' perceptions of safety (Kelloway, Mullen, and Francis, 2006; Barling, Loughlin, and Kelloway, 2002). Leadership style—specifically transformational leadership—contributes to sustaining a culture of safety. Transformational leaders transform organizations by motivating followers to transcend their own self-interest to improve performance through organizational learning and innovation (Grant, 2012; Garcia-Morales, Jimenez-Barrionuevo, and Gutierrez-Gutierrez, 2012). A study by McFadden and colleagues (2015) provides empirical evidence that safety is connected to the chief executive officer's transformational leadership style and is related to continuous quality improvement (CQI) initiatives. A transformational leadership style has a positive association with both perceived safety climate and employee participation in safety (Clarke, 2013). Therefore, it is likely that transformational leadership practices of chief nursing officers contribute to achieving clinical quality and sustaining a culture of safety in an organization (Clavelle, Drenkard, Tullai-McGuinness, and Fitzpatrick, 2012).

Nursing leadership is essential for improving and sustaining a culture of safety (Kerfoot, 2010). Alignment of senior leadership, managers, and front-line bedside nursing staff is crucial to sustain a culture of safety in an organization. The leadership of nurse managers and bedside nurses contributes to patient safety. "It is only through consistency, collaboration, dialogue, and continued conversation between nurse managers that we will achieve excellence in patient safety" (Kerfoot, 2006, p. 274). Nurse managers at the unit level work to ensure consistency and reliability of processes and procedures between clinical units to decrease the risk of error. Nurse managers sustain a culture of safety by actively listening to bedside nurse suggestions for improving patient safety (Turunen, Partanen, Kvist, Miettinen, and Vehviläinen-Julkunen, 2013). Consequently, bedside nursing staff is engaged in a culture of safety and willing to report errors and learn from them without fear. In an HRO, leading and sustaining a culture of safety is both a shared responsibility and the individual duty of every member of the organization (Riley, 2009).

INFRASTRUCTURE AND RESOURCE INVESTMENT

Infrastructure and resource investment must support the priorities, goals, and strategic plans of the organization. This requires an executive team that is committed to investing resources to build the infrastructure to support quality and safety within the organization. Members of the organization at all levels must be engaged in the quality and safety infrastructure. A human factors engineer is an excellent support professional to help build and sustain internal structures to support a culture of quality and safety. Human factors engineering is a discipline that takes into account human strengths and limitations in the design of interactive systems that involve people, tools and technology, and work environments to ensure safety, effectiveness, and ease of use (AHRQ, 2014). Allocating budgetary resources for human factors engineers to focus on how systems work in actual practice with real human beings in place and then designing systems that optimize safety and minimize risk of error in complex environments helps sustain a culture of safety within an organization. Human factors engineers help to improve safety by using tools and techniques such as usability testing, forcing functions, standardization, and resiliency efforts.

The internal governance or committee structure of an organization should be designed to support quality and safety. For example, a quality and safety committee chaired by a clinical leader is a structure that links the senior executive team and direct care–level team within an organization. This committee provides oversight to all quality and safety initiatives within an organization. Membership is interprofessional in nature and may include physicians, nurses, pharmacists, patient safety managers, infection prevention members, and patient experience members. Other infrastructure committees that contribute to sustaining a culture of safety include peer review committees, credentials committees, pharmacy and therapeutics committees, infection control committees, and medical executive committees. In addition, there are key infrastructure roles that sustain a culture of safety. Patient safety officers, risk managers, clinical documentation analysts, patient experience or customer services experts, and case managers are all part of the infrastructure of sustaining a culture of safety within an organization (Rovinski-Wagner and Mills, 2014).

The importance of workforce engagement with quality and safety priorities cannot be overstated. All employees must be empowered and engaged in ongoing vigilance (IOM, 2003). Safety is acknowledged as the responsibility of all employees. Experts closest to the bedside should lead performance-improvement processes that promote integration and standardization of workflow safety concepts within and across the organization (Shabot et al., 2013). Clinical staff should feel comfortable voluntarily reporting errors through an effective event- or error-reporting system without fear of punitive action. According to the AHRQ patient safety network (AHRQ, 2014), a robust event reporting system has the following four key attributes:

- The institution must have a supportive environment for event reporting that protects the privacy of staff who report occurrences.

- Reports should be received from a broad range of personnel.

- Summaries of reported events must be disseminated in a timely fashion.

- A structured mechanism must be in place for reviewing reports and developing action plans.

In a culture of safety, all who work within the organization are actively involved in identifying, reporting, and resolving safety concerns and are empowered to take action to prevent an adverse event (Spath, 2000). Creating these attitudes and behaviors among all employees requires ongoing communication, adoption of non-hierarchical decision-making practices, empowering employees to adopt innovative practices to enhance patient safety, and an organizational commitment to employee training and education (IOM, 2003).

DATA ANALYSIS AND FEEDBACK

Sustaining a culture of safety requires an organization to view multiple sources of data, aggregate that data into something meaningful, generate reports for action, and provide feedback to employees when appropriate (Wachter, 2012). Measurement provides information and feedback to both leadership and clinicians about organizational culture and clinical outcomes. Sustaining a culture of safety requires that clinical outcome data be tracked, measured, analyzed, and shared with employees (Rovinski-Wagner and Mills, 2014). In addition, the measurement and analysis of the work environment can help predict whether safety outcomes will be positive or negative. Mardon and colleagues (2010) reported an inverse relationship between safety culture and adverse events. The more positive a culture of safety, the fewer adverse event occurrences. Sustaining a culture of safety requires the review of multiple sources of data. According to Wachter (2012), types of data that should regularly be reviewed include the following:

- Data from the voluntary incident reporting system

- Data from trigger tools (and results of subsequent chart reviews)

- Data drawn from real-time surveillance systems, such as those for certain healthcare-associated infections

- Key outcome data such as risk-adjusted mortality and readmission rates

- Key process and structural data (for example, hand hygiene rates, appropriate use of checklists)

- Serious reportable events

- Serious patient complaints

- Data drawn from executive rounding and caregiver focus groups

Safety problems that can be measured by rates, such as catheter-associated urinary tract infection (CAUTI) or central line–associated bloodstream infection (CLABSI) rates, should be analyzed in depth when rates spike above prior baselines and compared to local, regional, and national benchmarks. Rates must be shared with employees throughout the organization to design and implement action plans to improve patient outcomes. Feeding results of quality and safety data analysis back to the reporters and those at the point of care is crucial to sustaining a culture of safety. Results can be shared at both the unit and organizational level through leadership rounding, safety huddles, and quality and safety dashboards, as well as through committees.

TRANSPARENCY

Transparency is increasingly necessary to improve the quality and safety within a highly reliable organization. *Shining a Light: Safer Health Care Through Transparency*, by the National Patient Safety Foundation's Lucian Leape Institute, defines transparency as "the free, uninhibited flow of information that is open to the scrutiny of others" (2015, p. xii). Transparency is the free flow of information between clinicians and patients, among clinicians themselves, among healthcare organizations, and between healthcare organizations and the public. Transparency promotes accountability, catalyzes improvements in quality and safety, promotes trust and ethical behavior, and facilitates patient choice. By being candid with both patients and clinicians, healthcare organizations can promote their leaders' accountability for safer systems, better engage clinicians in improvement efforts, and engender greater patient trust (Kachalia, 2013).

HROs practice transparency through sharing and open communication of information about hazards, errors, and adverse events among clinicians to improve systems of care. All members of the organization must be provided with the ability to report and discuss errors without fear of punishment or embarrassment within a Just Culture. Individuals are held accountable for their own behaviors and practices; they are not held accountable for flaws in the system. Organizational strategies that foster transparency include the following:

- **Building an organizational culture that reinforces the importance of quality and safety:** This includes a morning safety huddle and leader walking rounds.

- **Reporting safety concerns:** This includes a protected process for reporting safety concerns (Dixon and Shofer, 2006).

- **Ensuring that data is shared at the front lines of care:** For example, the organization might display the number of days since the last sentinel event and the last employee injury on the organizational intranet.

- **Designing robust processes for measurement and analysis of safety concerns:** Organizations must regularly review multiple sources of data (Wachter, 2012).

■ **Providing multiple feedback mechanisms to organization members:** This includes peer observation, coaching, routine review of complication rates, and use of tests and procedures.

■ **Holding employees accountable for their behaviors and actions:** Organizations must conduct and share the results of RCAs to learn and improve.

All members of the team must feel they can openly and honestly share information with each other. Staff must be empowered to speak up and stop the line if they see an unsafe practice (Kemper and Boyle, 2009). Communication and teamwork are crucial to achieving high reliability within an organization and sustaining a culture of safety. Effective communication and teamwork are aimed at creating a common mental model (Leonard, Graham, and Bonacum, 2004). Communication failures are one of the leading causes of inadvertent patient harm. Analysis of 1,725 sentinel events reported to The Joint Commission (TJC) from 2013 through the second quarter of 2015 revealed that communication failure was identified as one of the root causes of 1,395 events, or 81% (TJC, 2015). TeamSTEPPS and crew resource management (CRM) are teamwork systems designed to improve communication and teamwork skills among healthcare professionals. The goal is to produce highly effective medical teams that optimize the use of information, people, and resources to achieve the best clinical outcomes for patients, thus eliminating barriers to quality and safety (AHRQ, 2014; Sculli et al., 2013).

PROFESSIONALISM AND ACCOUNTABILITY

Professionalism with accountability is necessary to maintain and sustain a culture of safety (Dupree, Anderson, McEvoy, and Brodman, 2011). According to Merriam-Webster dictionary, *professionalism* is the conduct, aims, or qualities that characterize or mark a profession or a professional person (n.d.). Professional qualities include the skill, good judgment, and polite behavior that are expected from a person who is trained to do a job well. Accountability is the quality of being accountable, especially for an obligation, or a willingness to accept responsibility or to account for one's actions (Merriam-Webster, n.d.). Unfortunately, the conduct of all healthcare professionals does not always reflect behaviors that exemplify professionalism and accountability (Porto and Lauve, 2006). The Joint Commission leadership standard provides evidence of the need to focus on professionalism and the importance of creating an effective process to address behaviors that threaten a culture of safety. Disruptive behaviors have been shown to cultivate medical error and adverse events (Rosenstein and O'Daniel, 2005).

It is critical to create a context of respect. When respect is the cultural norm, employees are more likely to communicate to other members and generate a shared interpretation of the situation (Sutcliffe, 2011). According to Christianson and Sutcliffe (2009), when people interact with trust, honesty, and self-respect there is an increased likelihood that people will speak up about issues of concern, share their perspectives, and ask questions of others. They conclude that whenever one or more of these components is missing, an adverse event is more likely to occur. An organization must insist on civility for all interactions (Blouin, 2013). "Verbal outbursts, condescending attitudes, refusing to take part in assigned duties or respond to legitimate questions in a timely manner, and physical threats create breakdowns in the teamwork, communication, and collaboration necessary to deliver safe patient care" (Blouin, 2013, p. 38). In a culture of safety, the leaders of the organization, as well as employees, are clear about what is acceptable and unacceptable behavior. There is accountability. There is no difference in expectations regarding conduct and accountability for members of different disciplines, such as medicine and nursing, because differential treatment of disciplines inherently leads to a distrust of leadership (Dupree et al., 2011). Blouin (2013) recommends the following strategies to mitigate or prevent disruptive behaviors among medical, nursing, pharmacy, support, therapy, and administrative staff:

- Hold all team members accountable for modeling desired behaviors at all levels and across all departments and settings.

- Enforce a code of conduct consistently and equitably for all disciplines and settings.

- Educate all healthcare team members about professional behaviors including communication skills.

- Establish a comprehensive approach to address intimidating and disruptive behaviors that includes a zero-tolerance policy to reduce the fear of retribution against those reporting disruptive behaviors.

- Develop a system to detect and receive reports of unprofessional conduct.

- Develop a process to determine if, how, and when disciplinary actions should be taken.

- Develop a process for offenders to demonstrate empathy with and apologize to patients, families, and staff that are involved in or witness disruptive behavior.

Strategies to address disruptive behaviors must be comprehensively deployed and applied consistently across individuals, disciplines, shifts, and locations to develop trust and confidence in reporting safety concerns (Chassin and Loeb, 2011).

SUMMARY

An HRO provides safe care and is intentionally designed to reduce error while achieving exceptional performance in quality and safety. Building and sustaining a culture of safety is challenging and requires considerable commitment, focus, and energy from the organization. Strategies to maintain the gains within a culture of safety require intense focus, strong leadership, effective communication, teamwork, data-based practices, analysis of errors, a culture of safety and continuous learning, improvement processes, and ongoing evaluation of outcomes.

This commitment to sustaining gains spans from the boardroom to the bedside and everything in between. Safety is everyone's responsibility in an HRO.

KEY POINTS

- Three barriers that stand in the way of changing an organization are failure to see, failure to move, and failure to finish. Sustaining change requires the organization to understand the nature of each of these barriers and make the needed adjustments to break through each barrier.

- The commitment of leadership to safety is crucial and is needed from all organizational leaders from the boardroom to the bedside, as well as management.

- Infrastructure and resource investment must support the priorities, goals, and strategic plans of the organization. This requires an executive team that is committed to investing resources to build the infrastructure to support quality and safety within the organization. Members of the organization at all levels must be engaged in the quality and safety infrastructure within the organization.

- Sustaining a culture of safety requires an organization to view multiple sources of data, aggregate that data into something meaningful, generate reports for action, and provide feedback to employees when appropriate.

- HROs practice transparency through sharing and open communication of information about hazards, errors, and adverse events among clinicians to improve systems of care.

- Professionalism and accountability are the cornerstones of a highly reliable culture of safety. An organization must insist on civility for all interactions.

REFERENCES

Agency for Healthcare Research and Quality (AHRQ). (2014). Patient safety primer: Safety culture. Retrieved from http://psnet.ahrq.gov/primer.aspx?primerID=5

Agency for Healthcare Research and Quality (AHRQ). (n.d.). TeamSTEPPS: Strategies and tools to enhance performance and patient safety. Retrieved from http://teamstepps.ahrq.gov/about-2cl_3.htm

Barling, J., Loughlin, C., and Kelloway, E. K. (2002). Development and test of a model linking safety-specific transformational leadership and occupational safety. *Journal of Applied Psychology, 87*(3), pp. 488–496.

Benn, J., Koutantji, M., Wallace, L., Spurgeon, P., Rejman, M., Healey, A., and Vincent, C. (2009). Feedback from incident reporting: Information and action to improve patient safety. *Quality and Safety in Health Care, 18*(1), pp. 11–21.

Black, J. S., and Gregersen, H. (2008). *It starts with one: Individuals change organizations* (3rd ed.). Upper Saddle River, NJ: FT Press.

Blouin, A. S. (2013). High reliability: Truly achieving healthcare quality and safety. *Frontiers of Health Services Management, 29*(3), pp. 35–40.

Blouin, A. S., and McDonagh, K. J. (2011). A framework for patient safety, part 2, resilience, the next frontier. *Journal of Nursing Administration, 41*(11), pp. 450–452.

Boehm, H., and Bonnel, W. (2010). The use of peer review in nursing education and clinical practice. *Journal for Nurses in Staff Development, 26*(3), pp. 108–115.

Carroll, R. (2009). *Risk management handbook for health care organizations*. San Francisco, CA: Jossey-Bass.

Chassin, M. R., and Loeb, J. M. (2011). The ongoing quality improvement journey: Next stop, high reliability. *Health Affairs, 30*(4), pp. 559–568.

Christianson, M. K., and Sutcliffe, K. M. (2009). Sensemaking, high-reliability organizing, and resilience. In P. Croskerry, K. S. Cosby, S. M. Schenkel, and R. L. Wears (Eds.), *Patient safety in emergency medicine* (pp. 27–33). Philadelphia, PA: Lippincott Williams and Wilkens.

Clarke, S. (2013). Safety leadership: A meta-analytic review of transformational and transactional leadership styles as antecedents of safety behaviors. *Journal of Occupational and Organizational Psychology, 86*(1), pp. 22–49.

Clavelle, J. T., Drenkard, K., Tullai-McGuinness, S., and Fitzpatrick, J. J. (2012). Transformational leadership practices of chief nursing officers in Magnet organizations. *The Journal of Nursing Administration, 42*(10 Suppl), pp. S3–S9.

Dixon, N. M., and Shofer, M. (2006). Struggling to invent high-reliability organizations in health care settings: Insights from the field. *Health Services Research, 41*(4 Part 2), pp. 1619–1632.

Dupree, E., Anderson, R., McEvoy, M. D., and Brodman, M. (2011). Professionalism: A necessary ingredient in a culture of safety. *The Joint Commission Journal on Quality and Patient Safety, 37*(10), pp. 447–455.

Fields, D. M. (2006). Perfect storm. *BizEd*, January/February, pp. 34–37.

Garcia-Morales, V. J., Jimenez-Barrionuevo, M. M., and Gutierrez-Gutierrez, L. (2012). Transformational leadership influence on organizational performance through organizational learning and innovation. *Journal of Business Research, 65*(7), pp. 1040–1050.

Garner, J. K. (2015). Implementation of a nursing peer-review program in the hospital setting. *Clinical Nurse Specialist, 29*(5), pp. 271–275.

Grant, A. M. (2012). Leading with meaning: Beneficiary contact, prosocial impact, and the performance effects of transformational leadership. *Academy of Management Journal, 55*(2), pp. 458–476.

Heenan, M., Khan, H., and Binkley, D. (2010). From boardroom to bedside: How to define and measure hospital quality. *Healthcare Quarterly, 13*(1), pp. 55–60.

Hershey, K. (2015). Culture of safety. *Nursing Clinics of North America, 50*(1), pp. 139–152.

Hilliard, M. A., Sczudlo, R., Scafidi, L., Cady, R., Villard, A., and Shah, R. (2012). Our journey to zero: Reducing serious safety events by over 70% through high-reliability techniques and workforce engagement. *Journal of Healthcare Risk Management, 32*(2), pp. 4–18.

Huggett, J., and Moran, C. (2007). RAPID decision-making: What it is, why we like it, and how to get the most out of it. Retrieved from http://www.bridgespan.org/getattachment/ae740499-bc96-430a-838b-62b53098c7fe/RAPID-Decision-Making-what-it-is-why-we-like-it.aspx

Imai, M. (2012). *Gemba Kaizen: A commonsense approach to a continuous improvement strategy* (2nd ed.). New York, NY: McGraw Hill.

Institute for Healthcare Improvement (IHI). (2008). Getting boards on board: Engaging governing boards in quality and safety. Retrieved from http://www.ihi.org/resources/Pages/Publications/GettingBoardsonBoard.aspx

Institute of Medicine (IOM). (1999). To err is human: Building a safer health system. Washington, DC: The National Academies Press.

Institute of Medicine (IOM). (2001). *Crossing the quality chasm: A new healthcare system for the 21st century*. Washington, DC: The National Academies Press. Retrieved from http://www.nap.edu/openbook.php?record_id=10027

Institute of Medicine (IOM). (2003). *Keeping patients safe: Transforming the work environment of nurses*. Washington, DC: The National Academies Press.

Institute of Medicine (IOM). (2010). *The future of nursing: Leading change, advancing health*. Washington DC: The National Academies Press.

International Atomic Energy Agency. (2006). *Fundamental safety principles*. Vienna, Austria: International Atomic Energy Agency.

Ivers, N., Jamtvedt, G., Flottorp, S., Young, J. M., Odgaard-Jensen, J., French, S. D., … Oxman, A. D. (2012). Audit and feedback: Effects on professional practice and healthcare outcomes. *The Cochrane Database of Systematic Reviews, 6*.

Jha, A., and Epstein, A. (2010). Hospital governance and the quality of care. *Health Affairs, 29*(1), pp. 182–187.

The Joint Commission (TJC). (2013). Framework for conducting a root cause analysis and action plan. Retrieved from http://www.jointcommission.org/Framework_for_Conducting_a_Root_Cause_Analysis_and_Action_Plan

The Joint Commission (TJC). (2015). Sentinel event data root causes by event type 2004–2Q 2015. Retrieved from http://www. jointcommission.org/assets/1/18/Root_Causes_Event_Type_2004-2Q_2015.pdf

Joshi, M. S., and Hines, S. C. (2006). Getting the board on board: Engaging hospital boards in quality and patient safety. *Joint Commission Journal of Quality and Patient Safety, 32*(4), pp. 179–187.

Kachalia, A. (2013). Improving patient safety through transparency. *New England Journal of Medicine, 369*(18), pp. 1677–1679.

Kelloway, E. K., Mullen, J., and Francis, L. (2006). Divergent effects of transformational and passive leadership on employee safety. *Journal of Occupational Health Psychology, 11*(1), pp. 76–86.

Kemper, C., and Boyle, D. K. (2009). Leading your organization to high reliability. *Journal of Nursing Management, 40*(4), pp. 14–18.

Kerfoot, K. (2006). Reliability between nurse managers: The key to the high-reliability organization. *Nursing Economics, 24*(5), pp. 274–275.

Kerfoot, K. M. (2010). Good is not good enough: The culture of low expectations and the leader's challenge. *Pediatric Nursing, 36*(4), pp. 216–217.

Kimsey, D. B. (2010). Lean methodology in health care. *AORN Journal, 92*(1), pp. 53–60.

Kubiak, T. M., and Benbow, D. W. (2009). *The certified Six Sigma black belt handbook* (2nd ed.). Milwaukee, WI: ASQ Quality Press.

Leonard, M., Graham, S., and Bonacum, D. (2004). The human factor: The critical importance of effective teamwork and communication in providing safe care. *Quality and Safety in Health Care, 13*(Suppl 1), pp. i85–i90.

Mardon, R. E., Khanna, K., Sorra, J., Dyer, N., and Famolaro, T. (2010). Exploring relationships between hospital patient safety culture and adverse events. *Journal of Patient Safety, 6*(4), pp. 226–232.

McFadden, K. L., Stock, G. N., and Gowen, C. R. (2015). Leadership, safety climate, and continuous quality improvement: Impact on process quality and patient safety. *Health Care Management Review, 40*(1), pp. 24–34.

Merriam-Webster. (n.d.). Professionalism. Retrieved from http://www.merriam-webster.com/dictionary/professionalism

Merriam-Webster. (n.d.). Accountability. Retrieved from http://www.merriam-webster.com/dictionary/accountability

National Patient Safety Foundation's Lucian Leape Institute. (2015). Shining a light: Safer health care through transparency. Retrieved from http://c.ymcdn.com/sites/www.npsf.org/resource/resmgr/LLI/Shining-a-Light_Transparency.pdf

National Quality Forum (NQF). (2004). Hospital governing boards and quality of care: A call to responsibility. Retrieved from http://www.ihi.org/resources/pages/publications/hospitalgoverningboardsandqualityofcareacalltoresponsibility.aspx

Oster, C. A. (2011). Guiding principles for evidence-based practice. In J. Houser and K. S. Oman (Eds.), *Evidence-based practice: An implementation guide for healthcare organizations* (pp. 83–109). Burlington, MA: Jones & Bartlett Learning.

Patel, S. (2010). Achieving quality assurance through clinical audit. *Nursing Management, 17*(3), pp. 28–35.

Porto, G., and Lauve, R. (2006). Disruptive clinician behavior: A persistent threat to patient safety. *Patient Safety & Quality Healthcare*. Retrieved from http://www.psqh.com/julaug06/disruptive.html

Pronovost, P. J., Demski, R., Callender, T., Winner, L., Miller, M. R., Austin, J. M., … National Leadership Core Measures Work Groups. (2013). Demonstrating high reliability on accountability measures at the Johns Hopkins Hospital. *The Joint Commission Journal on Quality and Patient Safety, 39*(12), pp. 531–544.

Reason, J. (1990). *Human error*. Cambridge, UK: Cambridge University Press.

Reason, J. T. (1997). *Managing the risks of organizational accidents*. Farnham, UK: Ashgate Publishing Company.

Riley, W. (2009). High reliability and implications for nursing leaders. *Journal of Nursing Management, 17*(2), pp. 238–246.

Roberts, K., Madsen, P., Desai, V., and Van Stralen, D. (2005). A case of the birth and death of a high reliability healthcare organisation. *Quality and Safety in Health Care, 14*(3), pp. 216–220.

Rosenstein, A. H., and O'Daniel, M. (2005). Disruptive behavior & clinical outcomes: Perceptions of nurses & physicians. *Nursing Management, 36*(1), pp. 18–28.

Rovinski-Wagner, C. and Mills, P. D. (2014). Patient safety. In P. Kelly, B. A. Vottero, and C. A. Christie-McAuliffe (Eds.), *Introduction to quality and safety education for nurses core competencies* (pp. 95–130). New York, NY: Springer Publishing Company.

Sculli, G. L., Fore, A. M., West, P., Neily, J., Mills, P. D., and Paull, D. E. (2013). Nursing crew resource management: A follow-up report for the Veterans Health Administration. *Journal of Nursing Administration, 43*(3), pp. 122–126.

Shabot, M. M., Monroe, D., Inurria, J., Garbade, D., and France, A. C. (2013). Memorial Hermann: High reliability from board to bedside. *The Joint Commission Journal on Quality and Patient Safety, 39*(6), pp. 253–257.

Simon, R. W., and Canacari, E. G. (2012). A practical guide to applying lean tools and management principles to health care improvement projects. *AORN Journal, 95*(1), pp. 85–100.

Six Sigma. (n.d.). Statistical Six Sigma definition. Retrieved from http://www.isixsigma.com/new-to-six-sigma/statistical-six-sigma-definition/

Spath, P. (2000). Does your facility have a "patient-safe" climate? *Hospital Peer Review, 25*(6), pp. 80–82.

Sutcliffe, K. M. (2011). High reliability organizations (HROs). *Best Practice & Research Clinical Anaesthesiology, 25*(2), pp. 133–144.

Tschannen, D., and Lee, E. (2012). The impact of nursing characteristics and the work environment on perceptions of communication. *Nursing Research and Practice, 2012*.

Turunen, H., Partanen, P., Kvist, T., Miettinen, M., and Vehviläinen-Julkunen, K. (2013). Patient safety culture in acute care: A web-based survey of nurse managers' and registered nurses' views in four Finnish hospitals. *International Journal of Nursing Practice, 19*(6), pp. 609–617.

The W. Edwards Deming Institute. (2015). The Plan, Do, Study, Act (PDSA) cycle. Retrieved from https://www.deming.org/theman/theories/pdsacycle

Wachter, R. (2012). *Understanding patient safety* (2nd ed.). New York, NY: McGraw Hill Education/Medical.

Wachter, R. M., and Shojania, K. G. (2004). *Internal bleeding: The truth behind America's terrifying epidemic of medical mistakes* (2nd ed.). New York, NY: Rugged Land Books.

Warren, K. (2008). Quality improvement: The foundation, processes, tools and knowledge transfer techniques. In E. R. Ransom, M. S. Joshi, and D. B. Nash (Eds.), *The healthcare quality book vision, strategy and tools* (2nd ed.) (pp. 63–83). Chicago, IL: Health Administration Press.

Womack, J., and Jones, D. T. (2003). *Lean thinking: Banish waste and create wealth in your corporation.* New York, NY: Productivity Press Publishing.

Woods, D. D. (2006). Essential characteristics of resilience. In E. Hollnagel, D. D. Woods, D. D. and N. Leveson (Eds.), *Resilience engineering: Concepts and precepts* (pp. 21–34). Farnham, UK: Ashgate Publishing Ltd.

ASSIMILATION INTO PRACTICE ACROSS THE CONTINUUM

CHAPTER 17

THE USE OF HRO CONCEPTS TO IMPROVE PAIN MANAGEMENT AND SAFETY

Nan Davidson, MA, RN, CNS-BC

Traditional strategies to improve hospital safety have been structured on a framework of systematic, orderly steps or processes. The movement to apply high reliability organization (HRO) concepts to healthcare quality efforts highlights the value of effective interdisciplinary teams—specifically, teams that are organized around a common purpose to proactively seek problems and engage in clinical work to resolve them at the unit and organizational level. Although this project started several years ago, it is an exemplar that demonstrates the successful application of this quality and has achieved lifesaving outcomes that have been sustained over time.

The purpose of this patient-safety initiative was to improve pain effectiveness and decrease preventable opioid-induced oversedation events as identified by naloxone rescue utilization. The goal was to infuse new knowledge and translate into practice evidence-based strategies to prevent opioid-induced oversedation by trending and classifying respiratory depression events.

> Never doubt that a small group of thoughtful, committed citizens can change the world; indeed, it's the only thing that ever has.
>
> —Margaret Mead

HROs have the unique ability to "quickly coalesce around an issue and then disseminate change as a new normal" to achieve substantial outcomes (Samuels, 2010, p. 474). It seems basic, but the success of this project has been the passion of each team member. So, too, has been the creation of thoughtful, immediate change that would protect the patient from opioid harm. This sense of urgency was not haste but motivated the team to share their expertise to identify the best strategy that would have the greatest anticipated effect.

Another key aspect of HROs is the ongoing monitoring of a specific patient outcome to measure the impact of new interventions. Again, it seems basic, but HROs follow identified outcomes with an appetite for making a difference. They make adjustments to the quality plan in a timely manner to ensure that efforts are trending toward the desired outcome. In this case, it was to prevent patient harm and even death due to opioids. HROs recognize that the commitment of team members is more influential than any identified process. In other words, participants want to identify problems, create meaningful interventions, and track immediate outcomes to determine success. That was the hallmark characteristic of this project and team.

Active teams and the ability to design system barriers to prevent harm to the patient are at the core of HRO hospitals. HROs recognize the potential for human error and design processes to compensate for them to consistently produce desired outcomes (Riley, 2009).

Two primary characteristics define HRO organizations:

- **HROs look for problems:** They operate on the premise that safety issues exist, and they design strategies to find them.

- **HROs thrive on the impact of clinical expertise and collaboration:** They have established specialty groups to act on identified problems or safety issues. Teams engage in collaboration that extends beyond traditional conversation and sharing of ideas. They are built on relationships that are trusting and intertwined to bring to the surface the best possible solutions. Solutions are not only grounded in science. There is also consideration for their realistic application at the bedside.

HROs are committed to change and activate quickly when care practices are found deficient (Samuels, 2010). This pain-management effectiveness and safety project is an example of the successful application of these concepts.

ADVANCED PRACTICE NURSE, CLINICAL NURSE SPECIALIST ROLE IN HROS

The pain effectiveness and opioid safety project began in 2006 when a bedside nurse asked, "Why do we seem to have a lot of oversedation and respiratory depression in our postoperative patients?" This was a perfect opportunity to initiate an evidence-based practice (EBP) project that partnered the clinical nurse specialist (CNS) with the unit nursing staff. In addition, because the safety issue was recognized as a problem by the bedside staff, it created an ideal environment for any needed change to occur. This project remains ongoing and continues to identify opportunities to translate new knowledge into practices that make a significant impact on patient safety.

The CNS role has consistently been present and participated in quality activities to advance the practice of nursing to provide optimal patient care. As is characteristic of HROs, central to CNS practice is the desire to find problems or potential failures in patient care, to identify risk, and to ask questions to uncover issues. The CNS brings an "informed curiosity" that is needed to identify barriers and behaviors that contribute to near-miss events in complex situations (Ebright, 2014, p. 192). Their ability to interpret individual case- or system-level data and their knowledge of organizational culture are imperative to the development of innovations that influence outcomes. In addition, the CNS supports an HRO culture through fostering collaborative relationships and improving interdisciplinary communication (McKeon, Oswaks, and Cunningham, 2006).

HROs recognize that improvements in patient safety require a switch from the focus on individual care providers as the sole cause of error to consideration of the complex systems in which they work. CNS education emphasizes problem-solving strategies at the patient, nurse, and organizational levels (Ebright, 2014). The educational preparation of the CNS and the unique blend of core competencies of patient care provider, educator, consultant, and researcher have placed them in leadership roles in hospitals. Further, the CNS skills of communicator and change agent have put the CNS in a distinct position to lead successful and sustained patient-safety and quality improvements (Morrison, 2000; LaSala, Connors, Pedro, and Phipps, 2007; Finkelman, 2013).

THE PAIN TEAM

Identifying which professionals to have at the table for any issue or project is the most important aspect of quality improvement and change management. Diligent thought must be put into member selection to ensure that the goals of the team are met. Central to team membership is a shared interest in the topic. For HROs, membership goes beyond those who are just interested in a topic to those who hold a true passion for resolving safety issues or any other problems at hand. In this case, team members were those who had a heartfelt interest in making pain management more effective and safe. They were invested in providing their expertise to the group and provided strategy development that was imperative to making a collective impact on pain safety. As a whole, the interdisciplinary team was responsible for reviewing data, identifying improvement strategies, and facilitating practice change.

The pain team was organized with membership that included hospital-based professionals responsible for pain management throughout the continuum of perioperative care. The CNS, quality director, and physician served as coleaders of the team. The CNS's primary role was to collect and analyze data, identify gaps between practice and what the evidence stated, and work collaboratively with the interdisciplinary team to make practice changes to improve opioid safety. The quality director's primary role was to analyze and interpret data. In addition, the quality director helped to synthesize data and present it in a format that was meaningful and helpful to draw conclusions and to interpret impact from any strategies that were activated by the team. The physician leader played a key role in providing a medical perspective to issues. Further, this role partnered with the physician community and medical executive committee to provide administrative support of needed practice change.

Beyond these three facilitation roles, critical to team membership were disciplines that could offer expertise in pain management and safety. These included a surgeon and medical physician who practiced on the unit, an anesthesiologist, and a pharmacist. Further, and basic to any change-management project, it was critical to include persons directly involved with the patients' pain. The membership of bedside nurses and other disciplines, including physical and occupational therapists, provided a full range of care providers who offered important perspectives on patient pain. In addition, it was important to include manager- and director-level persons who could provide the formal authority to help facilitate any needed practice change. Although this membership list may seem large, we deliberately selected one representative from each of the identified stakeholder groups and kept the core membership at 15. This number ensured meaningful and focused discussion. It also allowed for the efficient reaching of consensus on data interpretation and the identification of relevant strategies that would have an impact on pain safety.

METHODOLOGY

The automated medication dispensary system monthly report was used to identify patients who had experienced an opioid-induced oversedation and respiratory depression event that required naloxone. From this report, each patient chart was reviewed to ensure that the need for naloxone was due to opioid use rather than something else, such as epidural itching, or to rule out opioid cause for mental status change. A monthly retrospective cluster analysis was completed to classify and trend naloxone rescue events based on the nearest premorbid event. The nearest premorbid event was defined as "what was the most likely cause or contributing factor" that triggered the need for naloxone rescue. For example, when this project started, the nearest premorbid events clustered around higher opioid dosing when the nurse started with a higher dose in the range order, which triggered the need for rescue. Another cluster early on was the concurrent dosing of opioid with other sedating medications like Valium, Ativan, or Phenergan. Over time, the clusters have changed and most recently included inconsistent sedation assessment before and after administering pain medication.

Month/Year:															
Patient/MR# Procedure Age Ht/Wt	**Date of event — POD**	**MD RN**	**Pain Level**	**Trigger to Intervene**		**Nearest Premorbid Event**			**Narcan dose**	**Unit**	**Response Outcome (Remained on floor or transferred to ICU)**	**Type of anes**	**Time in PACU (min)**	**Time PACU to event (min)**	**Comments** **Harm Category** No harm=remained on floor Harm = transfer to ICU or death
				Sed Sx?	**Resp Sx? RR/Quality/ Pulse Ox**	**Drug Time**	**Dose**	**Route**							

Data collection: Opioid induced oversedation/respiratory depression requiring naloxone.

Figure 17.1 Opioid-induced oversedation/respiratory depression requiring naloxone.

Each event was reviewed and data collected, including patient characteristics, symptoms, drug, dose, route, timing, patient care unit, and outcome. (Refer to Figure 17.1.) These data points were recorded and trended to identify clusters and opportunities to improve safety. For this project, emphasis was placed on monthly analysis of data. Timely review of naloxone rescue events was critical to identify safety issues as they were occurring. When a trend, or cluster, of events was identified, the information was presented to the pain team. There was not a benchmark or threshold that determined whether a trend or cluster was occurring. The existence of as few as one or two unsafe nearest premorbid events was considered a cluster and brought to the pain team for interpretation and recommendation for any practice change.

Once a safety issue was identified, the literature was reviewed to identify whether there was a gap between our current practice and the evidence. If a gap was present, the process of translation of new practice changes to protect patients while on opioid therapy was triggered. The Iowa Model of Evidence-Based Practice to Promote Quality Care was used when evaluating the strength of the literature and to determine the feasibility of making any practice change (Titler et al., 2001). The Plan, Do, Check, Act quality improvement model was used to carry out and reevaluate impact of changes on an ongoing basis (see Figure 17.2).

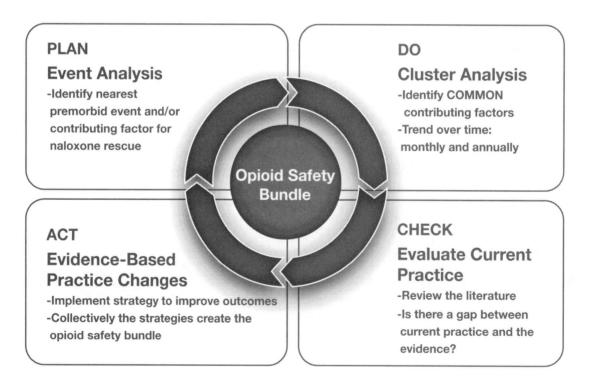

Figure 17.2 Opioid safety cycle analysis using the Plan, Do, Check, Act quality improvement model.

Over the past 10 years, EBP changes in the clinical setting have included the following:

- Establishment of an opioid fractionation policy (Pasero, Manworren, and McCaffery, 2007; Pasero and McCaffery, 1994)

- Continuous pulse oximetry the first 24 hours postoperatively and while on PCA pump (D'Arcy, 2008; Hagle, Lehr, Brubakken, and Shippee, 2004; Pasero and McCaffery, 1994)

- Fentanyl patch screen program (Food and Drug Administration [FDA], 2005)

- Sedation assessment using a sedation scale (Ely et al., 2003; Nisbet and Mooney-Cotter, 2009; Pasero and McCaffery, 2002)

- Established sleep apnea screening and monitoring program (Gross et al., 2006; Paje and Kremer, 2006)

- Limited sedating antiemetic utilization to high surveillance areas (Pasero, 2009; Pasero and McCaffery, 1994)

- Development of a pain order set to streamline opioid selection and dosing (Krenzischek, Dunwoody, Polomano, and Rathmell, 2008; Pasero et al., 2007)

- Development of the pain assessment card (Akyol, Karayurt, and Salmond, 2009; Beck et al., 2010; DuPree et al., 2009; Gupta, Daigle, Mojica, and Hurley, 2009; Jamison et al., 1997; Quinlan-Colwell, 2009)

- Further education on the nursing role in monitoring sedation levels while on opioids (Ely et al., 2003; Hagle et al., 2004; Nisbet and Mooney-Cotter, 2009; Pasero, 2009; Pasero and McCaffery, 2002)

The translation of each new practice strategy occurred in a variety of ways, depending on the needed change. Early changes required policy and procedure development, the establishment of pharmacy dosing parameter limits, and the identification of high-risk screening criteria by nursing and pharmacy. Later strategies have focused on practitioners coming together to gain consensus on standardizing safe opioid choices and dosing. In addition, recent activity has focused on pain assessment and the critical role nurses play in preventing opioid safety events by serially monitoring sedation levels when administering opioid. Education and tools to aid in conversations about pain with patients have been disseminated.

For example, in 2011–2012, the cluster analysis revealed safety issues around inadequate pain assessment and lack of monitoring of sedation level to prevent opioid-induced respiratory depression. The gap analysis revealed inadequate staff knowledge of pain-rating scales and their application at the bedside. Further, there was a significant lack of knowledge that sedation precedes opioid-induced respiratory depression. Staff nurses did not realize their role in assessing sedation levels before and after giving opioids. Consistent with HRO teams, the pain team went beyond simple educational strategies, like in-servicing, to address the identified knowledge deficits. Instead, it strived to be more creative and to provide more tangible tools for the nurse to use with the patient at the bedside. As a result, the process of infusing new knowledge into practice to address these two specific target areas was initiated.

To start, a tool to enhance pain assessment was designed with the intent to enhance conversation between the patient and nurse about pain. The development of the pain card provided an evidence-based assessment tool for the nurse to use and communicate with patients about pain. (See Figure 17.3.) The pain card is a two-sided clinical tool. The front side describes the hospital's commitment to pain management. In addition, a highlighted section addresses expectations for pain management. Finally, the front side discusses side effects of pain medication. The reverse side of the pain card consists of four pain-rating scales—a numeric rating scale, a verbal descriptor scale, a color analog scale, and a faces pain scale—to be individualized for the patient. This side of the pain card also includes a section that describes how the patient will be asked to participate in pain assessment and tactics for managing pain. This was designed to encourage open discussion between the nurse and patient regarding measurement, expectations, and effectiveness of the patient's pain regimen.

To address the knowledge deficit of nurses with regard to their role in preventing opioid-induced oversedation, a "Fast Facts: 5 Minute Inservice" sheet was developed. It included specific education essential for the safe monitoring of patients while on opioids (see Figure 17.4). The "Fast Facts" sheet is educational content for staff that is clinically focused and evidence-based. Content is limited to one page and is designed to be a self-directed inservice that is emailed directly to the bedside nurse. In addition, each manager can discuss or deliver the content at unit meetings and post it on bathroom doors or unit education bulletin boards. Each "Fast Facts" was archived in a unique location within the electronic policy management system. The purpose of creating an education folder within this system was to allow staff to have continual access to just-in-time educational materials.

Consistent with HRO teams, it was the goal to not only disseminate education about the important role nurses play to ensure opioid safety, but also to ensure behavior change at the bedside that would affect outcomes. The team wanted to guarantee that nurses knew how to perform a proper sedation assessment before and after opioid administration. To address this, the CNS went to each unit meeting and skills fair to teach, talk about, and demonstrate the sedation assessment procedure. The importance of pairing sedation and pain assessment was emphasized. Again, this level of unit and staff engagement mirrors HRO team behavior. In other words, team-member engagement and passion to affect outcomes drive the work that is required to ensure staff understanding and action to, in this case, prevent opioid-induced respiratory depression and preserve patient life.

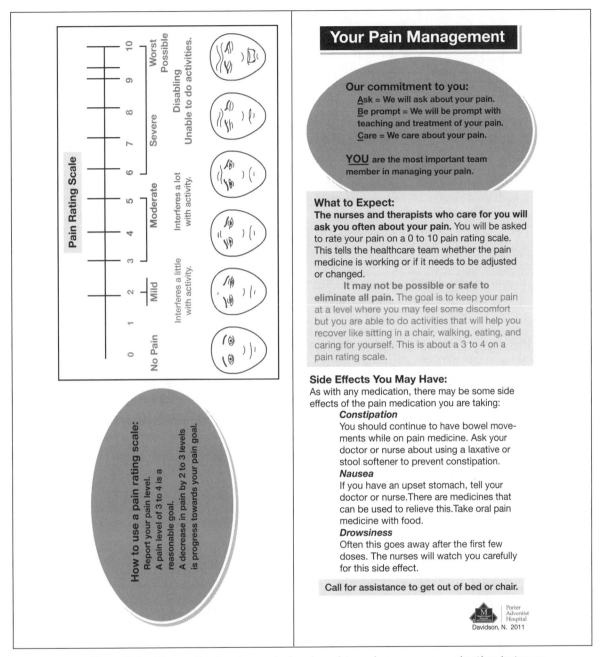

Figure 17.3   The patient pain card, developed to enhance communication between the patient and nurse when assessing pain.

Opioid Safety
Fast Facts – 5 Minute Inservice
Staff education content at your fingertips.
Vol. 4 Issue 2 April, 2014

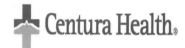

Preventing Opioid Induced Oversedation:
Using the Richmond Agitation Sedation Scale With Safety Guidelines

Nan Davidson, RN, MA, CNS-BC & Lorna Prang, RN, MS, CCRN, CNS, CCNS

Patient safety is an essential aspect of opioid therapy. Respiratory depression is the most serious side effect associated with opioid administration. *SEDATION PRECEDES OPIOID-INDUCED RESPIRATORY DEPRESSION.*

Patients are NOT: awake and not breathing!

- Increase in sedation level is an early warning sign of respiratory compromise and requires consideration for:
    - adjustment of opioid or other sedating medication
    - more frequent monitoring, and/or
    - rescue intervention as appropriate.
- Nursing plays a key role in preventing respiratory depression by performing serial assessment of the patient's sedation level.
- Use a standardized, evidence-based sedation assessment scale
    - to ensure clear communication and appropriate interventions among health care providers for various levels of sedation and that translates to all clinical settings.

Risk Factors for Opioid Induced Over-Sedation and Respiratory Depression

Patients are at highest risk for opioid-induced over-sedation during the first 24 hours of opioid therapy. In addition the following patient categories are at risk:

Populations at risk for opioid induced respiratory depression
- Opioid naïve patients
- Obstructive Sleep Apnea (OSA)
- Use of continuous rate on PCA
- Smoker
- Post surgery: upper abdominal or thoracic
- Concurrent use of benzodiazepines or sedating anti-emetics
- Age >65: especially low weight &/or with co-morbidities
    - Age >65: especially low weight &/or with co-morbidities
    - 61-70 2.8 times higher risk
    - 71-80 5.4 times higher risk
    - >80 8.7 times higher risk
- Obesity
- PCA dosing per proxy
- Inadequate monitoring of sedation levels

How to do a Sedation Assessment using the RASS

When approaching the patient, first OBSERVE if they are alert, restless or agitated. (RASS Level 0 to +4).
If they are "Alert and Calm" it is safe to give opioid.
If the patient is not alert, then state the patient's name and ask them to "open their eyes and look at you". If the:

a. Patient awakens with sustained eye opening and eye contact (>10 seconds). (RASS level –1 or DROWSY) MAY CONTINUE PAIN REGIMEN BUT CAUTION GIVING ADDITIONAL OPIOID.

b. Patient awakens with eye opening and contact, but not sustained (<10 seconds. (RASS level –2 or Light Sedation). **CONSIDER STOPPING OPIOID** to maintain RASS at -1 or above.

c. Patient has any movement in response to voice but no eye contact. **(RASS level –3 or Moderate sedation). STOP OPIOID.** CALL RRT or CODE BLUE if indicated.

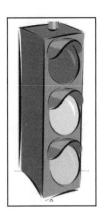
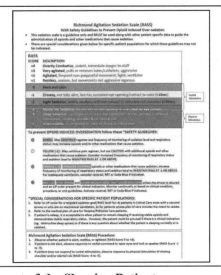

Assessment of the Sleeping Patient

Nurses often ask if they should awaken sleeping patients to determine level of sedation.

- If patient is asleep, it is acceptable to allow patient to remain sleeping if receiving stable opioids and demonstrates stable respiratory status. However, the patient must be aroused if there is a clinical indication (eg. obstructive sleep apnea) or if there is any question about whether the patient is sleeping normally or is sedated.
- It is reassuring to know that patients who are sleeping normally and have well-controlled pain will fall back to sleep after they are aroused for the sedation assessment.
  - If they do not fall back asleep, they may require further assessment because they may have pain. If they fall asleep after having a period of poor pain control, assess to be sure that what seems like sleep is not actual over sedation.

References

Ely, E. W. (2003). Monitoring sedation status over time in ICU patients: Reliability and validity of the Richmond Agitation-Sedation Scale (RASS). The Journal of the American Medical Association. 289(22), 2983-2991.

Jarzyna, D., Jungquist, C., Pasero, C., Willens, J., Nisbet, A., Oakes, L., Dempsey, S., Santangelo, D., Polomano, R. (2011). American society for pain management nursing guidelines on monitoring for opioid-induced sedation and respiratory depression. *Pain Management Nursing*. 12(3), 118-145.

Nisbet, A. T., Mooney-Cotter, Florence. (2009). Comparison of selected sedation scales for reporting opioid-induced sedation assessment. Pain Management Nursing, 10(3), 154-164.

Pasero, C. (2009). Assessment of sedation during opioid administration for pain management. Journal of PeriAnesthesia Nursing, 24(3), 186-190.

Pasero, C. (2009). Challenges in Pain Assessment. Journal of Perianesthesia Nursing. 24(1), 50-54.

Sessler, C.N., Gosnell, M., Grap, M.J., etal. (2002). The Richmond Agitation-Sedation Scale: validity and reliability in adult intensive care patints. American Journal of Respiratory Critical Care Medicine. 166:1338-1344.

The Joint Commission Sentinel Event Alert. Safe use of opioids in hospitals. Issue 49, August 8, 2012.

Figure 17.4 The "Fast Facts: 5 Minute Inservice" is a format for educational content to be distributed to staff by email.

These two practice-change examples reveal the deliberate effort that went into strategizing appropriate interventions for each safety cluster that was identified. Each strategy developed included careful review of the literature and thoughtful impact of application at the bedside. At times, ad hoc team members and subgroups were established to work on strategies to bring back to the pain team. Key stakeholders were kept intact to not only develop strategies and tools but also implement and make changes at the unit and care-provider level.

As with any successful change project, the time involved was justified. Each change project took an average of about 1 year. The practice changes have evolved over time and present today as an *opioid safety bundle*. The opioid safety bundle is a list of EBP changes made over time that collectively made an impact on naloxone rescue rate. (See Table 17.1.) In other words, not one single practice change has served to improve patient safety. Instead, collectively, each strategy has had a cumulative effect and has made a major impact on patient safety. The literature to support each EBP change is cited.

TABLE 17.1 THE OPIOID SAFETY BUNDLE

Premorbid Safety Events	EBP Change
Higher opioid dosing	2006: Implemented opioid fractionation policy (Pasero et al., 2007; Pasero and McCaffery, 1994)
First 24 hours after surgery	2006: Implemented continuous pulse oximetry in the first 24 hours after surgery and while on PCA pump (D'Arcy, 2008; Hagle et al., 2004; Pasero and McCaffery, 1994)
Fentanyl patch for acute pain	2007: Implemented fentanyl patch screen program (FDA, 2005)
Oversedation leading to respiratory compromise	2007: Implemented education on nursing assessment of sedation to prevent respiratory compromise using a sedation scale (Ely et al., 2003; Nisbet and Mooney-Cotter, 2009; Pasero and McCaffery, 2002)
Obstructive sleep apnea (OSA)	2008: Developed and implemented OSA screen and monitoring program (Gross et al., 2006; Paje and Kremer, 2006)
Concurrent opioid dosing with other sedating medications	2009: Limited sedating antiemetic utilization to high-surveillance areas (Pasero, 2009; Pasero and McCaffery, 1994)
Variability in order set opioid selections and routes	2010: Developed standardized pain order set used to streamline opioid choices and routes (Krenzischek et al., 2008; Pasero et al., 2007)
Ensure accurate pain, pulse oximetry, and sedation assessment and monitoring	2011: Developed and implemented the Porter pain card (Akyol et al., 2009; Beck et al., 2010; DuPree et al., 2009; Gupta et al., 2009; Jamison et al., 1997; Quinlan-Colwell, 2009)
	2012: Pulse oximetry and sedation assessment education (Booker, 2008; Clark, Giuliano, and Chen, 2006; DeMeulenaere, 2007; Ely et al., 2003; Hagle et al., 2004; Nisbet and Mooney-Cotter, 2009; Paragas, 2008; Pasero and McCaffery, 2002; Pasero, 2009; Valdez-Lowe, Ghareeb, and Artinian, 2009)

| Ensure accurate sedation assessment and monitoring | 2013–14: Paired pain and sedation assessment education and integration into electronic medical record (Ely et al., 2003; Hagle et al., 2004; Pasero, 2009; Pasero and McCaffery, 2002; Nisbet and Mooney-Cotter, 2009) |

METRICS

Application of HRO concepts—including establishing effective interdisciplinary teams, identifying problems, and creating a series of nets and barriers to prevent their occurrence—has positively affected the safety of patients on opioids. The application of a formal methodology to identify opioid safety opportunities for improvement and the implementation of new knowledge and EBP have reduced the incidence of preventable opioid-induced oversedation. Tracking for naloxone rescue has been completed on an annual basis since 2006. An example of how month-to-month tracking of naloxone events, using the fiscal year time frame, can be presented is shown in Figure 17.5. This display of data makes it easy to see which units or patient populations may have opioid safety problems. This level of tracking and display are consistent with HRO organizations that want to provide timely intervention when and where issues exist.

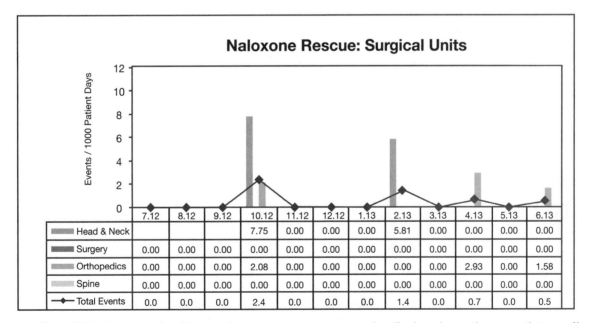

Figure 17.5 An example of how naloxone rescue events can be displayed month to month to easily identify patient populations or units where opioid safety problems may exist.

An example of how the outcome achievement—in this case, naloxone rescue rate—can be presented to communicate impact to leadership and staff is presented in Figure 17.6. Information is presented in a total hospital number and at the unit level for the postoperative surgical units, including general surgery, orthopedics, and spine. The head and neck patient population was new to the hospital in 2013 and added to the database at that time. In this snapshot of data, the overall hospital naloxone rescue rate has decreased from 1.46 (FY 2010) to 0.46 (FY 2013), a 68% decrease. Year-to-year data can be described as follows: from 1.46 (FY 2010) to 1.05 (FY 2011), a 28% decrease; from 1.05 (FY 2011) to 0.85 (FY 2012), a 19% decrease; and from 0.85 (FY 2012) to 0.46 (FY 2013), a 46% decrease.

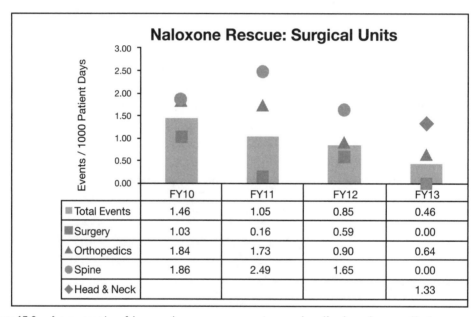

	FY10	FY11	FY12	FY13
■ Total Events	1.46	1.05	0.85	0.46
■ Surgery	1.03	0.16	0.59	0.00
▲ Orthopedics	1.84	1.73	0.90	0.64
● Spine	1.86	2.49	1.65	0.00
◆ Head & Neck				1.33

Figure 17.6 An example of how naloxone rescue rate can be displayed annually to present impact of practice changes over time.

DISSEMINATION

Dissemination of information and education to team members and staff was situational and occurred in a variety of ways depending on the needed practice change. Knowledge of the organizational structure and councils was critical to ensuring that relevant staff, as well as those who would be affected, had the right information to support the implementation of improvement activities. This included communication from the pain team through the shared governance structure that included a nurse practice council, a professional development council, and a policy and procedure committee.

In addition, knowledge of mechanisms (or how units have structured their communication with each other) and what technology the organization uses to communicate with staff was important. Examples of mechanisms of communication on the unit included the following:

- One-on-one conversations with staff.

- Setting up a learning station at each competency fair.

- Use of a communication tool labeled "Hot Topics." A hot topic is a limited piece of information that can be written on a small whiteboard at the nurse's station—for example, "Don't forget to assess sedation level before and after giving pain medicine!"

Examples of technology used in our organization included email, mass texting, a virtual bulletin board in the staff lounge, and a hospital website. Email communication was always used as a way to ensure that all staff had access to information. After the initial email was sent, texting, use of the unit-based virtual bulletin board, or use of the hospital website was considered.

SUMMARY

In an era of hospital transparency and focus on the elimination of any hospital-acquired injury, it is vital to not only establish a quality improvement initiative to enhance opioid safety but also to embrace the added value of applying concepts that are core to HRO organizations. This work provides hospitals with a foundation to support ongoing evidence-based quality-improvement activities required of HROs. Collectively, the EBP changes create a system that is designed to establish barriers between the hazard of opioid-induced oversedation and potential loss of the patient.

KEY POINTS

- Appreciate small things that go wrong. The HRO assumption is that small things that go wrong are early warning signs of safety issues that can uncover a problem where intervention is needed. Further, the value placed on interdisciplinary dialogue and passion to work together to put safety solutions into place is essential to affect outcomes. Close surveillance of naloxone rescue events acts as an early warning system to identify potential risk to patient safety for patients on opioids and other sedating medications.

- Identify a close surveillance trigger. Monthly cluster analysis of naloxone rescue data alerts organizations to potential harms, triggers timely review of current practice, and activates the translation of EBP changes that augment patient safety while on opioid therapy. These practice changes are incorporated into pain policies and guidelines, education, and ongoing quality-improvement activities.

■ Truly value the interdisciplinary team. The evolution of the opioid safety bundle over time was the direct result of interdisciplinary teamwork that is characteristic of HROs. The adverb *truly* is added as a descriptor because it emphasizes the value, to the fullest degree, of the importance of the team. It is not just a group that gets together randomly to talk about problems or issues. It is a group that is deliberately assembled and has the knowledge, skills, and attitudes of an effective team. Team members have a clear and common purpose. They can compensate for each other and manage conflict well. They understand each other's roles and how they fit together. They anticipate each other's communication. They trust each other's intentions. Most importantly, they strongly believe in the team's collective ability to succeed and affect outcomes (Baker, Day, and Salas, 2006). They *truly* believe in their power to affect change and safety. It may seem unachievable to organize such a group, but it is not. The critical component is leadership that understands the importance of these key qualities and selects team members suitable to achieve what otherwise would not be achievable.

REFERENCES

Akyol, O., Karayurt, O., and Salmond, S. (2009). Experiences of pain and satisfaction with pain management in patients undergoing total knee replacement. *Orthopedic Nursing, 28*(2), pp. 79–85.

Baker, D. P., Day, R., and Salas, R. (2006). Teamwork as an essential component of high-reliability organizations. *Health Services Research, 41*(4), pp. 1576–1598.

Beck, S. L., Towsley, G. L., Berry, P. H., Lindau, K., Field, R. B., and Jensen, S. (2010). Core aspects of satisfaction with pain management: Cancer patients' perspectives. *Journal of Pain and Symptom Management, 39*(1), pp. 100–115.

Booker, R. (2008). Pulse oximetry. *Nursing Standard, 22*(30), pp. 39–41.

Clark, A. P., Giuliano, K., and Chen, H. M. (2006). Pulse oximetry revisited: "But his O(2) was normal!" *Clinical Nurse Specialist, 20*(6), pp. 268–272.

D'Arcy, Y. (2008). Keep your patient safe during PCA. *Nursing, 38*(1), pp. 50–55.

DeMeulenaere, S. (2007). Pulse oximetry: Uses and limitations. *The Journal for Nurse Practitioners, 3*(5), pp. 312–317.

DuPree, E., Martin, L., Anderson, R., Kathuria, N., Reich, D., Porter, C., and Chassin, M. R. (2009). Improving patient satisfaction with pain management using Six Sigma tools. *The Joint Commission Journal on Quality and Patient Safety, 35*(7), pp. 343–350.

Ebright, P. (2014). Patient safety. In J. S. Fulton, B. L. Lyon, and K. L. Goudreau (Eds.), *Foundations of clinical nurse specialist practice* (2nd ed.) (pp. 183–197). New York, NY: Springer Publishing Company.

Ely, E. W., Truman, B., Shintani, A., Thomason, J. W., Wheeler, A. P., Gordon, S., … Bernard, G. R. (2003). Monitoring sedation status over time in ICU patients: Reliability and validity of the Richmond Agitation-Sedation Scale (RASS). *Journal of the American Medical Association, 289*(22), pp. 2983–2991.

Finkelman, A. (2013). The clinical nurse specialist: Leadership in quality improvement. *Clinical Nurse Specialist, 27*(1), pp. 31–35.

Food and Drug Administration (FDA). (2005). Safety warnings regarding use of fentanyl transdermal (skin) patches. Retrieved from http://www.fda.gov/Drugs/DrugSafety/PostmarketDrugSafetyInformationforPatientsandProviders/ucm051739.htm

Gross, J., Bachenberg, K. L., Benumof, J. L., Caplan, R. A., Connis, R. T., Coté, C. J., … American Society of Anesthesiologists Task Force on Perioperative Management. (2006). Practice guidelines for the perioperative management of patients with obstructive sleep apnea: A report by the American Society of Anesthesiologists Task Force on Perioperative Management of patients with obstructive sleep apnea. *Anesthesiology, 104*(5), pp. 1081–1093.

Gupta, A., Daigle, S., Mojica, J., and Hurley, R. W. (2009). Patient perception of pain care in hospitals in the United States. *Journal of Pain Research, 2009*(2), pp. 157–164.

Hagle, M. E., Lehr, V. T., Brubakken, K., and Shippee, A. (2004). Respiratory depression in adult patients with intravenous patient-controlled analgesia. *Orthopedic Nursing*, 23(1), pp. 28–29.

Jamison, R. N., Ross, M. J., Hoopman, P., Griffin, F., Levy, J., Daly, M., and Schaffer, J. L. (1997). Assessment of postoperative pain management: Patient satisfaction and perceived helpfulness. *The Clinical Journal of Pain*, 13(3), pp. 229–236.

Krenzischek, D. A., Dunwoody, C. J., Polomano, R. C., and Rathmell, J. P. (2008). Pharmacotherapy for acute pain: Implications for practice. *Journal of Perianesthesia Nursing*, 23(1), pp. S28–S42.

LaSala, C. A., Connors, P. M., Pedro, J. T., and Phipps, M. (2007). The role of the clinical nurse specialist in promoting evidence-based practice and effecting positive patient outcomes. *The Journal of Continuing Education in Nursing*, 38(6), pp. 262–270.

McKeon, L. M., Oswaks, J. D., and Cunningham, P. D. (2006). Safeguarding patients: Complexity science, high reliability organizations, and implications for team training in healthcare. *Clinical Nurse Specialist*, 20(6), pp. 298–304.

Morrison, J. D. (2000). Evolution of the perioperative clinical nurse specialist role. *AORN Journal*, 72(2), pp. 227–232.

Nisbet, A. T., and Mooney-Cotter, F. (2009). Comparison of selected sedation scales for reporting opioid-induced sedation assessment. *Pain Management Nursing*, 10(3), pp. 154–164.

Paje, D. T., and Kremer, M. J. (2006). The perioperative implications of obstructive sleep apnea. *Orthopedic Nursing*, 25(5), pp. 291–297.

Paragas, J. (2008). Keeping the beat with pulse oximetry. *Nursing*, 38(11), pp. 56hn1–56hn2.

Pasero, C. (2009). Assessment of sedation during opioid administration for pain management. *Journal of Perianesthesia Nursing*, 24(3), pp. 186–190.

Pasero, C., and McCaffery, M. (2002). Monitoring sedation: It's the key to preventing opioid-induced respiratory depression. *American Journal of Nursing*, 102(2), pp. 67–69.

Pasero, C. L., and McCaffery, M. (1994). Avoiding opioid-induced respiratory depression. *American Journal of Nursing*, 94(4), pp. 25–30.

Pasero, C., Manworren, R. C., and McCaffery, M. (2007). PAIN control IV opioid range orders for acute pain management. *The American Journal of Nursing*, 107(2), pp. 59–60.

Quinlan-Colwell, A. D. (2009). Understanding the paradox of patient pain and patient satisfaction. *Journal of Holistic Nursing*, 27(3), pp. 177–182.

Riley, W. (2009). High reliability and implications for nursing leaders. *Journal of Nursing Management*, 17(2), pp. 238–246.

Samuels, J. G. (2010). The application of high-reliability theory to promote pain management. *The Journal of Nursing Administration*, 40(11), pp. 471–476.

Titler, M. G., Kleiber, C., Steelman, V. J., Rakel, B. A., Budreau, G., Everett, L. Q., … Goode, C. J. (2001). The Iowa model of evidence-based practice to promote quality care. *Critical Care Nursing Clinics of North America*, 13(4), pp. 497–509.

Valdez-Lowe, C., Ghareeb, S. A., and Artinian, N. T. (2009). Pulse oximetry in adults. *The American Journal of Nursing*, 109(6), pp. 52–59.

CHAPTER 18

PEDIATRIC PATIENT SAFETY: UTILIZING SAFETY COACHING AS A STRATEGY TOWARD ZERO HARM

Sharon Sables-Baus, PhD, MPA, RN, PCNS-BC, CPPS

Everyone has probably heard the phrase, "Children are not little adults." But what does this mean in terms of pediatric patient safety? Are there differences in the ways we address, improve, and ensure the safety of pediatric patients when they receive healthcare that is different from adults?

Both adult and pediatric healthcare systems must operate in a constant state of vigilance to have the fewest number of errors occur. Yet due to the inherent complexities in pediatric healthcare delivery, a thorough understanding of those differences is necessary. To exemplify high reliability in a pediatric organization, this chapter focuses on how children are indeed different from adults and how one organization that specializes in the care of infants, children, adolescents, and young adults established an innovative patient safety culture program, including safety coaching, to avert harm (Pronovost et al., 2006; Weick and Sutcliffe, 2007).

> "
> I never cease to be amazed at the power of the coaching process to draw out the skills or talent that was previously hidden within an individual, and which invariably finds a way to solve a problem previously thought unsolvable.
>
> —John Russell
> "

HIGH RELIABILITY ORGANIZATIONS AND A CULTURE OF SAFETY

High reliability organizations (HROs) are distinguished by their effective management of the delivery of healthcare through organizational control of both hazard and probability while recognizing variability as a constant (Agency for Healthcare Research and Quality [AHRQ], 2008). This calls for a collective mindfulness of preoccupation with failure, reluctance to simplify, sensitivity to operations, commitment to resilience, and deference to expertise (Weick and Sutcliffe, 2007). What distinguishes a high-risk system are the factors that the system must control to ensure safety. Whether it is the environment, the healthcare system itself, or the patient, all are constantly changing and challenging the reliability of the system to deliver safe care. A culture of safety is fundamental for avoiding patient harm (Reason, 1997). In a culture of safety, everyone is encouraged to work toward patient safety and to take action as necessary.

A culture of safety is more complex to articulate when caring for children than when caring for adults. Children differ from adults anatomically, physiologically, immunologically, psychologically, developmentally, and metabolically. These differences are in a constant state of change.

Often, the term *children* is used to cover all age groups from birth to age 19. However, there are five different age groups within that span:

- Newborns (1 to 28 days)
- Infants (up to 12 months)
- Children (1 to 10 years)
- Adolescents (10 to 19 years)
- Young adults (20 to 39 years)

Forrest and colleagues (1997) conceptualized unique issues for children compared to adults as the four Ds: developmental change, dependency, differential epidemiology, and demography. The demography changes affecting pediatric populations are constant. We are seeing unprecedented gains in child survival and an increasing life expectancy. Financing of child health services (the fifth D, dollars)—although more of an external characteristic—is different as well. Many healthcare dollars for children focus on promoting prevention, early screening, and early intervention.

PEDIATRIC SAFETY

Professionals who care for pediatric patients in both acute and primary care settings must have a working knowledge of patient safety to prevent injury to children, although research in pediatric ambulatory settings is limited. Pediatric professionals must advocate for studies that examine risks that are unique to children to eliminate avoidable harm in any setting in which medical care is rendered to children. Standardized nomenclature provides consistency between interdisciplinary teams and can facilitate multisite studies. Currently, there is no standard nomenclature for pediatric patient safety that is widely used.

PEDIATRICS AS A SPECIALTY

Pediatrics is a medical specialty focusing on the prevention, diagnosis, and treatment of infants, children, and adolescents. The primary aims of those working in pediatric settings are to provide preventive health maintenance for healthy children and medical care for those who are seriously or chronically ill. Those who specialize in pediatrics work to reduce infant and child mortality, control infectious disease, foster healthy lifestyles, and ease the day-to-day difficulties of children and adolescents with chronic conditions.

Pediatrics as a specialty recognizes that genetic, biological, social, and environmental influences affect the developing child. Abraham Jacobi (1830–1919) is referred to as the "father of pediatrics" because he broke new ground in the scientific and clinical investigation of childhood diseases. Lillian Wald (1867–1940) founded the Henry Street Settlement in New York City, which provided nursing and social work pediatric services. In 1909, President Theodore Roosevelt called the first White House Conference on Children, which focused on the care of dependent children. As a result of this conference, the U.S. Children's Bureau was established in 1912 and placed under the Department of Health, Education and Welfare (now the Department of Health and Human Services). This marked the beginning of a period of scientific and clinical investigation into infant mortality.

Since those early days, other federal programs have been established that have an impact on children such as Medicaid; Women, Infants and Children (WIC); and the Education for All Handicapped Children Act (Public Law 94-142), which was passed in 1975. This law provides support to states and local governmental entities to protect the rights of, meet the individual needs of, and improve the results for infants, toddlers, children, and youth with disabilities and their families. This landmark law is currently enacted as the Individuals with Disabilities Education Act (IDEA), as amended in 1997.

The same genetic, biological, social, and environmental influences that affect the developing child and are recognized in the field of pediatrics make for challenges in ensuring safe health-care for children. Pediatric healthcare professionals are well aware that care of children cannot be inferred from care of adults. Children go through distinct periods of development as they move from infants to young adults. During each of these stages, multiple changes in the development of the brain take place. What occurs and approximately when these developments take place are genetically determined. However, environmental circumstances—such as hospitalization and exchanges with key individuals, such as nurses, within that environment—have significant influence on how each child benefits from each developmental event. Constant change in development, growth, and environment place children at increased risk for adverse safety events when receiving healthcare in our current system.

Parents of children are also experiencing change in development, either personally or as parents. Families are in a continual state of adjustment as children grow and develop. It is this dynamic quality of both family and child that makes provision of safe care for children so difficult and so very different from adult care. The philosophy of family-centered care recognizes the importance of family in a child's life. As such, the term *partnering with families* has arisen in pediatric healthcare. The dynamic nature of development of both the child and his or her parents leads to the need for dynamic partnership. There is a need to support families in their natural caregiving and decision-making roles by building on their unique strengths and acknowledging their expertise in caring for their child, even when that child is hospitalized. Families can play a pivotal role in safety, advocating for their children and monitoring their child's progress through acute illness, but they may need to be taught ways to do so. The single most important way parents can help prevent errors is to be an active member of their child's healthcare team (Conway et al., 2006; Kuo et al., 2012).

PEDIATRIC HEALTH SYSTEMS AND POLICY

Health systems must also be dynamic. They must be able to respond rapidly and appropriately to the changing physical, emotional, mental, and social development of infants, toddlers, children, and youth. Systems must be in place to enhance the experience of care. Children are at a greater risk of medical errors due in part to dynamic developmental physiology, size and weight, dependency on parents and other care providers, and different pathophysiology and epidemiology of medical conditions from adults (Bearer, 1995). Pediatric healthcare is in a state of constant transformation as children's hospitals routinely question, probe, and improve the way they deliver care. HROs recognize variability as a constant and are focused on minimizing that variability and its effects to ensure patient safety (Reason, 1997).

Patient safety in the pediatric arena may be defined as preventing injury to children caused directly by the healthcare system. Seminal policy statements from the American Academy of Pediatrics have led the way to identification of and strategies to affect patient safety. The

American Academy of Pediatrics (AAP) published "Principles of Patient Safety in Pediatrics" in 2001 (Lannon et al., 2001). In 2003, it published "Prevention of Medication Errors in the Pediatric Inpatient Setting" (Stucky, American Academy of Pediatrics Committee on Drugs, and American Academy of Pediatrics Committee on Hospital Care, 2003). In 2007, "Patient Safety in the Pediatric Emergency Care Setting" was published (Committee on Pediatric Emergency Medicine, American Academy of Pediatrics, Krug, and Frush). From these policies, efforts to improve patient safety and prevent errors have developed. It is well recognized that most errors in pediatric care are "systems errors related to equipment, complex processes, fragmented care and lack of standardized procedures" (Lannon et al., 2001, p. 1473). Despite active detection, errors will occur in systems as complex as pediatric healthcare (Dougherty and Simpson, 2004).

PEDIATRIC ERRORS AND NEAR MISSES: MEDICATIONS AND IDENTIFICATION

The purpose of instilling a culture of safety is to ensure no harm in all areas where pediatric patients can be seen, including ambulatory settings, behavioral health settings, home care, and hospitals. Patient safety goals should also be instilled in Critical Access Hospitals (CAHs), which are hospitals that are located in rural areas that have no more than 25 beds and keep patients fewer than 96 hours. Two areas of safety culture emphasis that require different approaches from those seen in adult care are prevention of errors related to medications and patient identification.

The Use of Medications

When it comes to medications, special considerations to prevent a medical error and patient harm must be made for children. Children pose special challenges to the medication-processing system at all stages (Takata, Taketomo, Waite, and California Pediatric Patient Safety Initiative, 2008). Ordering medications typically involves more calculations in pediatrics compared with adult medicine because weight-based dosing is needed for virtually all drugs. You may recall how the actor Dennis Quaid's newborn twins nearly died after receiving 1,000 times the prescribed dose of a blood thinner (Grant, 2010). Children are at a greater risk for medication errors due to different epidemiology of medical conditions and development-related issues with communication and swallowing.

Medication errors affect the pediatric age group in all settings: outpatient, inpatient, emergency department, and at home. For example, caregivers of young children frequently measure doses of liquid medications incorrectly. Medication errors can occur at all stages in medication use: when calculating weight-based doses, when transcribing or placing orders into the computerized physician order entry (CPOE) system, when dispensing, and when administering. Some children, particularly those with chronic illnesses and on multiple medications, may be at special risk of medication errors. One study found an increased error rate in analgesics and antimicrobials for overweight/obese (BMI ≥ 85th percentile) patients 5 to12 years of age (Miller, Johnson, Harrison, and Hagemann, 2010). Many medications for children are given in ambulatory care settings, in schools, in childcare settings, and in the home, which increases the risk for errors in calculation. Errors associated with medications are believed to be the most common type of pediatric medical error and are a significant cause of preventable adverse events.

Proper Identification of Patients

In addition to pediatric medication errors, accurate and consistent placement of a patient identification (ID) band is needed to reduce errors associated with patient misidentification. Patient identification is the cornerstone of patient safety. Identification bands have become an important area of focus when it comes to hospital patient safety and also workflow efficiency (Phillips, Saysana, Worley, and Hain, 2012). The use of barcode technology for patient identification is a growing trend at many healthcare organizations.

There are many reasons an ID may not be placed on a pediatric patient, such as small size of the extremities, especially in the neonate, or the child taking it off. Still, the lack of an identification band leads to inability to correctly identify the patient. Even if the ID band is in place, a small band may make scanning a challenge. Making multiple armbands and placing them on a clipboard for ease of scanning is called a *workaround*. Workarounds place the patient at risk for harm. With barcoding, as with any technology, the key to success lies in helping nurses and clinicians confirm patient identification with the greatest possible ease and reliability.

PEDIATRIC ERRORS AND NEAR MISSES: COMMUNICATION

Effective communication among healthcare professionals is challenging due to a number of interrelated dynamics (Nagelkerk et al., 2014). Ineffective communication among healthcare professionals is one of the leading causes of medical errors and patient harm (Leonard, Graham, and Bonacum, 2004; Lyndon, 2006). There must be optimal communication among interprofessional team members as well as team collaboration. Children have limited voice and rely on skilled, collaborative teamwork for the safe delivery of quality care.

The growing body of literature on safety and error prevention reveals that ineffective or insufficient communication among team members, including patients and their families, is a significant contributing factor to adverse events (Bartlett, Blais, Tamblyn, Clermont, and MacGibbon, 2008; Coté, Notterman, Karl, Weinberg, and McCloskey, 2000; Cullen et al., 1997; Gandhi et al., 2003). One method organizations can use to enhance communication and teamwork is bedside reporting. Bedside reporting, or rounding, may well increase patient involvement, enhance patient knowledge of their own care, increase teambuilding among staff, and prevent adverse events.

One unique way to encourage caregivers to hear their patients' voices is for interdisciplinary rounding to be delivered and recorded at the bedside in real time (Hain, Ng, Aronow, Swanson, and Bolton, 2009; Kau et al., 2008). This ensures that patients and their families are involved in their care. System-wide change to bedside rounding has been shown to improve patient satisfaction with nursing and physician care, decrease length of stay, decrease patient safety issues, and increase nurse satisfaction with nurse/physician communication (Gonzalo, Chuang, Huang, and Smith, 2010; Phipps et al., 2007).

Disparate healthcare providers' ability to work well in teams has added to the complexity of healthcare delivery and is a central factor in patient harm (Dekker, 2012; Frankel, Leonard, and Denham, 2006). A transformation in culture may be needed to improve patient safety and prevent errors by developing a focus on systems and not on individuals. There needs to be a culture of sharing and open discussion of errors so that contextual data about the error can be collected and evaluated. Peer review and legal protections should be extended to encourage participation. In addition, information discussed during patient safety reviews should be undiscoverable in civil or criminal courts.

Preventable errors in pediatrics, such as errors attributable to changes in patient weight and physiologic maturation, should be monitored closely so that systems can be developed to prevent these types of errors in the future. Information technology has great potential to minimize such errors, but human error—even with the best technology—is always possible. High reliability practices that acknowledge human factors and the intricacies of pediatric populations must be developed, and outcomes must be measured to prevent harm.

PEDIATRIC ERRORS AND NEAR MISSES: SYSTEMS AND INDIVIDUALS

Pediatric patient safety must take into account harm to children caused not only directly by the healthcare system but also by an individual working within that system. The Institute of Medicine's (IOM) report "To Err Is Human: Building a Safer Health System" (IOM, 1999) has generated a focus on preventable harm in healthcare organizations. The notion that harm can be prevented and that errors leading to harm are not inevitable is indeed a view that children and their families would agree is worthwhile. A culture of safety transforms healthcare organizations toward the reduction or elimination of preventable harm where it is identified. A *Just Culture*—a term coined by Sidney Dekker (2012)—is an organizational culture where the focus is on balancing learning from errors or near misses with accountability for consequences. A system fostering a rich reporting culture must be created to capture accurate and detailed data for both harm and near misses.

An environment that supports a systems-focus approach and takes into account individual accountability may promote a culture of safety. Healthcare professionals can play an important role in helping their colleagues acquire motivation to change their behavior. Coaching is a form of inquiry-based learning characterized by collaboration (Dickerson, Koch, Adams, Goodfriend, and Donnelly, 2010; Duff, 2013). Individual coaching is a well-accepted educational method in fields such as sports, music, and business. Coaching experts argue that feedback and skill practice through on-the-job coaching yield improved performance, regardless of the level of expertise of the person being coached. However, the role of coaching in the healthcare industry has not been well studied.

SAFETY COACHING

True culture change requires constant reinforcement. Constant reinforcement of the culture of safety within a system may be achieved through the use of safety coaches (Harton and Ingram, 2013). In one organization that specializes in the care of infants, children, adolescents, and young adults, a safety coaching program was implemented as part of the journey to do no harm.

In this program, individuals in all the healthcare professions either self-select or are nominated for the role of safety coach by their peers. The culture of safety at both the systems and the individual level are emphasized. The training underscores the healthcare system's mental model on patient safety. A shared mental model can be defined as "a mechanism whereby humans generate a description of system purpose and form, explanation of system functioning and observed system states and prediction of future system states" (Rouse and Morris, 1986, p. 360). Mental models that take into account contextual elements have been studied in the effectiveness of air traffic controllers (Smith-Jentsch, Mathieu, and Kraiger, 2005). In one study examining mental models on safety in industry, the authors found that when variables influencing safety are considered within a framework of safe work behaviors, managers and employees share a similar mental model (Prussia, Brown, and Willis, 2003). The program ensures that safety coaches are introduced to the system's model to do no harm, and participants are encouraged to share in the model by acknowledging their own behaviors that can have an effect on a patient's care, including behaviors that affect the system.

The coaches begin with an all-day training, including didactic education on recognizing triggers and opportunities to coach, as well as role-playing scenarios to practice coaching skills. Triggers to coach include safety practices such as the following:

- Introductions of staff to each other and to patients and their family members
- Pause to care
- Advancing research and clinical practice through close collaboration (ARCC)
- I am *c*oncerned; I'm *u*ncomfortable; this is a *s*afety issue (CUS)
- Situation, background, assessment, recommendation (SBAR)
- Read back/repeat back

Triggers also include safety bundles, such as for the following:

- Adverse drug events

- Catheter-associated urinary tract infections (CAUTIs)

- Falls

- Patient identification

- Pressure ulcers

- Surgical site infections

- Ventilator associated pneumonia (VAP)

- Venous thromboembolism (VTE)

- Central line–associated bloodstream infection (CLABSI)

Safety coaches are in-the-moment coaches, working side by side with staff. They are responsible for keeping safety first and foremost in the staff's minds. One endeavor of the safety coach is to observe peers engaged in patient care. Observing for inconsistency in safety practices, such as noticing a co-worker taking a medication into the wrong patient room but stopping before it is given (near miss), the safety coach must recognize that the person may not realize his or her lapse in following the correct procedure or may have developed a workaround due to problems encountered with the system or organization. The coach must not only notice the lapse in performance but also be able to talk with the person about near misses as well as recognize and encourage good practice in real time (Barach and Small, 2000). For example, using open-ended questions to encourage the nurse to talk about the experience of obtaining the medication may prompt the sharing of a workaround that he uses that led to the near miss.

In the safety coach training program, the safety coach is taught to use a framework to structure feedback called the Situation-Behavior-Impact (SBI) Feedback Tool (Weitzel, 2003). This helps people understand precisely the behavior on which the safety coach is commenting and why. When the impact of the behavior on others is shared, the person being coached is given time to reflect on his or her actions and to think about what he or she needs to change. An example of safety coaching using the SBI format is as follows:

- **Situation (S):** A new RN is working on a very busy medical unit when a seasoned RN (safety coach) notices her entering a patient room without using the antiseptic foam. The nurse (safety coach) approaches the new nurse to ask about the incident and uses an open-ended questioning technique about her understanding of what hand hygiene means to her.

- **Behavior (B):** The new nurse is at first taken aback, but with the supportive communication strategies used by the safety coach, she acknowledges that she was intent on entering the room only to deliver linen. Since she was not going to touch the patient, she did not think it was necessary to use the hand antiseptic before entering.

■ **Impact (I):** After the nurse (coach) listened to the new nurse's understanding of what it means to follow proper hand hygiene, she did an excellent job of providing the new nurse with the proper education around hand-hygiene protocol and how it is very important to provide safe care for all patients and perform the hand-hygiene protocol fully. The new RN was extremely grateful for the education and thanked the nurse (coach) for her approach. The new RN had no idea that she was not following hand-hygiene protocol.

When a safety coach approaches a peer engaging in unsafe practice, the coach must recognize that ambivalence on the part of the staff member is normal. Safety coaches use open-ended questions as well as the skill of reflective listening so staff hear their own words as opposed to those of the safety coach. The coach then helps the staff member to develop a discrepancy between current behaviors or the status quo and what the person would like things to look like in the future. Importantly, this discrepancy needs to be based on what is important to the staff member, not to the coach. That way, the person begins to hear his or her own reasons for changing. For example, when a staff member is asked by the safety coach about not turning the patient, yet charting that the patient was turned every 2 hours, the conversation begins with the open-ended question, "Tell me about what was going on today with your patient in room 202." The nurse may respond that he was rushed all day and wanted to get home on time, so when he did his charting, he quickly documented what he did. He may seem ambivalent at first. He may share that he did not notice that he had charted incorrectly. He may go on to say that he feels very responsible to chart only the cares he provides. The safety coach can begin with, "I hear you say that that you are a responsible nurse and take charting seriously." The coaching goes on from that point, always reflecting what the nurse shares to clarify meaning and eventually discussing what the nurse may put into place to help prevent this error in the future.

Rolling with resistance is a strategy that honors where the staff member is in terms of thinking, feeling, and acting (Burke, Arkowitz, and Menchola, 2003). Rather than push for change, the coach understands that the solutions reside within the staff member. In the preceding example, the coach must not engage the nurse directly about the falsified charting or the nurse may resist the conversation. Rolling with his resistance to discuss the situation is important. Seeking information about what was going on during charting and then asking him what he can do in the future to avoid the mistake honors his ability to find the solution. Finally, the coach supports self-efficacy by understanding that the staff member's beliefs about his or her ability to change are directly related to that person's capacity to change. The coach may state, "I have seen you provide safe care and chart thoroughly on patients prior to this instance. I have faith that you can implement the strategies you shared so that your charting in the future will reflect only the cares you have completed."

Empathy is a skill that permits the safety coach to promote behavior change, especially when ambivalence on the part of the staff member is encountered. For example, studies have shown that hand-washing compliance is abysmal in many hospitals (Pittet, Mourouga, and Perneger, 1999; Voss, Widmer, and Pittet, 2003). Suppose a safety coach views a co-worker coming out of a patient room without using alcohol spray, which is against hospital policy and does not align with the shared mental model of safety in the organization. The coach would first inquire about an opportunity to talk with the employee. The coach would be curious, using active listening and open-ended questions to find out why the employee did not wash his or her hands. The coach would then facilitate a discussion focusing on helping the employee see the contradictions between what he or she wants to do (keep the patient safe from harm) and what he or she is actually doing (not washing his or her hands). The coach will promote a belief that the person can change by identifying previous successful experiences and focusing on the employee's skills. Thus, core to the coach-staff relationship is the coach's strong belief in the staff member's ability to decide when and how to make desired changes.

Safety coaches fill the need for a non-punitive, safe, and blame-free strategy for healthcare professionals to describe actual or potential errors. Safety coaching has been shown to be an effective safety strategy in industries such as construction, aviation, and nuclear power, and may prove beneficial in healthcare settings. If the safety coach structures discussions with staff so that they allow for exploration of the near miss and seek staff resolution to change their behavior, healthcare may be improved. Safety coaches should use objective measurement to determine how to report the situation as either a near miss or actual harm so reports are accurate.

The events, both actual and near misses, include details of the event obtained through the coaching process, and are recorded using the available hospital system. This data is available for use in unit-specific dashboards that unit managers and safety coaches can share with staff. Thus, the circle of finding and addressing system or individual errors, actual or potential, is completed. The process supports staff involvement in a culture of safety, which is fundamental for avoiding patient harm.

SUMMARY

We can realistically acknowledge that children are different from adults and that the approaches to eliminate serious harm for children may indeed be different from those of the adult. However, we must admit that there is opportunity to learn from other industries. As long as the approaches are science-based, we may be able to borrow strategies from other industries outside of healthcare. Safety coaching, borrowed from the construction industry, is becoming a strategy for experienced pediatric nurses to use to ensure safe care for pediatric patients. Continued work is needed to infuse safety practices into the everyday work of pediatric clinicians, and safety coaching may be the best approach. Rigorous evaluation systems must be deployed and developed so that the risk of errors to children can be further reduced or eliminated.

KEY POINTS

- Children are not little adults. There are differences in the ways we must address, improve, and ensure the safety of pediatric patients.

- Errors in pediatric care are due to systems errors related to equipment, complex processes, fragmented care, and lack of standardized procedures and/or failure on the part of the healthcare worker to do no harm.

- Children and their environments are dynamically changing and pose special challenges, especially in medication-processing systems and deficiencies in the accurate and consistent placement of patient IDs.

- A system fostering a rich reporting culture must be created to capture accurate and detailed data for both harm and near misses.

- HROs use safety coaching to avert harm. This aids in organizational control of both hazard and probability thanks to a preoccupation with failure.

REFERENCES

Agency for Healthcare Research and Quality (AHRQ). (2008). Becoming a high reliability organization: Operational advice for hospital leaders. Retrieved from http://archive.ahrq.gov/professionals/quality-patient-safety/quality-resources/tools/hroadvice/hroadvice.pdf

Barach, P., and Small, S. D. (2000). Reporting and preventing medical mishaps: Lessons from non-medical near miss reporting systems. *BMJ, 320*(7237), pp. 759–763.

Bartlett, G., Blais, R., Tamblyn, R., Clermont, R. J., and MacGibbon, B. (2008). Impact of patient communication problems on the risk of preventable adverse events in acute care settings. *Canadian Medical Association Journal, 178*(12), pp. 1555–1562.

Bearer, C. F. (1995). How are children different from adults? *Environmental Health Perspectives, 103*(Suppl. 6), pp. 7–12.

Burke, B. L., Arkowitz, H., and Menchola, M. (2003). The efficacy of motivational interviewing: A meta-analysis of controlled clinical trials. *Journal of Consulting and Clinical Psychology, 71*(5), pp. 843–861.

Committee on Pediatric Emergency Medicine, American Academy of Pediatrics, Krug, S. E., and Frush, K. (2007). Patient safety in the pediatric emergency care setting. *Pediatrics, 120*(6), pp. 1367–1375.

Conway, J., Johnson, B., Edgman-Levitan, S., Schlucter, J., Ford, D., Sodomka, P., and Simmons, L. (2006). Partnering with patients and families to design a patient-and family-centered health care system: A roadmap for the future: A work in progress. *Institute for Patient- and Family-Centered Care*. Retrieved from http://www.ipfcc.org/pdf/Roadmap.pdf

Coté, C. J., Notterman, D. A., Karl, H. W., Weinberg, J. A., and McCloskey, C. (2000). Adverse sedation events in pediatrics: A critical incident analysis of contributing factors. *Pediatrics, 105*(4), pp. 805–814.

Cullen, D. J., Sweitzer, B. J., Bates, D. W., Burdick, E., Edmondson, A., and Leape, L. L. (1997). Preventable adverse drug events in hospitalized patients: A comparative study of intensive care and general care units. *Critical Care Medicine, 25*(8), pp. 1289–1297.

Dekker, S. (2012). *Just Culture: Balancing safety and accountability* (2nd ed.). Farnham, UK: Ashgate Publishing Company.

Dickerson, J. M., Koch, B. L., Adams, J. M., Goodfriend, M. A., and Donnelly, L. F. (2010). Safety coaches in radiology: Decreasing human error and minimizing patient harm. *Pediatric Radiology, 40*(9), pp. 1545–1551.

Dougherty, D., and Simpson, L. A. (2004). Measuring the quality of children's health care: A prerequisite to action. *Pediatrics, 113*(1), pp. 185–198.

Duff, B. (2013). Creating a culture of safety by coaching clinicians to competence. *Nurse Education Today, 33*(10), pp. 1108–1111.

Forrest, C. B., Simpson, L., and Clancy, C. (1997). Child health services research. Challenges and opportunities. *JAMA, 277*(22), pp. 1787–1793.

Frankel, A. S., Leonard, M. W., and Denham, C. R. (2006). Fair and just culture, team behavior, and leadership engagement: The tools to achieve high reliability. *Health Services Research, 41*(4), pp. 1690–1709.

Gandhi, T. K., Weingart, S. N., Borus, J., Seger, A. C., Peterson, J., Burdick, E., … Bates, D. W. (2003). Adverse drug events in ambulatory care. *New England Journal of Medicine, 348*(16), pp. 1556–1564.

Gonzalo, J. D., Chuang, C. H., Huang, G., and Smith, C. (2010). The return of bedside rounds: An educational intervention. *Journal of General Internal Medicine, 25*(8), pp. 792–798.

Grant, M. (2010). Dennis Quaid's quest. *AARP The Magazine*, September/October.

Hain, P. B., Ng, C. S., Aronow, H. U., Swanson, J. W., and Bolton, L. B. (2009). Improving communication with bedside video rounding. *The American Journal of Nursing, 109*(11 Suppl.), pp. 18–20.

Harton, B. B., and Ingram, S. W. (2013). Ready for lift off: Implementing a safety coach initiative. *Nursing Management, 44*(5), pp. 40–45.

Institute of Medicine (IOM). (1999). To err is human: Building a safer health system. Washington, DC: National Academies Press.

The Joint Commission. (2015). National patient safety goals. Retrieved from http://www.jointcommission.org/standards_information/npsgs.aspx

Kau, E. L., Baranda, D. T., Hain, P., Bolton, L. B., Chen, T., Fuchs, G. J., and Ng, C. S. (2008). Video rounding system: A pilot study in patient care. *Journal of Endourology, 22*(6), pp. 1179–1182.

Kuo, D. Z., Houtrow, A. J., Arango, P., Kuhlthau, K. A., Simmons, J. M., and Neff, J. M. (2012). Family-centered care: Current applications and future directions in pediatric health care. *Maternal and Child Health Journal, 16*(2), pp. 297–305.

Lannon, C. M., Coven, B. J., Lane France, F., Hickson, G. B., Miles, P. V., Swanson, J. T., … National Initiative for Children's Health Care Quality Project Advisory Committee. (2001). Principles of patient safety in pediatrics. *Pediatrics, 107*(6), pp. 1473–1475.

Leonard, M., Graham, S., and Bonacum, D. (2004). The human factor: The critical importance of effective teamwork and communication in providing safe care. *Quality & Safety in Health Care, 13 Suppl. 1*, pp. i85–i90.

Lyndon, A. (2006). Communication and teamwork in patient care: How much can we learn from aviation? *Journal of Obstetric, Gynecologic, and Neonatal Nursing, 35*(4), pp. 538–546.

Miller, J. L., Johnson, P. N., Harrison, D. L., and Hagemann, T. M. (2010). Evaluation of inpatient admissions and potential antimicrobial and analgesic dosing errors in overweight children. *The Annals of Pharmacotherapy, 1*(44), pp. 35–42.

Nagelkerk, J., Peterson, T., Pawl, B. L., Teman, S., Anyangu, A. C., Mlynarczyk, S., and Baer, L. J. (2014). Patient safety culture transformation in a children's hospital: An interprofessional approach. *Journal of Interprofessional Care, 28*(4), pp. 358–364.

Phillips, S. C., Saysana, M., Worley, S., and Hain, P. D. (2012). Reduction in pediatric identification band errors: A quality collaborative. *Pediatrics, 129*(6), pp. e1587–e1593.

Phipps, L. M., Bartke, C. N., Spear, D. A., Jones, L. F., Foerster, C. P., Killian, M. E., … Thomas, N. J. (2007). Assessment of parental presence during bedside pediatric intensive care unit rounds: Effect on duration, teaching, and privacy. *Pediatric Critical Care Medicine, 8*(3), pp. 220–224.

Pittet, D., Mourouga, P., and Perneger, T. V. (1999). Compliance with handwashing in a teaching hospital. Infection control program. *Annals of Internal Medicine, 130*(2), pp. 126–130.

Pronovost, P. J., Berenholtz, S. M., Goeschel, C. A., Needham, D. M., Sexton, J. B., Thompson, D. A., … Hunt, E. (2006). Creating high reliability in health care organizations. *Health Services Research, 41*(4), 1599–1617.

Prussia, G. E., Brown, K. A., and Willis, P. G. (2003). Mental models of safety: Do managers and employees see eye to eye? *Journal of Safety Research, 34*(2), pp. 143–156.

Reason, J. T. (1997). *Managing the risks of organizational accidents*. Farnham, UK: Ashgate Publishing Company.

Rouse, W. B., and Morris, N. M. (1986). On looking into the black box: Prospects and limits in the search for mental models. *Psychological Bulletin, 100*(3), pp. 349–363.

Smith-Jentsch, K. A., Mathieu, J. E., and Kraiger, K. (2005). Investigating linear and interactive effects of shared mental models on safety and efficiency in a field setting. *Journal of Applied Psychology, 90*(3), pp. 523–535.

Stucky, E. R., American Academy of Pediatrics Committee on Drugs, and American Academy of Pediatrics Committee on Hospital Care. (2003). Prevention of medication errors in the pediatric inpatient setting. *Pediatrics, 112*(2), pp. 431–436.

Takata, G. S., Taketomo, C. K., Waite, S., and California Pediatric Patient Safety Initiative. (2008). Characteristics of medication errors and adverse drug events in hospitals participating in the California Pediatric Patient Safety Initiative. *American Journal of Health-System Pharmacy, 65*(21), pp. 2036–2044.

Voss, A., Widmer, A., and Pittet, D. (2003). Hand antisepsis: Evaluation of a sprayer system for alcohol distribution. *Infection Control and Hospital Epidemiology, 24*(9), p. 637.

Weick, K. E., and Sutcliffe, K. M. (2007). *Managing the unexpected: Resilient performance in an age of uncertainty* (2nd ed.). San Francisco, CA: Jossey-Bass.

Weitzel, S. R. (2000.) *Feedback that works: How to build and deliver your message*. Greensboro, NC: Center for Creative Leadership.

CHAPTER 19

APPLYING HIGH RELIABILITY PRINCIPLES ACROSS A LARGE HEALTHCARE SYSTEM TO REDUCE PATIENT FALLS

Noreen Bernard, MS, RN, NEA-BC

Healthcare organizations strive to reduce patient falls and aspire to have fall rates of zero. Fall prevention is an important clinical focus in patient safety. Countless interventions, tools, fall-prevention programs, increased use of sitters, and a variety of nursing practices are implemented across the United States in an effort to keep patients safer (Adams and Kaplow, 2013).

This chapter describes a large, multi-hospital system's dedication to fall prevention through the use of high reliability organization (HRO) principles. Further, it reviews change management and the impact on cultural transition as a related and relevant element of transforming an organization to be highly reliable. The cultural transformation in this project was driven through the use of empowerment, innovation, and nurse-led initiatives. Presented is a background of the organization, problem selection, description

> "Transformation is about picking something bigger than us, and that we think we cannot do, and then going after it.
>
> —*Bruce Avolio*"

of the project team, project design, pilot study results, toolkit development and deployment, post-project results, monitoring plans, and project expansion, with the purpose of sharing highly reliable fall-reduction practices. A discussion of the project related to HRO principles, including project strengths and lessons, summarizes the clinical challenge to innovatively transform a system-wide culture of patient safety.

An HRO focuses on exceptional safety in patient care delivery through specific training to minimize errors and work toward a defect-free environment (Riley, 2009). Collaborative, team-oriented care delivery is an effective method for achieving high reliability. Further, when those with the closest line of sight to the patient direct the clinical care, safety and effectiveness improve significantly because of the relevant knowledge of those professionals. Standardization of clinical practice supports decreased variation in the delivery of patient care and improved performance outcomes. As this multi-hospital system evaluated the historically unimproved and inconsistent fall rates, a council of clinical nurses determined that a new approach was needed to improve patient safety.

BACKGROUND

At the beginning of the project, the healthcare system described in this chapter was composed of 13 acute care hospitals spanning an entire state, including rural facilities. At the end of the project, the healthcare system supported 15 hospitals across two states. The company structure is a faith-based, nonprofit healthcare organization. It is the fourth largest private employer in the primary state, employing more than 20,000 associates. Approximately 5,500 are nurses, with an overall baccalaureate preparation rate of 55%. Of the current nurses, 24% hold specialty certifications. The nursing leadership structure is deeply rooted in shared leadership across the whole system as well as in the individual facilities. At the system level, there are councils composed of members and leaders of the local shared governance councils. This structure ensures connectivity among local hospitals and drives standardization across the system. All system-level councils (nursing practice, professional development, and advanced practice nursing) report to the nursing executive council, composed of the chief nursing officer (CNO) from each hospital and the chief nurse executive for the system.

At the system and local levels, the nursing practice council consults, recommends, designs, and implements evidence-based, standardized nursing practice, policies, procedures, clinical documentation, and clinical equipment changes. It further initiates nursing practice projects and leads those projects from commencement to completion. The system nursing practice council priorities, activities, decisions, recommendations, and work outcomes are approved by the system-level nursing executive council.

NURSING PRACTICE COUNCIL MEMBERSHIP

It is important to clearly describe the composition of the system-level nursing practice council. It is composed of facility nursing practice council nurse leaders who are direct care providers. These nurse leaders typically spend 90% of their working hours providing direct clinical care. This structure clearly depicts shared leadership and nurse empowerment. Membership on the council also includes the system chief nurse executive, a representative from the system professional development council, a member from the advanced practice nursing council, members from the patient safety team, and nursing informatics representation. The role of the council is to support the overall company nursing vision of achieving national distinction in nursing excellence.

The system nursing practice council was formed in 2010. At its initiation, the council conducted a needs assessment in collaboration with the nursing executive council and identified an opportunity to improve fall rates across the system. The ability for nurses to affect a nurse-sensitive indicator in a formal manner sends clear messaging about the application of nursing expertise in developing an HRO. The concept of deference to experts is made clear in Riley's (2009) discussion on important HRO elements, as well as the role of the nurse leader in supporting empowerment as a method to create an HRO.

CONCEPTUAL MODEL TO ADDRESS CHANGE

A framework for change management was present at the initiation of this work. The executive sponsors of the system nursing practice council embraced John Kotter's model of change management as a typical framework to approach nursing practice changes. The steps of the model are as follows:

1. Establish a sense of urgency.

2. Create the guiding coalition.

3. Develop a vision and strategy.

4. Communicate the change vision.

5. Empower employees for change.

6. Generate short-term wins.

7. Consolidate gains and produce more change.

8. Anchor new approaches in the culture (Gupta, 2011).

These eight steps were evident in the work of the nursing practice council (the guiding coalition) throughout this project.

FALL-RATE MONITORING AND OWNERSHIP OF THE PROBLEM

Leaders in HROs pay attention to the weak signals, the research, and the available data, and take initiative to find opportunities to prevent deaths and injuries (Kerfoot, 2003). When assessing the problem of unimproved fall rates across the system, another problem was identified: The ownership of fall data and accountability resided in the quality departments in most of the hospitals. So the first challenge became the handoff of fall prevention over to nursing.

Before this project, the quality department primarily monitored clinical outcomes, with an interface to nursing. While this relationship historically was acceptable, fall rates remained unchanged, thereby demonstrating a sense of urgency and a need for change. The quality department had direct contact with the fall data, while the nursing department was peripherally connected to the data. Therefore, it was only minimally aware of the potential safety improvement opportunities. According to HRO organizing principles, deference to expertise is essential. Decision-making must migrate to the people with the most expertise, regardless of rank in the organization (Sutcliffe, 2011). Thus, the decision to shift the ownership of falls reduction out of the quality department and over to nursing aligned with HRO principles.

During the transition of falls ownership, as well as ongoing, collaboration with the quality department was essential for success. Clinical nurses from each hospital, along with other council members, were empowered and charged to reduce falls through standardized nursing practice. This began a journey of culture change with the transition to standardized nursing practice and accountability to reduce patient falls. Achieving uniformity in the delivery of nursing care ensures high reliability through stable processes with low variation (Riley, 2009).

PROJECT TEAM

Several initial steps were taken in this project. First, development of an effective team ensured that the right knowledge, skills, and attitudes were in place to transform fall prevention across a large healthcare system. Effective team characteristics include team leadership, backup behavior, performance monitoring, communication, trust, and team orientation (Riley, 2009). The decision was made to use the system-level nursing practice council (front-line clinical nurses) as the guiding coalition because the council membership already represented diverse perspectives.

PROJECT DESIGN

The first step in organizing the project was to gather the nursing practice council members, as well as representatives from quality departments, to participate in a rapid decision-making event. A Six Sigma black belt facilitated the session. Before the event, the team conducted a literature review on fall prevention and gathered a list of current hospital-level nursing practices. The fall-prevention programmatic information from other health systems, as well as studies on fall-reduction programs, demonstrated variety in effective clinical interventions for fall reduction (Barker, Kamar, and Berlowitz, 2009; Butcher, 2013; DiBardino, Cohen, and Didwania, 2012; Fonda, Cook, Sandler, and Bailey, 2006; Kim, Mordiffi, Bee, Devi, and Evans, 2007; Lovallo, Rolandi, Rossetti, and Lusignani, 2010). Further, a literature review of the scope of the problem of falls was included at the outset of the session (Lueckenotte and Conley, 2009; Oliver, Healey, and Haines, 2010). At the event, a falls data review was also conducted to understand the baseline metrics. Lastly, cultural readiness was evaluated as positive for proceeding with the project.

During the event, the team discovered extensive variation in nursing interventions and assessments for fall prevention. Subsequently, a wide range of fall rates existed. The team determined there was a clear need to change the fall risk assessment tool as well as related nursing interventions and practices. For example, the existing fall risk assessment tool scored patients as high, moderate, or low risk for falls. Two years of baseline data indicated that 270 out of 510 falls, or 53%, were rated as moderate risk. Yet, patients rated as high fall risk did not fall as often as those with moderate risk scores. Similarly, qualitative feedback from clinical nurses before the rapid decision-making event informed the team that the existing fall-prevention protocols simply provided too many interventions for a nurse to select when designing the patient care plan.

The team agreed to conduct two pilot studies—one to look at fall-prevention interventions and the other to develop a standardized fall risk assessment tool. A pilot project design and methodology ensued, along with the development of typical project plan elements such as metrics, timelines, and communication. This was not a formal research study but a clinical practice project. The pilot project was broken into two phases, discussed in the next sections.

OUTCOMES

Two sets of outcomes were evaluated before determining the final nursing-practice changes. The first, described in phase one of the pilot study, involved fall-prevention interventions. Each hospital submitted a proposal to test one or more nursing interventions, which team members believed would reduce falls in their organization. The outcomes of that first phase are described in the next section. The second set of outcomes that were assessed pertained to the fall-assessment instrument. Two specific areas of interest were the focus of phase two. First, did the Hendrich II™ tool provide impactful accuracy during the fall risk assessment stage of planning patient care? Second, how easy or difficult was the tool to use? The results from this part of the pilot are provided after the results from phase one.

PHASE ONE OF THE PILOT STUDY AND RESULTS

The first phase focused on nursing interventions related to fall prevention. One goal of the project team was to ensure that the work in the project was engaging, fun, and rewarding. Thus, the team agreed to a friendly, professional contest. Each hospital was directed to submit proposals to pilot evidence-based fall-prevention interventions. A total of 12 submissions were received for the intervention pilots. The nursing practice council reviewed the submissions to ensure alignment and thoroughness of pilot methodologies, data collection, communication plans, and general implementation approaches. After the pilot launched, the nursing practice council diligently monitored the falls data each month from each hospital.

The data from the first phase of the pilot project demonstrated a range of 30% to 50% quantitative reduction in total falls at the end of the first phase of the pilot, with significant improvement in falls with injury. The interventions tested—which were primarily singular interventions rather than bundles of interventions—were evidence-based. Two matching time periods were compared to measure the impact of using evidence-based interventions. These included 6 months of fall data before the intervention pilot project and 6 months of fall data during the intervention pilot project. The council wanted to ensure similar time frames were compared to decrease potential variables in the data sets. The time frame used was January to June to account for seasonal effects.

Designing high reliability processes includes the concept of healthcare bundles (Riley, 2009). Inspired by the reduction in fall rates, the nursing practice council chose to bundle key nursing interventions that were substantiated by documented reductions in fall rates during the pilot. The recommended basic bundle of nursing interventions for patients scoring as high risk included the following:

- Toileting every 2 hours during the day shift
- Toileting every 4 hours during the night shift
- Use of properly fitting non-slip footwear
- Activation of bed or chair alarm
- Instruction to call for assistance to get up
- Patient and family education about how to ensure safety

Other fall-prevention interventions are presented in the revised falls policy and procedure document as adjunct options to this bundle should nursing assessment indicate a need for additional interventions.

Fall-Prevention Intervention Guidelines for Low-Risk Patients

A safe patient care environment is essential for all patients at all times. Fall-prevention interventions are organized based on the Hendrich II™ assessment-scoring tool (Hendrich, 2007; Hendrich, Bender, and Nyhuis, 2003).

Low-risk patients are those patients who have a fall-risk score between 0 and 4 points. For these patients, fall-prevention interventions include maintaining a safe care environment by doing the following:

- Removing excess equipment, supplies, and furniture from rooms and hallways
- Coiling and securing excess electrical and telephone wires
- Ensuring dry flooring
- Restricting window openings

In addition, basic safety interventions such as the following should be provided:

- Orienting patients to their surroundings, such as the bathroom location, bed controls, and call light
- Keeping the bed in the lowest position during use
- Keeping the bed's top two side rails up
- Securing locks on beds, stretchers, and wheelchairs
- Keeping floors free of clutter and obstacles, with special attention paid to the path between the bed and the bathroom/commode
- Placing the call light and other frequently needed objects within reach
- Answering call lights promptly
- Encouraging patients and visitors to call for assistance
- Displaying special instructions for vision- and hearing-impaired patients
- Ensuring adequate lighting, especially at night
- Using properly fitted non-skid footwear

Fall-Prevention Intervention Guidelines for High-Risk Patients

High-risk patients are those patients who score 5 or more on the Hendrich II™ fall risk assessment tool. These patients should receive the previously listed low-risk interventions (Hendrich,

2007; Hendrich et al., 2003). In addition, they should receive high-risk interventions. These include the following:

- Instituting a flagging system, such as a yellow color code. Place a fall risk magnet or other designated identification outside the patient room and/or in another appropriate and visible area within the room, and place a designated colored wristband on the patient.

- Setting a minimum 2-hour toileting schedule during daytime hours and a minimum 4-hour toileting schedule during nighttime hours.

- Remaining with the patient when toileting as appropriate per clinical judgment.

- Activating audible bed/chair alarm per clinical judgment.

Other fall-prevention interventions to consider include the following:

- Hourly rounding

- Using all four side rails for beds with an air overlay

- Using the assistance of trained caregivers when transporting patient

- Notifying the receiving area of a patient's high fall-risk status

- Locating the patient in a room with the best visual access to the nursing station

- Using a low bed

- Using protective devices such as hipsters, helmets, and gait belts

- Using 24-hour supervision/sitter

- Using physical and/or occupational therapy evaluation

- Using physical restraint or an enclosed bed only with a licensed independent practitioner (LIP) authorized order and adherence to restraint policies

PHASE TWO OF THE PILOT STUDY AND RESULTS

The fall risk assessment pilot was scheduled in the second phase of the project. In this phase, four nursing units piloted the Hendrich II Fall Risk Model™, which research from the literature review indicated was an effective fall-prevention program. Previously, a different assessment tool was used to score patients as high, moderate, or low risk for falls. The four nursing units, located in four different facilities, included a telemetry unit, an intensive care unit, a general medical/surgical unit, and an inpatient rehabilitation unit. Throughout this phase, a strong partnership with informatics was formed to plan for potential electronic medical record (EMR) redesigns to accommodate assessment and intervention practice changes that might emerge as a result of this project.

The tool was piloted for 60 days, and qualitative data was gathered using a five-point scale nurse survey inquiring about the accuracy (see Figure 19.1) and ease of use of the Hendrich II Fall Risk Model™ (see Figure 19.2). The survey was administered to 194 nurses; 120 responded, for a response rate of 62%. Nurses who scored the tool as inaccurate indicated there had been a lack of education on how to properly use the assessment tool. As per change management evidence, the neutral and inaccurate responders may also represent nurses who were resistant to change.

Perception of Assessment Tool Accuracy

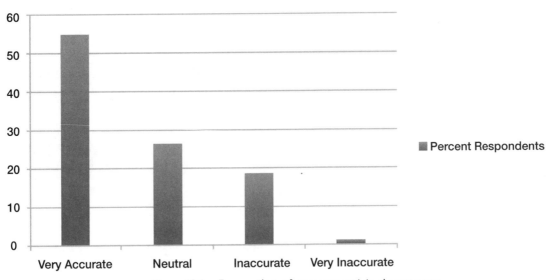

Figure 19.1   Perception of assessment tool accuracy.

Ease of Assessment Tool Use

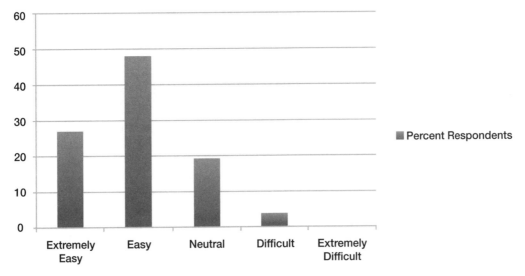

Figure 19.2   Ease of assessment tool use.

Among the respondents, 77% reported the assessment tool as extremely easy or easy to use, and 19% rated the tool's simplicity as neutral. Only 4% rated it as difficult, and no respondents rated it as extremely difficult to use.

Both phases of the pilots represented Kotter's (Gupta, 2011) sixth stage of change management. The generation of short-term wins using pilot studies is an extremely effective way to socialize future nursing practice changes, identify areas to make improvements, and develop future processes with the lessons learned from the trial.

TOOLKIT DEVELOPMENT AND DEPLOYMENT

Based on the pilot intervention and assessment tool results, the system-level nursing practice council (project core team), with approval and support of the nursing executive council, voted to implement the Hendrich II Fall Risk Model™ and a standardized fall-prevention nursing intervention bundle. The deployment strategy was to design a comprehensive toolkit that could be used to ensure a standardized project implementation. The toolkit was developed by subject matter experts within the healthcare system and contained the following elements for deployment of the standardized nursing practices:

- Executive summary outlining the project objectives

- Communication plan containing collateral such as an elevator speech, a company-wide memo, posters, and handouts

- Documentation guidelines and expectations, including EMR assessment and intervention screen changes

- Education plan, including inservice materials, online learning modules, evidence from professional journals, competency validation tools, and bedside orientation packet for contingent labor and float staff

- Outcome metrics tracking plan

- Specific nursing practice changes outlined in handouts

- Revised comprehensive fall-risk assessment, prevention, and management policy

- Post-fall assessment algorithm

- References and evidence

Deployment of the toolkit included a unified timeline for implementation. The nursing practice council designed an intranet website where the toolkit could reside and be accessible at any time by any associate. The system-wide professional development council assisted with the deployment of the education and recommended ongoing fall prevention education as an annual learning requirement for all clinicians and as an essential part of orientation of new employees.

A hard copy notebook of all the toolkit materials was produced to conduct on-the-job training for outside contract labor and float pool staff. Well-trained personnel and continuous learning are characteristics of HROs (Sutcliffe, 2011).

POST GO-LIVE RESULTS, MONITORING PLAN, AND PROJECT EXPANSION

Post go-live data indicated a reduction in falls with injury of 58.5% in the first quarter after implementation of the standardized nursing intervention bundle and the Hendrich II Fall Risk Model™. Subsequently, an overall 21% reduction in falls with injury resulted at the end of the first year of implementation. Total falls and falls with injury occurrences continue to decrease. While the exact cost avoidance dollars were not calculated for this initial set of data, there is a significant positive impact to the organization and patient safety.

The system-wide nursing practice council, in collaboration with the system executive nursing council (composed of chief nursing officers), monitor falls, falls with injury, and fall rates monthly. As a result of this project, the post-fall assessment algorithm is used across the system at the hospital level. Similarly, the entire healthcare system is using the Upright® Fall Prevention Program for ongoing mandatory education, fall prevention programmatic improvements, and application of tools in the ambulatory and outpatient care settings of this system (Heindrich, 2007; Heindrich et al., 2003).

Future expansion of this project may include a comparison of work culture variables, such as nursing satisfaction, with patient falls. According to Choi and Boyle (2013), higher nursing workgroup job satisfaction is directly correlated to fewer patient falls in acute care settings. Another comparison point looks at patient perspectives about falling, which could be extrapolated through patient satisfaction data for patients who have experienced falls and those who have not fallen (Carroll, Dykes, and Hurley, 2010).

DISCUSSION

Several demonstrations of HRO principles have emerged in this project.

- The focus on patient safety became critical to clinical nurses due to the repositioning of responsibility for fall prevention and monitoring to clinical nurses. An emphasis on the role of leadership is also highlighted in this project, with nursing leaders being charged with ensuring that a culture of safety is the top priority in this healthcare system.

- A team approach is clearly a key step in creating an HRO (Riley, 2009). This project includes system-wide partnership from the nursing department, informatics, quality, leadership, communications/marketing, advanced practice nursing council, and the professional development council (composed of education leaders across the system). Without multidisciplinary collaboration, it is more difficult to create a culture of consistent, reliable patient safety.

- Ongoing monthly discussion of fall data and prevention efforts, including the use of the toolkit, ensures that communication is valued, with deference to the expert clinical nurses who have a direct line of sight to the patient. These discussions occur on both the system nursing practice council and local nursing practice council to ensure vertical and horizontal communication. The ongoing partnership with patient safety officers, nurse leaders, advanced practice nurses, nurse executives, and other clinical departments such as physical therapy, pharmacy, and others ensures that all viewpoints are valued.

- The fall committees at each hospital are interdisciplinary, so unit practices remain guided by an interprofessional approach.

- The new hire, incumbent annual, and all other education is mandatory for all disciplines and includes non-clinical employees as well.

The importance of decreasing clinical variability to gain improved clinical outcomes is key (Riley, 2009). Improving clinical outcomes clearly has positive cost reduction and cost avoidance figures related to it as well. This project represents the successful implementation of high reliability concepts with positive patient safety outcomes.

Using a shared leadership model is an innovative method for facilitating nursing practice change implementation. Further, teaching clinical nurses how to successfully manage change has immeasurable positive lessons. The change management model used in this design followed Kotter's (Gupta, 2011) recommended steps. When nurses lead nursing initiatives (deference to expertise), true ownership and accountability for nursing practice occurs. This ensures the highest possible success rate with the implementation of nursing practice changes.

PROJECT STRENGTHS

A primary strength of this project was the use of Kotter's model of change management. The right processes support getting the right results (Riley, 2009). Before the onset of the project, there was a sense of urgency to reduce falls. The discovery of unchanging fall rates, inconsistency of nursing practice, and peripheral involvement of nurses in preventing falls prompted nursing leadership, via the system nursing practice council, to prioritize the standardization of fall prevention care for a system of 13 hospitals.

The guiding coalition was the system-wide nursing practice council with added participants such as patient safety officers, advanced practice nurses, nurse leaders, and informatics professionals. A direct line to hospital-based nursing practice councils and falls committees provided bench strength through the entirety of this project.

The vision and strategy for innovation was deferred to the experts—the front-line, clinical nurses who had the best knowledge of how to keep patients from falling. The vision for decreasing patient falls was initially set by a clinical nurse who had a passion for improving patient safety. She was instrumental in maintaining inspiration and energy for the project team throughout the project. Strategically, teaching clinical nurses how to identify a need for change through a rapid decision-making session—then teaching them how to manage a 2-year project, how to measure outcomes, how to conduct ongoing monitoring, and how to communicate and deploy the changes—was the plan for sustainability and hard-wiring.

Communicating the change to support the vision and standardization of nursing practice was essential and remains ongoing. As stated, a comprehensive toolkit for the change in nursing practice was developed for deployment. Within that toolkit was a communication plan, which included a short elevator speech and other collateral to help inform constituents of the changes. Before project results and final implementation decisions, the strength of the guiding coalition included a lengthy time period by which to socialize the work of the system nursing practice council. Through the pilot projects and ongoing communication, the vision to reduce patient falls across 13 hospitals was woven into the social fabric of the organizations, which is essential for the adoption and sustainability of a change.

Employees in the process were highly empowered. The clinical nurses on the initial project team chose to use the pilot project submission process as a competition to not only challenge nurses to submit their best ideas but to also make the project fun. According to Gupta (2011), playful activities serve as incentives for people to innovate and commit to a change.

Short-term wins were generated through the phase one pilot project. When clinicians recognized the positive impact on the reduction of patient falls for which they were responsible, excitement and enthusiasm built, thus supporting culture change.

Stage seven of the Kotter model of change includes consolidating gains and generating more innovation (Gupta, 2011). Publicizing success facilitates interest and gains more buy-in while decreasing resistance to change. In this particular project, initial successes were shared at an international evidence-based practice conference as well as locally in the annual company nursing report.

The final stage of Kotter's change model is to ensure sustainability of the change. The monthly monitoring of falls data, ongoing education and training, and incorporation of the Hendrich II Fall Risk Model™ algorithm into a new electronic medical record system are examples of how the results of this project are hard-wired into the culture of the organization. Calculating the return on investment of the project is also a significant method to ensure executive interest and support for the redesigned, standardized nursing practice across the system (Spetz, Brown, and Aydin, 2015).

LESSONS LEARNED

A few lessons were learned during this project. The most noticeable was the knowledge and skill set deficit that exists in clinical nurses regarding how to use HRO concepts and change management to scientifically transform nursing practice. This includes knowledge deficits in the following:

■ Mentoring on how to conduct an evidence-based literature review

■ How to assess existing clinical data

■ How to plan and implement a major change project

■ How to use research and evidence to drive practice choices

■ How to successfully sustain a major change project

Several opportunities for mentoring existed during this project. Subject matter experts graciously gave their time and energy to provide the necessary education and coaching along the way.

Another surprise was the extensive variation in how local (hospital-based) data is shared with clinical nurses. Delays in reporting the data, discussing the data, and determining steps for unit-level improvements exist and are an area for opportunity for any organization. During the initial phase of this project, these challenges affected the ability of nursing practice council representatives to effectively report fall data at monthly council meetings. After project completion, this challenge was mitigated by online access to monthly falls data.

A continued challenge is the variation in philosophy about fall prevention among the local entities and units. Despite the literature, this project, and the continued focus on fall rates, individual nurses and nurse leaders who are unfamiliar with the project continue to explore alternative nursing practices to reduce falls in their department. Ongoing communication and firmness to ensure standardized practice are essential to prevent deviation from project recommendations. Nursing leadership has a critical role to play in ensuring a culture of patient safety, which includes adherence to standardized workflows and behaviors. Similarly, project team members who still reside in the organization have a key role in sustaining the interest in and attention to preventing patient falls.

While achieving a zero fall rate in a hospital seems daunting, especially in a large healthcare system, it is the right goal and the right vision to create a culture of patient safety. Further, this important work transforms an organization and the structures and processes by which better clinical outcomes can be achieved. Transformation of an organization can occur only through the selection of an opportunity that seems impossible and maintaining the pursuit of excellence, never giving up on the possibilities.

SUMMARY

The use of HRO strategies is an effective methodology for building a culture of nurse-led initiatives to improve patient safety. The use of evidence-based data is essential to guide clinical nurses in designing nursing practice changes. Further, development and deployment of an implementation toolkit for nursing practice changes is a useful approach to ensuring full transition. Lastly, ongoing monitoring and process improvement sustains the gains and assists with the hard-wiring of the new nursing practice changes.

KEY POINTS

- Empowering clinical nurses to redesign nursing care delivery to improve fall rates is a practical application of HRO principles.

- Teaching clinical nurses how to assess evidence, access the clinical expertise of colleagues, and use data to make important nursing practice decisions is a journey that positively affects clinical outcomes, such as reduced patient falls.

- Planning change through the use of a substantiated change management model is most effective to sustained fall reduction.

- Using an interprofessional approach to fall prevention facilitates development of an HRO that demonstrates patient safety.

- Standardizing a fall-assessment instrument and corresponding nursing interventions reduces clinical variation and creates an environment where clinical outcomes can be equally compared across several entities in a large healthcare system.

- Shared leadership models of decision-making are not only possible across multiple facilities but also may be more effective than other strategies when implementing significant change.

- Reducing the number of falls not only improves patient safety but also results in significant cost avoidance for the organization.

REFERENCES

Adams, J., and Kaplow, R. (2013). A sitter-reduction program in an acute health care system. *Nursing Economics, 31*(2), pp. 83–89.

Barker, A., Kamar, J., and Berlowitz, D. (2009). Bridging the gap between research and practice: Review of a targeted hospital inpatient fall prevention programme. *Quality & Safety in Health Care, 18*(6), pp. 467–472.

Butcher, L. (2013). The no-fall zone. *Hospitals & Health Networks, 87*(6), pp. 26–30.

Carroll, D. L., Dykes, P. C., and Hurley, A. C. (2010, November). Patients' perspectives of falling while in an acute care hospital and suggestions for prevention. *Applied Nursing Research, 23(4)*, pp. 238–241.

Choi, J., and Boyle, D. K. (2013). RN workgroup job satisfaction and patient falls in acute care hospital units. *Journal of Nursing Administration, 43*(11), pp. 586–591.

DiBardino, D., Cohen, E. R., and Didwania, A. (2012). Meta-analysis: Multidisciplinary fall prevention strategies in the acute care inpatient population. *Journal of Hospital Medicine, 7*(6), pp. 1–7.

Fonda, D., Cook, J., Sandler, V., and Bailey, M. (2006). Sustained reduction in serious fall-related injuries in older people in hospital. *The Medical Journal of Australia, 184*(8), pp. 379–382.

Gupta, P. (2011). Leading innovation change: The Kotter way. *International Journal of Innovation Science, 3*(3), pp. 141–149.

Hendrich, A. (2007). Predicting patient falls. *American Journal of Nursing, 107*(11), pp. 50–58.

Hendrich, A. L., Bender, P. S., and Nyhuis, A. (2003). Validation of the Hendrich II Fall Risk Model™: A large concurrent case/control study of hospitalized patients. *Applied Nursing Research, 16*(1), pp. 9–21.

Kerfoot, K. (2003). Attending to weak signals: The leader's challenge. *Nursing Economics, 21*(6), pp. 293–295.

Kim, E. A., Mordiffi, S. Z., Bee, W. H., Devi, K., and Evans, D. (2007). Evaluation of three fall-risk assessment tools in an acute care setting. *Journal of Advanced Nursing, 60*(4), pp. 427–435.

Lovallo, C., Rolandi, S., Rossetti, A. M., and Lusignani, M. (2010). Accidental falls in hospital inpatients: Evaluation of sensitivity and specificity of two risk assessment tools. *Journal of Advanced Nursing, 66*(3), pp. 690–696.

Lueckenotte, A. G., and Conley, D. M. (2009). A study guide for the evidence-based approach to fall assessment and management. *Geriatric Nursing, 30*(3), pp. 207–216.

Oliver, D., Healey, F., and Haines, T. P. (2010). Preventing falls and fall-related injuries in hospitals. *Clinics in Geriatric Medicine, 26*(4), pp. 645–692.

Riley, W. (2009). High reliability and implications for nursing leaders. *Journal of Nursing Management, 17*(2), pp. 238–246.

Spetz, J., Brown, D. S., and Aydin, C. (2015, January). The economics of preventing hospital falls: Demonstrating ROI through a simple model. *The Journal of Nursing Administration, 45*(1), pp. 50–57.

Sutcliffe, K. M. (2011). High reliability organizations (HROs). *Best Practice & Research Clinical Anaesthesiology, 25*(2), pp. 133–144.

CHAPTER 20

MAGNET RECOGNITION PROGRAM® MODEL COMPONENT SYNTHESIS WITH HRO

Jean Beckel, DNP, RN, MPH, CNML

AN OVERVIEW OF THE MAGNET RECOGNITION PROGRAM® AND MAGNET® COMPONENTS

Magnet® designation is the highest international health-care recognition for excellence in the delivery of nursing services, the promotion of quality supporting professional practice, and the dissemination of nursing best practices.

The American Nurses Credentialing Center (ANCC) (2013) Magnet Recognition Program® grew out of a 1983 American Academy of Research study. Researchers sought to identify work environment characteristics that would promote the recruitment and retention of highly qualified registered nurses. The research outcomes recognized 41 hospitals for having 14 features distinguishing their ability

> So never lose an opportunity of urging a practical beginning, however small, for it is wonderful how often in such matters the mustard-seed germinates and roots itself.
>
> —Florence Nightingale

to attract and retain nurses (resulting in use of the term *Magnet hospitals*). These characteristics, which have become known as the 14 "Forces of Magnetism," are as follows:

- Quality of nursing leadership

- Organizational structure

- Management style

- Personnel policies and programs

- Professional models of care

- Quality of care

- Quality improvement

- Consultation and resources

- Autonomy

- Community and the hospital

- Nurses as teachers

- Image of nursing

- Interdisciplinary relationships

- Professional development

Forces of Magnetism is copyrighted material of the American Nurses Credentialing Center. All rights reserved. Reproduced with the permission of the American Nurses Credentialing Center.

In 1990, based on the 1983 study, the American Nurses Association (ANA) created the Magnet Hospital Recognition Program for Excellence in Nursing Services™. The ANCC became the coordinating body, and formal standards for application documents were established. The year 1994 marked the first time a healthcare organization was designated a Magnet hospital. By 1998, Magnet recognition had expanded to long-term care facilities. In 2000, it became recognized internationally. The name was officially changed to the Magnet Recognition Program in 2002.

Hospitals seeking Magnet designation submit an application and documentation supporting the presence of structures, processes, and outcomes addressed in the Magnet application manual standards. Successful scoring of the documents within a defined range of excellence results in a site visit appraisal, with the Commission on Magnet Recognition making a final determination related to Magnet designation based on all facets of the application process.

In 2007, following a statistical analysis of Magnet appraiser team scores, a new Magnet conceptual model was introduced. The Magnet Model (see Figure 20.1) incorporates the 14 Forces of Magnetism, grouping them into five components:

- Transformational Leadership
- Structural Empowerment
- Exemplary Professional Practice
- New Knowledge, Innovations & Improvements
- Empirical Outcomes

The oval encircling these components represents the global nature of nursing and healthcare. The empirical outcomes component is integrated into the other four, illustrating accountability for demonstrating the impact of professional nursing practice related to all components.

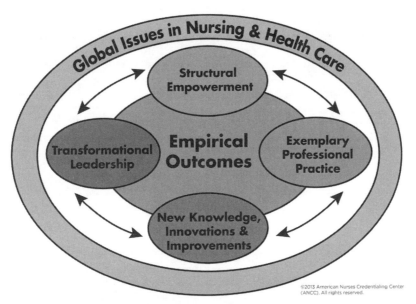

Figure 20.1 Magnet® Model showing the five key components.

The Magnet Recognition Program has evolved over the past 25 years, providing opportunity for focused research related to organizational and patient outcomes and comparing differences in outcomes between Magnet and non-Magnet healthcare organizations. (See Table 20.1.) Much of the initial Magnet research targeted nurse perception of the practice environment, while more recent research has focused on quantifying the impact of Magnet designation on patients, nurses, and the organization (Drenkard, 2010). Magnet healthcare organizations experience lower mortality, failure-to-rescue, falls, hospital-acquired pressure ulcers, and read-mission rates. Nurses in Magnet healthcare organizations demonstrate higher levels of overall staffing, nurse education, and professional nursing certification, and lower levels of turnover, burnout, nurse needle-stick injuries, and musculoskeletal injuries. These outcomes show that Magnet designation has a positive influence on organizational work and safety environment.

TABLE 20.1   DIFFERENCES FOUND IN MAGNET HEALTHCARE ORGANIZATION ENVIRONMENTS

Patient Outcomes in Magnet Healthcare Organizations	Nursing Outcomes in Magnet Healthcare Organizations
14% lower mortality rates (McHugh et al., 2013)	Decreased turnover and vacancy (Jones and Gates, 2007; Upenieks, 2003)
12% lower failure-to-rescue rates (McHugh et al., 2013)	13% lower "high burnout" rate (Kelly, McHugh, and Aiken, 2011)
Lower readmission rates (Smith, 2013)	Increased nurse satisfaction (Upenieks, 2002)
5–10.3% lower patient fall rates (Lake, Shang, Klaus, and Dunton, 2010; Unruh, 2008)	18% lower job dissatisfaction (Upenieks, 2002)
Decreased hospital-acquired pressure ulcers (Bergq-uist-Beringer et al., 2013; Choi, Bergquist-Beringer, and Staggs, 2013)	Lower average number of patients per nurse (Kelly et al., 2011)
Increased patient safety (Armstrong and Laschinger, 2006; Hughes, Chang, and Mark, 2009)	For each 1.0 patient decrease in staffing ratio, a resulting 9% decrease in patient mortality (Aiken et al., 2011)
Increased patient satisfaction (Smith, 2013)	More highly educated nurses (Kelly et al., 2011)
	For every 10% increase in bachelors-prepared nurses, a 5% decrease in patient mortality and failure to rescue (Aiken et al., 2011)
	More certified nurses (Kelly et al., 2011)
	Better work environment (Brady-Schwartz, 2005)
	Lower rates of nurse needle-sticks and musculoskeletal injuries (Aiken, Sloane, and Klocinski, 1997)

Examination of the Magnet Model component characteristics (ANCC, n.d.) provides the foundation for synergistic relationships with high reliability organization (HRO) principles. These characteristics are as follows:

■ **Transformational Leadership:** Although all nurses are leaders within the organization, it is senior leaders who set strategic and professional practice direction. Nursing leaders are involved in setting organizational priorities and influence decisions that affect the organization beyond the scope of nursing. Visionary leaders are visible advocates for nursing and lead the organization to desired future states.

■ **Structural Empowerment:** Internal and external relationship building is encouraged. Alignment of mission, vision, values, and strategic plans with structures and processes supporting active nurse presence and communication flow drive the organization to identify and achieve desired outcomes. Nursing has a voice in organizational communication and decision-making through shared governance structures and quality improvement processes.

■ **Exemplary Professional Practice:** There is autonomous top-of-license practice in a collegial interprofessional environment, with nursing practice based on demonstrated competency. Clinical nurses use trended data to drive decision-making and improve outcomes. Benchmarking of organizational and unit data to national databases provides a lens for performance evaluation. Benchmarking is evidence of the shift in focus by national quality organizations and by Magnet to demonstrate the impact and value of nursing within the organization. Nurses have a key function in coordination and continuity of care.

■ **New Knowledge, Innovations & Improvements:** Nursing input is valued and sought in the design of care delivery models, workspace, and patient care technology. There is a recognition of the professional responsibility to apply evidence to practice and patient care and to further develop nursing science through participation in nursing research.

Table 20.2 summarizes Magnet component characteristics.

TABLE 20.2 MAGNET COMPONENT CHARACTERISTICS

Transformational Leadership	Structural Empowerment	Exemplary Professional Practice	New Knowledge, Innovations & Improvements
Vision	Innovative environment	Understanding of the role of nursing	Contribution to nursing practice
Strategic	Strong professional practice	Autonomous practice based on competence	Redesign
Influence	Living out mission, vision, and values to achieve outcomes	Application of nursing role with patients, families, communities, and interprofessional teams	Redefine
Clinical knowledge	Strong collaborative relationships and partnerships	Nurse partnerships to deliver patient-/person-centered care	New models of care

continues

TABLE 20.2   MAGNET COMPONENT CHARACTERISTICS   (CONTINUED)

Transformational Leadership	Structural Empowerment	Exemplary Professional Practice	New Knowledge, Innovations & Improvements
Strong expertise related to professional nursing practice	Development, direction, and empowerment to achieve outcomes	Nurses ensure continuity of care, internal and external to organization	Visible contributions to the science of nursing
Listen	Outreach to improve community health	Incorporation of specialty standards and regulations into practice	Application of existing new knowledge
Challenge	Shared governance	Use of internal and external experts to improve practice	Support for and participation in nursing research
Influence organizational change with impact beyond nursing	Involvement in unit and organizational decision-making councils	Involvement in professional practice model development, implementation, and evaluation	Results of nursing research shared inside and outside the organization
Advocate for nursing research	Participation in professional organizations	Use of resources to address ethical issues	Evaluation of evidence related to practice
Align resources with organizational and unit goals	Support for nursing professional development and certification	Participation in nurse recruitment and retention	Application of existing evidence in nursing practice
Lead through change	Nursing education for non-nurses to enter nursing career	Lead interprofessional activities to improve care and educate patients and families	Nursing influence in the design of technology to enhance the patient experience and work environment
Leadership development at all levels of nursing	Support to improve nurse teaching experience	Support for nurse autonomy in shared governance structure	Nursing influence in the design of space and workflow to enhance nursing practice and the environment
Use trended data to support care delivery	Facilitation for transition into new nursing roles	Improved nurse workplace safety	Innovation supported and encouraged
CNO and leader visibility and accessibility	Support to improve preceptor expertise	Proactive management of risk and errors and evaluation of patient safety data	Nursing integral to provision and improvement of patient care
Clinical nurse input influences change in nursing practice, the nurse practice environment, and the patient experience	Support for nurse participation in community healthcare outreach	Use of trended data to improve care and acquire resources	

| Transform the organization to meet the future | Recognition of nurse contribution to organization's strategic priorities | Outperformance of external benchmarks on RN satisfaction, patient satisfaction with nursing, and nurse-sensitive quality indicators (injury falls, hospital-acquired pressure ulcers, catheter-associated urinary tract infections, and central line–associated bloodstream infections) |

Environments that integrate the characteristics of these Magnet components robustly support professional practice, accountability, collegiality, collaboration, and trust.

SYNERGY BETWEEN MAGNET® COMPONENTS AND HRO PRINCIPLES

Weick and Sutcliffe (2007) examined risk, resilience, and results to more deeply analyze the five HRO principles they defined. Their work encourages organizations to integrate performance evaluation, use incremental changes to develop new methods, and constantly seek improvement. They advocate for environments that are highly alert to variation, able to quickly apply what is learned, and strive for effective and efficient service provision.

In this section, traits shared by HROs are examined, examples in practice are illustrated, and each trait is related to the Magnet® Model components and characteristics. Both HROs and Magnet recognition relate to the overarching culture present within each organization. This culture reflects the influence of history, mission, vision, values, strategic goals, current leadership, community relationships, and a multitude of other factors. Organizational culture is demonstrated in how each individual aligns his or her behavior within the practice framework and delivery of care to those served. Those served include patients, family members, visitors, co-workers, internal colleagues, and community members within the organizational service area. It also includes those not often considered by employees, such as local or state organizations, faith-based communities, service providers (for example, home care agencies, emergency medical services, and interpreter services), and regulatory agencies. Culture is embedded within the organization, and both HRO principles (Gamble, 2013) and Magnet component characteristics drive culture change to optimize clinical, practice environment, and community outcomes.

HRO PRINCIPLE 1: PREOCCUPATION WITH FAILURE

It is much more difficult to speak the truth than people commonly imagine.

—Florence Nightingale

There is a tendency for healthcare organizations to ignore or overlook failures and focus on successes. But preoccupation with failure—especially small failures—is key. Preoccupation with failure is demonstrated in the ability of each employee within the organization to maintain environmental vigilance through constant attentiveness and to openly share concerns, however minor they may seem. Hospitals promote this trait through the encouragement of near-miss reporting, the recognition of employees whose reports prevent harm to patients, and the support of the use of lean process improvement and failure mode effect analysis. These practices identify potential failures and provide the opportunity to address and correct structures and processes. Near misses are recognized as opportunities to improve rather than ignored with the belief that current checks and balances will catch future failures. Desired outcomes are linked to organizational strategic goals and staff behavior.

EXAMPLE

An 83-year-old male was admitted to the surgical floor following hip replacement surgery. Surgical blood loss resulted in a drop in hemoglobin. The physician ordered administration of one unit of blood. The nurse followed hospital procedures to obtain and hang the blood. After 15 minutes, the nurse assessed the patient's blood pressure and noted a decrease from his baseline. The patient denied any other symptoms, but the nurse was concerned. The nurse stopped the blood, notified the charge nurse, and called the physician. The nurse was aware that this patient's ACE inhibitors had been known to cause hypotension with a transfusion and was concerned that the blood pressure decrease could indicate an impending transfusion reaction. A CBC was ordered and obtained, with normal results. The physician ordered continuation of blood administration. The nurse sent the first blood bag to lab for a transfusion workup and ordered a new bag of blood, which was administered without blood pressure decrease or any other sign of transfusion reaction. In this example, the nurse acted on her preoccupation with failure, even though this patient's response to the blood transfusion fell outside the "usual" scope of transfusion reaction symptoms. This nurse knew that a transfusion reaction to the blood would be detrimental to the patient. She kept the patient's safety at the center of her concern and persisted in action based on her assessment of the situation, to the benefit of the patient.

Synergy with Magnet Recognition Program® Components

Achieving an organizational environment that is preoccupied with failure requires the establishment of trust relationships. Leadership alignment with the vision of elimination of patient harm is crucial to enculturation of both HRO and Magnet characteristics (Chassin and Loeb, 2013). Leaders establish key metrics that are used to measure outcomes. These metrics are communicated to the front-line staff, allowing them to articulate the impact of their practice on these outcomes. Transformational leaders create shared governance structures and communication systems, demonstrating the value of nurse and employee input. Leaders model connectivity, yet demand accountability for professional nursing practice within the scope of licensure. Clear communication of and demonstrated follow-through related to leadership expectations establish a safe environment for reporting actual or potential concerns. This drives employees to deeply examine their practice and the practice environment. Autonomous nursing practice in a collegial interprofessional environment establishes a functional team focused on doing the right thing in the right way. This promotes practice questions, examination of evidence, and potentially the generation of new nursing knowledge through research. Failure to rest on past laurels and consistently seeking improvement become accepted as expected behavior. When this is communicated to nursing preceptors, new graduate nurses, newly hired experienced nurses, and nurses transferring into specialty practice settings, transition to practice becomes a true learning experience—for both existing staff and new hires. Fresh eyes are given permission to examine prevailing practices, determine evidence supporting current or revised practice, and participate in change processes to improve patient care delivery.

HRO PRINCIPLE 2: RELUCTANCE TO SIMPLIFY

> *Another frequent error is to inquire whether one cause remains, and not whether the effect which may be produced by a great many different causes, not inquired after, remains.*
>
> —*Florence Nightingale*

Complexity theory involves understanding complex relationships influencing the present state and holds that complex problems need simple solutions (Lindberg, Nash, and Lindberg, 2008). Multiple methods exist to analyze potential influences and determine problem sources, such as diverse checks, adversarial reviews, and the cultivation of multiple perspectives. Use of these methods differentiates HROs from those who surmise the cause of existing problems, apply "quick fix" temporary solutions or "one size fits all" solutions that miss the heart of the issue, and experience the re-emergence of the problem at a later date. HROs resist the urge to simplify during problem-solving, providing an opportunity to identify the source of presenting problems and use focused, simple solutions. This allows them to solve the right problem in the right way. Recognition of crucial information available upon completion of more in-depth analysis allows for appropriate application of resources.

EXAMPLE

Continuous analgesia delivery (CAD) pumps are often used to deliver pain-relief medication to patients. The pumps used are designed with a low-volume alarm to alert nurses to needed patient and pump attention. In one hospital, nurses responded to the low-volume alert but continuously found no volume left to infuse in the medication cassette. They initially thought it was a pump programming error. One nurse persisted in her quest to find the answer to the empty cassettes, contacting the sales representative and then the vendor company. She found that the company assumed use of a 100-milliliter cassette in its CAD pump development and programmed the low-volume alert based on that delivery system. However, the hospital was using 50-milliliter cassettes. This resulted in the nurses finding empty cassettes when the low-volume alert sounded. The nurse elevated the concern to the vendor, and the pump programming was redesigned. In this seemingly simple example, we see a nurse who did not assume she knew the answer to the problem and was concerned for patient safety and alarm management. Action related to reluctance to simplify is sometimes likened to "a dog with a bone." This nurse grabbed the bone and did not let go until she found the answer and solved the problem that was causing the presenting symptoms.

Synergy with Magnet Recognition Program Components

HRO traits and Magnet characteristics are interwoven into the organizational culture of safety. Transformational leaders clearly communicate patient and staff safety goals. Development of a culture of continuous learning does the following:

- Promotes evaluation of actual and near-miss falls

- Promotes the use of multi-pronged delivery methods for patient and staff education

- Promotes the interdisciplinary review of medications, equipment, footwear, and patient toileting (Quigley and White, 2013)

Structural empowerment provides event evaluation processes that seek to identify all possible influences, unravel the complexities surrounding the event, learn from process variation, and enhance safety capacity. Development of more robust interdisciplinary process improvement systems leverages expertise and provides a forum for sharing diverse perspectives. The result is thoughtful and intentional development of cohesive, exemplary, professional, evidence-based practices (EBPs) that elevate practice and patient outcomes.

HRO PRINCIPLE 3: SENSITIVITY TO OPERATIONS

In dwelling upon the vital importance of sound observation it must never be lost sight of what observation is for. It is not for the sake of piling up miscellaneous information or curious facts, but for the sake of saving life and increasing health and comfort.

—Florence Nightingale

Mindfulness of discriminatory detail provides a setting with built-in early warning systems. The Agency for Healthcare Research and Quality (AHRQ) (Hines, Luna, Lofthus, Marquardt, and Stelmokas, 2008) contends that a constant state of mindfulness is required to both create and sustain a highly reliable system able to produce exceptionally safe and consistently high-quality care. Sensitivity to operations strengthens organizational ability for early identification of potential errors and actual errors. The absence of assumptions establishes an environment where each employee can focus on what is done and how it is done. Constant vigilance through observation of processes allows for evaluation of what might be accomplished through improvement and how that improvement could happen. Dynamic work environments invite employee feedback—not in the format of complaints about things the individual doesn't like, but as an employer/employee partnership supporting work environment and outcome enhancement.

> **EXAMPLE**
>
> Inpatient psychiatric units often care for patients at high risk for self-harm or harm to others. All staff practicing in this environment are responsible for patient and employee safety. Information related to safety risks is included in new-hire orientation. One morning, a nurse on the inpatient adult psychiatric unit found a laboratory tourniquet in a trash can. The nurse removed the tourniquet and then communicated with the laboratory to identify the employee responsible for drawing patient blood tests that morning. The laboratory recognized that this was a new hire. The event was used to support employee learning. While safety information was provided—and indicated as understood—at orientation, application of that safety information in the specific clinical setting became a true employee learning experience. Increased reporting of "good catch" or "near-miss" events signals development of a robust organizational safety environment. Transparency and accountability in event reporting indicate employees are growing in sensitivity to operations.

Synergy with Magnet Recognition Program Components

Transformational leaders foster transparency in communication, building organizational knowledge and employee engagement in living out the mission, vision, and values. Shared governance structures function as conduits of information flow. Employees are empowered to actively dialogue with leaders, identifying and contributing to improvement initiatives. Implementation of lean, failure mode effect analysis, and/or transforming care at the bedside processes invites point-of-care staff participation in proactive assessment processes with strong reliance on data-driven performance management. Magnet organizations and HROs actively work to overcome the challenge of establishing a safe actual and potential error-reporting climate. Engagement of employees in practice environment evaluation and improvement initiatives drives application of evidence, generation of new nursing knowledge, and emergence of exemplary professional practice.

HRO PRINCIPLE 4: COMMITMENT TO RESILIENCE

Nothing but observation and experience will teach us the ways to maintain or bring back the state of health.

—*Florence Nightingale*

Resilience implies the ability to bounce back from an occurrence. HROs develop methods to identify and manage risk. These may include the use of report cards, dashboards, and real-time reporting systems to provide alerts based on variation from expectations. In conjunction with these early warning systems, a paradigm of failure as a learning opportunity prevails, building a creative atmosphere where employees feel freer to report, act, improvise, and improve the organization. Professional development for leaders and staff enhances each individual's ability to assess situations and act based on overall calculated risk and organizational—rather than personal—benefit. The organization's mission and strategic goals provide the foundation for personal actions and responsiveness.

EXAMPLE

A hospital is known for treating spinal injuries and has developed treatment processes based on standards of care. An interdisciplinary team was initiated to assess improvement opportunities in care processes related to injuries requiring spinal decompression. The team evaluated current practices, finding each area treating the patient was operating within current standards of practice. But they believed the time of 10.5 hours from patient onset of symptoms to operative spinal decompression could be improved. The team focused on improving communication by doing the following:

- A spinal alert was incorporated into the rapid response team procedures.
- Communication algorithms were developed and implemented to better coordinate movement of the patient through various treatment areas.
- Processes for patient access to the MRI and physician reading of MRI results were fine-tuned.
- Nurse education enhanced nurses' ability to recognize symptoms potentially requiring operative spinal decompression.

Following implementation of these process changes, the time from patient onset of symptoms to operative spinal decompression was decreased from 10.5 hours to 7.5 hours. Comprehensive evaluation of patient services removed the silos that can develop and brought key stakeholders together with a united vision. Implementation of changes tested system response and allowed implementation of interventions providing the best response for the patient. The team demonstrated resilience in improving patient care capability through the application of untested strategies and then making changes as needed to those strategies to develop the best outcome possible.

Synergy with Magnet Recognition Program Components

Professional nursing practice is interwoven within the Magnet components and provides a solid foundation for practice autonomy and individual actions. Willingness to actively take risks and run the risk of failure is balanced with actions defined by the scope of practice and based on the professional practice model. Personal responsibility and professional accountability are cornerstones for practice decisions. The organization nurtures a nimble practice environment with the ability to respond quickly to internal and external influences. Nurses do this through the application of evidence to practice and coordination of the interdisciplinary team's approach to the plan of care, including unique patient and family needs. The voice of nursing is perceived as crucial, and nurse participation is sought in shared governance and improvement initiatives. Clinical staff is encouraged to test changes, evaluate results, and learn to respond appropriately to success and failure. The mantra "that's the way we have always done it" is actively discouraged through implementation of EBP projects and nursing research. Transformational leaders foster point-of-care understanding of organizational strategic goals to provide a foundation for employee decision-making and develop an environment that supports risk-taking while minimizing catastrophic results of that risk-taking.

HRO PRINCIPLE 5: DEFERENCE TO EXPERTISE

What cruel mistakes are sometimes made by benevolent men and women in matters of business about which they can know nothing and think they know a great deal.

—*Florence Nightingale*

Historically hierarchical healthcare organizations often demonstrate deference to executive-level leadership for input on decision-making. HROs may retain a hierarchical structure, but there is recognition and exploitation of rich point-of-care employee expertise resources. This is exhibited through the implementation of processes that routinely bring leaders into closer proximity with front-line staff at the point of care and generate opportunity for the exchange of information. These processes may include leadership rounding, employee forums, and improvement initiatives like the Robert Wood Johnson Foundation/Institute for Healthcare Improvement Transforming Care at the Bedside program. Leaders rely less on the employee's length of service to determine expertise than on the attributes of curiosity, creativity, and openness to change. All staff are invited to respectfully question current practices and suggest interventions to improve environment and outcomes. Needleman and Hassmiller (2009) advocate for hospitals to recognize the potential contributions of front-line staff to benefit from their insight and improve quality and care delivery efficiency.

EXAMPLE

A medical unit in a large hospital provided care to a wide variety of increasingly complex patients. With growing numbers of isolation and high-risk patients, staff knew handwashing was essential to staff and patient safety. The unit gathered an interdisciplinary team to evaluate options for improvement of bedside care. A staff nurse facilitated the team and guided members in the use of rapid cycle change processes. Over a few months the team successfully implemented the following:

- The installation of two hallway handwashing sinks with signage to explain the benefits to staff and patients (suggested by a clinical nurse)

- The purchase and placement of a second wastebasket in each patient room to decrease the need for staff to walk to throw away medical waste (suggested by a nursing assistant)

- The installation of a consulting physician chair on the wall of each patient room so physicians could sit at eye level with the patient during their rounding visit (suggested by a clinical nurse)

In this example, the expertise of front-line staff was leveraged to make small but significant changes in the patient-care environment. Team members documented cost savings and improvement in the patient experience. Hospital leaders conceptually and financially supported the suggested improvements, sending a clear message to clinical staff that their expertise was recognized and appreciated.

Synergy with Magnet Recognition Program Components

Magnet healthcare organization characteristics include a tendency toward flatter organizational charts, decreasing the layers between clinical and executive staff. Transformational leaders are cognizant of the expertise of front-line staff and actively work to optimize information flow from the point of care to the executive level. Executive leaders advocate for nursing practice and patient care resources. Nurses at all levels are sought to participate in process evaluation and improvement initiatives, lead interdisciplinary teams, and coordinate continuity of patient care. Magnet healthcare organizations allocate necessary resources to support a culture of continuous improvement with front-line staff participating in decision-making. Shared governance structures are established to provide a forum for bidirectional communication between leaders and front-line staff. An environment of inquiry is created and nurtured. The response "that's the way we have always done it" is replaced with "could we be doing this in a different way to make it better for the patient, family, or staff?" Initiation of practice questions guides robust evaluation and application of evidence and best practices, which becomes a stepping stone to the generation of nursing research. Maturation of processes drives development of research questions by clinical nurses, with organizational support to pursue those questions for the improvement of patient care practices.

SUMMARY

> *Go your way straight to God's work, in simplicity and singleness of heart.*
> —*Florence Nightingale*

The Magnet® components and high reliability principles target cultural improvement and maturation, driving organizations to improved outcomes. Both acknowledge the role of transformational leaders as crucial to successful organizational integration. And through integration efforts of Magnet component characteristics and high reliability principles, organizations are driven to develop environments high in personal and professional accountability and integrity.

Neither Magnet designation nor the use of HRO principles is a mantle to be displayed by healthcare organizations. Both are visible only when embedded into the underlying culture and displayed through the actions of each individual employee. Inculcation of Magnet and high reliability principles enables an organization to optimize the internal work environment, patient experience, and patient outcomes. This places the organization in a stronger position with regard to the recruitment of skilled employees and the development of services that can be extended to the surrounding community and service area, providing benefits beyond the walls of the facility.

Organizational structures and processes that support the components of the Magnet Recognition Program® are compatible and synergistic with HRO principles. The result is organizations focused on strong leaders able to clearly communicate organizational vision, structures empowering each employee to participate in decision-making, development and implementation of exemplary professional practice, and application and generation of new knowledge in the practice arena. Examination of performance using benchmarked data supports an environment of continuous learning, evaluation, and improvement, evidenced in organizational outcomes.

KEY POINTS

■ Organizational structures and processes that support the components of the Magnet Recognition Program® are compatible and synergistic with HRO principles.

■ The Magnet® components and high reliability principles target cultural improvement and maturation, driving organizations to continuous learning and improved outcomes.

■ The roles of transformational leaders, integrity, and personal and professional accountability are crucial to both Magnet and HRO. Strong leaders clearly communicate organizational vision, structures empower participation in decision-making, exemplary professional practice is implemented, and new practice knowledge is generated and applied.

■ Magnet designation and HRO principles are visible only when embedded into the underlying culture and displayed through the actions of each individual employee.

■ Inculcation of Magnet and high reliability principles optimizes the internal work environment, patient experience, and patient outcomes.

REFERENCES

Aiken, L. H., Cimiotti, J. P., Sloane, D. M., Smith, H. L., Flynn, L., and Neff, D. F. (2011). The effects of nurse staffing and nurse education on patient deaths in hospitals with different nurse work environments. *Medical Care, 49*(12), pp. 1047–1053.

Aiken, L. H., Sloane, D. M., and Klocinski, J. L. (1997). Hospital nurses' occupational exposure to blood: Prospective, retrospective, and institutional reports. *American Journal of Public Health, 87*(1), pp. 103–107.

American Nurses Credentialing Center (ANCC). (2013). *2014 Magnet® Application Manual.* Silver Spring, MD: American Nurses Credentialing Center.

American Nurses Credentialing Center (ANCC). (n.d.). Announcing a new model for ANCC's Magnet Recognition Program®. Retrieved from http://www.nursecredentialing.org/MagnetModel

Armstrong, K. J., and Laschinger, H. (2006). Structural empowerment: Magnet hospital characteristics and patient safety culture: Making the link. *Journal of Nursing Care Quality, 21*(2), pp. 124–132.

Bergquist-Beringer, S., Dong, L., He, J., and Dunton, N. (2013). Pressure ulcers and prevention among acute care hospitals in the United States. *The Joint Commission Journal on Quality and Patient Safety, 39*(9), pp. 404–414.

Brady-Schwartz, D. C. (2005). Further evidence on the Magnet Recognition Program: Implications for nursing leaders. *Journal of Nursing Administration, 35*(9), pp. 397–403.

Chassin, M. R., and Loeb, J. M. (2013). High-reliability health care: Getting there from here. *The Milbank Quarterly, 91*(3), pp. 459–490.

Choi, J., Bergquist-Beringer, S., and Staggs, V. S. (2013). Linking RN workgroup satisfaction to pressure ulcers among older adults on acute care hospital units. *Research in Nursing & Health, 36*(2), pp. 181–190.

Cook, E. T. (1913). *The life of Florence Nightingale, volume 2* (p. 406). London, UK: Macmillan and Co, Limited.

Drenkard, K. (2010). The business case for Magnet. *The Journal of Nursing Administration, 40*(6), pp. 263–271.

Gamble, M. (2013). 5 traits of high reliability organizations: How to hardwire each in your organization. *Becker's Hospital Review.* Retrieved from http://www.beckershospitalreview.com/hospital-management-administration/5-traits-of-high-reliability-organizations-how-to-hardwire-each-in-your-organization.html

Hines, S., Luna, K., Lofthus, J., Marquardt, M., and Stelmokas, D. (2008). Becoming a high reliability organization: Operational advice for hospital leaders. *Agency for Healthcare Research and Quality*. Retrieved from http://archive.ahrq.gov/professionals/quality-patient-safety/quality-resources/tools/hroadvice/hroadvice.pdf

Hughes, L. C., Chang, Y., and Mark, B. A. (2009). Quality and strength of patient safety climate on medical-surgical units. *Health Care Management Review, 34*(1), pp. 19–28.

Jones, C. B., and Gates, M. (2007). The cost and benefits of nurse turnover: A business case for nurse retention. *The Online Journal of Issues in Nursing, 12*(3).

Kelly, L. A., McHugh, M. D., and Aiken, L. H. (2011). Nurse outcomes in Magnet and non-Magnet hospitals. *The Journal of Nursing Administration, 41*(10), pp. 428–433.

Lake, E. T., Shang, J., Klaus, S., and Dunton, N. E. (2010). Patient falls: Association with hospital Magnet status and nursing unit staffing. *Research in Nursing & Health, 33*(5), pp. 413–425.

Lindberg, C., Nash, S., and Lindberg, C. (2008). *On the edge: Nursing in the age of complexity*. Seattle, WA: CreateSpace.

McHugh, M. D., Kelly, L. A., Smith, H. L., Wu, E. S., Vanak, J. M., and Aiken, L. H. (2013). Lower mortality in Magnet hospitals. *Medical Care, 51*(5), pp. 382–388.

Needleman, J., and Hassmiller, S. (2009). The role of nurses in improving hospital quality and efficiency: Real-world results. *Health Affairs, 28*(4), pp. w625–w633.

Nightingale, F. (1992). *Notes on nursing: What it is, and what it is not* (pp. 60–76). Philadelphia, PA: Lippincott Williams and Wilkins.

Quigley, P. A., and White, S. V. (2013). Hospital-based fall program measurement and improvement in high reliability organizations. *Online Journal of Issues in Nursing, 18*(2).

Smith, S. A. (2013). Magnet hospital status impact on mortality, readmission, and patient reported quality of care (doctoral dissertation). University of Hawaii on Manoa.

Unruh, L. (2008). Nurse staffing and patient, nurse, and financial outcomes. *The American Journal of Nursing, 108*(1), pp. 62–71.

Upenieks, V. V. (2002). Assessing differences in job satisfaction of nurses in Magnet and non-Magnet hospitals. *The Journal of Nursing Administration, 32*(11), pp. 564–576.

Upenieks, V. V. (2003). The interrelationship of organizational characteristics of Magnet hospitals, nursing leadership, and nursing job satisfaction. *The Health Care Manager, 22*(2), pp. 83–98.

Weick, K. E., and Sutcliffe, K. M. (2007). *Managing the unexpected: Resilient performance in an age of uncertainty* (2nd ed.). San Francisco, CA: Jossey-Bass.

CHAPTER 21

ACHIEVING HRO: THE ROLE OF THE BEDSIDE SCIENTIST IN RESEARCH

Alma Jackson, PhD, RN, COHN-S

Patient care and safety are at the forefront of high reliability organizations (HROs), which is exactly where the nurse is. In the past few years, checklists, bundles, clinical guidelines, and many other practices have emerged that assist in creating HROs and meeting a "target zero" goal for errors. No one knows as much about the smallest of details in the delivery of healthcare than bedside nurses. They are aware of the small things that can go wrong and the early warning signs of trouble. When working to create a safe protocol or practice change, the nurse is the one to ask. If you are in administration and wondering why nurses create workarounds that may compromise safety, ask the nurses. If you want a new process to succeed, then involve the nurses. If you want it to fail, then don't.

In 2010, the Institute of Medicine (IOM) released its report "The Future of Nursing: Leading Change, Advancing Health." This widely referenced report states that "nurses have great potential to lead innovative strategies to improve healthcare" (p. 95). It also states that nurses should practice to the fullest extent of their education. Now is the time to prepare nurses in the role of bedside scientist. Nurses are recognizing their critical role in evidence-based practice (EBP) and research. For nurses, not a day goes by without

> "Knowing is not enough; we must apply. Willing is not enough; we must do.
>
> —*Goethe*

performing evidence-based clinical bundles and hearing about new research that applies to practice. Nurses also have their own questions about why a task is done one way when clearly there is a better way to get the job done. Nursing has evolved from the days of training and doing to now asking why—why do we do things this way?

The airline industry is the leader in HROs. When accidents happen, the stakes are high. One retired airline captain stated that the difference in airline safety and healthcare is this: "When the airplane goes down, so do the crew. When an accident happens in healthcare, you are not going to die too." The stakes are still high, however—which is the reason behind the IOM's drive to save millions of lives through the implementation of key processes that have been documented to reduce the incidence of errors. More can be done to improve patient safety and quality care by fostering a research agenda within the organization that involves nurses examining their practices. This aligns well with the culture of HROs, where front-line staff are valued for their expertise.

A glimpse of what can happen with a bottom-up approach to safer patient care was evidenced in the Robert Wood Johnson Foundation's (2011) national program, "Transforming Care at the Bedside from 2003–2008." Designed as a quality improvement project for medical-surgical nursing units, this program gave front-line staff the ability to redesign processes. The deference to staff as the experts to come up with solutions resulted in a significant reduction in falls, discharge 30-day readmission rates, and number of codes. Staff turnover also decreased from 15.0 to 5.8%.

The literature is now replete with quality-improvement and EBP projects that have resulted in improvements in many measures. What is not as abundant is the research agendas of hospitals that have helped create an HRO, maintain its sustainability over time, while also promoting Magnet® and Joint Commission requirements. A strong research agenda that promotes a culture of inquiry is a win-win for the organization on many levels.

THE RESEARCH AGENDA

The benefits of a research-intensive organization are many. The culture of inquiry within an HRO is ideal for promoting the best in patient quality and safety. It also provides a research mechanism to study failures as well as best practices. A research agenda that is widely pervasive in the organization becomes interdisciplinary and innovative. A principal investigator and research team establish responsibility and sustainability. Interdisciplinary no longer means that the physician decides on the research and has the nurse collect the data. The nurse is a critical member of the research team because of his or her expertise in patient care. Infusing the organization with EBP through research involves supporting the bedside nurse scientist through four key components:

- Educating (or re-educating) nurses about research

- Creating a research council inclusive of bedside nurses

- Fostering research activities embracing the knowledge of the bedside nurse

- Creating the infrastructure that supports the bedside nurse

EBP VERSUS RESEARCH

There is a difference between EBP and research. The wealth of information about providing evidence-based care abounds. However, there are quite a few healthcare professionals who cannot define EBP. EBP uses the best evidence to direct patient care decisions and management. It consists of three things:

- Clinical expertise

- Patient preference

- Research

According to Polit and Beck, "Research is a systematic inquiry that uses disciplined methods to answer questions or solve problems. The ultimate goal of research is to develop, refine, and expand knowledge" (2012, p. 3). Research is a component of EBP.

Not every nurse knows research. This is a key problem with the three components of EBP. Not all EBP is trustworthy. The setup of the study may not have been done well, or it may not be replicable as a research study. How was the study done? Is the research article you just read worthy of a practice change? Tales from the field indicate that education is lacking. Practice changes have been implemented based on a review of a few research studies that are just not that good.

TALES FROM THE FIELD

A small rural hospital was investigating ways to reduce its incidence of pressure ulcers. During this time, the hospital had a sales representative display different products as well as provide two research articles about the products. The research was done by the manufacturer. The hospital also found three research articles relaying information about patient positioning in beds that was different from what the hospital was currently doing. The hospital began an intervention of changing patient positioning and using a product to protect bony prominences. In 3 months, there was no improvement.

In an urban hospital, success for decreasing pressure ulcers was demonstrated when a master's level nursing student initiated the use of a sacral pressure ulcer patch in the ICU. This student was currently taking her research class and had resources in both academia and the practice setting. Her study contained detailed inclusion criteria for eligible patients. The study also included patient rounding to check for the patch, on-site certified wound and ostomy nurses (CWON), and a visible chart in the break room for nurses to monitor progress. In 3 months the pressure ulcer rate was zero. The decline in rate to zero was almost immediate. The cost/benefit to the hospital was large and also immediate. As a nurse-sensitive indicator, long-term benefits included improved reimbursement from Medicare.

—Misty Novak, MS, RN, CWON

BARRIERS TO RESEARCH AGENDA IMPLEMENTATION

The difference between the two hospitals in the preceding "Tales from the Field" sidebar speaks to the barriers that prevent the implementation of an adequate research agenda. These differences are outlined in Table 21.1.

TABLE 21.1   DIFFERENCES BETWEEN RURAL AND URBAN HOSPITAL

Rural Hospital	Urban Hospital
Lack of databases and online libraries	Large online database through school
Lack of resources	On-site CWON and nurse scientist
Lack of knowledge	Master's nursing research project with academic resources

These are just a few of the barriers noted in the literature when setting a research agenda. They also include, but are not limited to, the following:

- Time

- Increased workload

- Difficulty recruiting and retaining staff

- Lack of prioritization to implement

- Lack of authority to change practice (Grant, Stuhlmacher, and Bonte-Eley, 2012; Hain and Kear, 2015)

- Other nurses

The barrier of other nurses is not often mentioned in the literature, but every nurse and manager knows that there is always pushback from someone—often another nurse or nurses, and usually more senior nurses. This also speaks to the importance of the culture of the HRO and the need to establish the infrastructure to support the bedside nurse scientist. Enthusiasm for research fades quickly when faced with negativity from peers and no support from management.

TALES FROM THE FIELD

We have so many changes in the ED where I work that are based on evidence. The most recent change has been our practice on medicating patients after intubation for pain and sedation. In 2013, the U.S. Society for Critical Care made changes to practice recommendations that include treating pain before sedating patients and using only light sedation rather than the heavy sedation we have traditionally relied on. In addition, the guidelines recommend using validated tools to measure pain, agitation, and sedation levels (Barr et al., 2013). Years of data collection show increased mortality and morbidity related to heavy sedation after intubation. Our nurses are used to heavily sedating agitated patients after they are intubated, and this has been a big practice change. We are still working hard on it. I educated all of our staff during our annual skills day and had a lot of pushback from some of our senior nurses. Our medical doctors (MDs) were educated at the same time by their emergency department (ED) medical director and by the newer ED MDs who were taught this practice change in their residency programs. We had a combined journal club with ED MDs and registered nurses (RNs) to discuss the changes before implementation. Currently we are collecting data to evaluate our use of the validated tools to measure sedation and pain. We are fortunate to have pharmacists in our ED and ED physicians who are committed to this practice change and are helping us drive it. Unfortunately, some of our nurses have been our biggest barriers to change, but we are working on it. It has been our strongest senior nurses who have been most resistant to the change. I am working as the clinical educator and try to go to the floor as much as I can to help the bedside RN with intubated patients to assist with this change.

—Sheila Desilet, RN

OVERCOMING BARRIERS

The problems identified as barriers have been overcome by many organizations as they pursue "target zero" safety for their HROs. Education is critical. This should first occur in academia, then in the facility's orientation. An organization that is active in research and EBP has diverse approaches to keep research and EBP at the forefront of the organization. These are discussed in more detail in the following sections.

EDUCATION

Many nurses are not educated in EBP or research and must become so to maintain control of their practice and remain active contributors to HROs. Educational sessions should be offered at work, in academia, and through various methods in the classroom or online.

Overcoming this barrier should begin in nursing school, where curriculum is included in research and EBP. Accredited schools are mandated to include this in the curriculum. However, there is a wide difference in the amount of education on the subject between the associate degree and the bachelor's degree. I have seen curriculum in an ADN program that includes a 2-hour lecture on research, and that is it! The BSN typically includes a semester-long course.

Students at this level often complain and ask why they need to know this "stuff that they will never use." Few students are aware of the pervasiveness of EBP in the workplace and understand the need to know. The end result is tuning out. They want to know how to do the skills needed to be a nurse, not a nurse scientist. Advanced practice nurses with master's degrees or higher have more education in the academic setting and are often required to complete their own quality improvement project, EBP project, or research project, depending on the program and type of degree.

ORIENTATION

HROs that wish to make research part of the culture need to include it in the orientation. Here is where the bedside nurse begins her initiation into the differences of a transparent organization that measures its metrics, challenges its beliefs, and values a fresh pair of eyes. The new employee should:

- Be oriented to available resources
- Be introduced to research committees and their mission
- Have educational opportunities explained
- Be invited to attend a research meeting
- Identify his or her strengths and weaknesses on the subject of research

Whether the employee is a new graduate or has been out of school for years, there should be some research refresher program for him or her to attend. The nature of the subject is complex and should be assessed routinely through research competencies or a research project. Continuing education offerings and an annual research and EBP conference are mechanisms to share information and outcomes while building relationships. Sharing data and metrics reveals many opportunities for bedside nurses to develop their skills in research to improve patient outcomes.

Orientation should also include background information in nurse-sensitive indicators and the value-based purchasing (VBP) domains, measures, and weights for each fiscal year as shared by the Centers for Medicare and Medicaid Services (CMS). Many nurses are never given this information nor have had it explained. However, they do like to see that what they do matters to the bottom line of the hospital. They also know (or should know) their role in good Hospital Consumer Assessment of Healthcare Providers and Systems (HCAHPS) scores.

This bottom-up approach to patient improvement worked well for the Robert Wood Johnson Foundation's "Transforming Care at the Bedside" program. Since then, there have been many nurse-led research studies that document positive outcomes. These are the studies led by the bedside nurse scientist with the assistance of a research team rather than the other way around—management conducting the study and telling the nurse what to do. There is a world of difference!

Table 21.2 provides a summary of just a few research projects I have seen developed by bedside nurses as they learn the process of nursing research. Nurses need not be intimidated by their lack of research knowledge or experience. That is the purpose of working as a team. Bedside nurse scientists can easily identify a research question that would promote quality and safety because they are the front-line staff. It is up to academia and the institution to help them develop the study, gather the data, and perform an analysis.

TABLE 21.2   EXAMPLES OF RESEARCH PROJECTS DEVELOPED BY BEDSIDE NURSES

Research Question	Facility
Does trimming PICC lines before insertion cause more or fewer adverse reactions in the neonatal population?	Large urban neonatal intensive care unit
If the nurses on the intensive care unit implement barcode medication administration, will patient safety increase and medication errors decrease?	Large urban intensive care unit
Will standardized protocols to streamline care processes in a small outpatient clinic reduce patient wait times and increase patient satisfaction?	Rural outpatient clinic
Will a nurse-driven urinary catheter removal protocol linked to physician insertion orders decrease the incidence of infection?	Rural medical-surgical unit

OFFERING A RESEARCH FELLOWSHIP

The infrastructure and desire to foster research within some organizations goes beyond mentoring to a formal research fellowship. The program goal is to assist bedside nurses to gain experience in performing a research study. Fellowships require significant resources on the part of the institution as well as time and commitment for the nurses involved. The use of resources becomes a driver to require applications with inclusion criteria such as, but not limited to, the following:

- Minimum BSN degree
- Minimum length of time at hospital
- Recommendations from supervisors
- Contract post fellowship to maintain employment

Although programs vary in length across the country, most continue through a period of 1 year. During this year, nurses meet monthly and are provided education in all research-related skills needed to develop and present or publish their own work. A variety of educational activities are required as well as mentoring and coaching. The hospital pays for the nurses to take the time off to attend the formal classes. When the fellowship is completed, these graduates become a resource to their fellow peers. The following "Tales from the Field" sidebar describes an example of a beginning research fellowship started by an RN finishing her master's degree in an urban community hospital.

TALES FROM THE FIELD

I'm so proud and excited to have this opportunity to help build such an important program. I was hired in January 2015 to help build the research program at our hospital. Each meeting I set up I tried to see how research would fit in with what they were trying to accomplish. When I had my first meeting with our CNO I wanted to bring something that would benefit all the nurses in our institution. As I was doing my own research online, I came across different articles about implementing a nursing research fellowship program. We are on the Magnet® journey, so I felt this would be a great way to demonstrate nurses practicing EBP. We sent out fellowship applications during nurse's week, and today I'm meeting with the educators who will be teaching different topics. We have two mentors who will each take a fellow to help with this process. Building this program will take a village to make it successful. The curriculum is based on a 12-month time period, and in the end the fellows will present their protocol and findings at a meeting for all associates to attend. I'm incredibly lucky that our CNO saw the value of this program and agreed to provide 4 hours per month paid time to each fellow. Literally, I only got through half of my speech and she said absolutely! This year will definitely be a learning process, and the hope is that we will continue to grow it each year with more fellows.

—Emily Tremlett, RN

BRIDGING THE GAP

As seen in the "Tales from the Field" sidebars, it takes a village to bring research and EBP to the forefront of an organization. I have seen redundancy in some organizations in which each department is in its own silo. Information is not shared, and department heads try to best each other in results. Competition and rework cost money and do not work! Research councils and research teams are instrumental in achieving results. One person cannot see or do all in complex healthcare organizations. The following sections contain examples of how effective HROs work.

THE RESEARCH COUNCIL

The mission of a research and EBP council is to help bridge the gap between research and practice. It promotes excellence in patient care and safety, which is a hallmark of HROs. The true mission of most councils is validating, identifying, and/or creating practices to achieve the best outcomes in patient care. Secondarily, councils serve as a means for teaching and learning.

Councils should largely consist of bedside nurses. These nurses are able to identify areas of concern and improvement from their units, creating opportunities for research. Representatives from other disciplines are also included. Councils are usually led by a doctorally prepared nurse researcher. Other members of the team can include the following:

- Chief nursing officer
- Quality director
- Magnet® coordinator
- Safety manager
- Medical librarian

It is the research council in most facilities that develops an event that displays research and EBP to its employees, either through poster displays of completed projects, educational conferences, or both. Acknowledging those who have worked on projects during the year is a motivational strategy that continues the momentum of research activity within the organization.

Other activities of the research council depend on the size of the facility as well as the council. These include the following:

- Assistance with mentoring
- Journal clubs
- Research evidence for policy and procedure development
- Education

THE RESEARCH TEAM

Effective HROs work with a team approach; so do effective research teams. One of my first experiences viewing the work of interdepartmental research teams was a trip to Cleveland Clinic's Research/EBP Symposium in the early 2000s. All stakeholders involved in a work process that developed a research/EBP poster or podium presentation were introduced. It was the first time I saw housekeeping and maintenance involved in a project as equal team players. In one study on infection control, they shared the processes for cleaning and maintenance, while the nurse scientist developed the project proposal. That type of forward thinking and the creation of inclusionary teams fostered buy-in for all team members as well as educating them as they moved forward in the process. There was also pride in creating a better solution to a problem.

A team consists of the following:

- A specific individual and interactive role

- A distributed set of necessary skills

- Shared and explicit purposes, information, goals, plans, protocols, and feedback mechanisms (Gordon, Mendenhall, and O'Connor, 2012, p. 81)

In this model, the research team is at the center of the activity, with communication between all parties. (See Figure 21.1.)

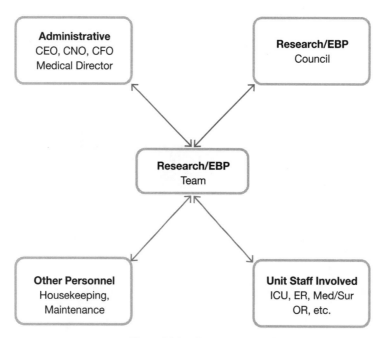

Figure 21.1 Research model.

At a minimum, the research/EBP team consists of the principal investigator, stakeholders involved in the process, and data collectors. In HROs, these members can communicate effectively in a safe environment without fear of retaliation. The following "Tales from the Field" sidebar illustrates what can happen in a non-HRO facility.

TALES FROM THE FIELD

A small rural hospital wanted to develop a perioperative protocol to improve patient outcomes for patients with diabetes. The diabetes nurse educator was made aware of the problem when reviewing the post-operative blood glucose of patients in the recovery room. These high levels can lead to problems with wound healing and infection as well as prolonged hospital stays. The project was led by the diabetes nurse educator and supported by the CNO. The research team also consisted of two nurses working in the perioperative area, a registered dietician, and a nurse academician who taught research. The team reviewed many excellent research studies as well as standards of care for anesthesiology. They spoke with orthopedic surgeons to garner support, as they were the first group to be involved in the protocol. They also spoke with anesthesiologists, who also seemed supportive.

When the team was ready to roll out the protocol, they presented it to the medical board. The first problem was that the CNO could not attend. However, they did not anticipate any problems because of the prior conversations between stakeholders. One physician (not a stakeholder) did not like the protocol and voiced his dislike loudly. The team was able to answer his questions regarding power analysis for sample size, blood glucose range, and a variety of other questions. During this time, you could feel a shift in the room. The anesthesiologist, who had supported the protocol, changed his mind and said he would rather have high glucose levels on his patients than have them bottom out and not wake up from surgery. In other words, he did not agree with the anesthesiology standards of practice. Then the orthopedic surgeon decided that his practice did not have enough patients to meet the sample number of patients. Finally, another physician asked if the patient was going to pay for the additional testing.

The physicians clearly had the "captain of the ship" mindset. They were going to support the one physician who did not agree, even if they had agreed prior to the meeting. Even if there had been a "do-over" with the CNO, the outcome would probably have been similar. This reflects the need for a culture change because progress was halted without it, even when all stakeholders were considered.

—Alma Jackson, PhD, RN, COHN-S

CREATING AN INFRASTRUCTURE THAT SUPPORTS THE BEDSIDE NURSE

As mentioned, it is often the nurses with whom we work who do not support change. When this happens, the culture of the HRO is such that support is given to the bedside nurse to implement the change to drive the research. Consider the following "Tales from the Field" sidebar.

TALES FROM THE FIELD

It was discovered that the cardio-thoracic ICU and the step-down unit were using sulfonylureas in the post op period. The incidence of hypoglycemia was highest on these units. For years, cardiac surgeons have used sulfonylureas during the post op period. They also did not feel that hypoglycemia described blood sugars below 70mg/dl. Rather, they believed hypoglycemia described blood sugars below 50mg/dl. The chief of endocrinology presented data to them showing why there should be concern for blood sugars less than 70mg/dl, the dangers of hypoglycemia post op cardiac surgery, and how sulfonylurea use was associated with hypoglycemia, especially when used with insulin. She was met with resistance, but both she and the inpatient diabetes team continued to present data to them. Even with backing from the pharmacy and therapeutics committee, the cardiac surgeons did not find cause to change practice. It wasn't until their colleagues from other institutions throughout our health system backed the research that they conceded to change their practice at my hospital. This whole process took 2½ years.

—Ann Hasse, RN

Two and half years to a process change that causes harm to patients is too long. It is evident that in the culture of the institution, the doctors viewed themselves similarly to airline pilots, who were not to be questioned because they knew everything. In HROs, this culture is unacceptable. The airline industry has averted many disasters with its culture change. Healthcare will do the same when the shift is made.

NURSING ROLE RESPONSIBILITIES TO MAINTAIN MOMENTUM

Throughout this chapter, we have made it clear that the bedside nurse is essential in creating a "target zero" for errors. They have their finger on the pulse of the process and are experts in patient care processes.

ROLES OF FRONT-LINE STAFF

It is the responsibility of the front-line staff to bring forward concerns, report near misses and incidents, and be open to creative opportunities for improvement in patient care. They also need to become more educated in the research process so they can become more active participants in developing a research project. Front-line staff should share responsibilities for journal clubs, serve as research project champions, and join research councils or research teams. If they qualify for the research fellowship, they should apply, participate, and be a mentor for others.

ROLES OF ADVANCED PRACTICE NURSES

Advanced practice nurses (APNs) have more academic education in research and should take a leadership role in mentoring. They can identify practice issues and concerns and recommend outcome measures that are important to monitor. For example, nurse practitioners (NPs) are responsible for following indicators specific to their practice such as symptom management, anticoagulation monitoring, and clinic wait time. They should determine appropriate data collection based on assessment, data, and metrics they observe. Other activities include the following:

- Lead role as a member of the research council
- Lead role as a member of a research team
- Present at the facility research conference as well as nationally
- Mentor nurses in practice issues, outcomes, and metrics

ROLE OF THE DOCTORALLY PREPARED NURSE

The doctorally prepared nurse has had multiple research courses in a PhD program and at a minimum one research course in a DNP program. It is usually a PhD-prepared nurse who holds a position of nurse scientist. Many hospitals now employ nurse scientists who possess both research skills and clinical expertise. Their role is to facilitate research in the institution through program development and education, mentoring, grant writing and review, presentations at conferences, and research committee participation. In essence, they are the research champions of the facility and are highly valued in HROs.

Either a DNP or a PhD-prepared nurse can lead a research council. They can serve as principal investigators, search for and develop grants, and assist in educating other nurses in the research process. Some facilities do not have the funds or an individual who fits the job description of a doctorally prepared nurse. In this case, they often use colleagues from academia to help support their research efforts.

SUMMARY

HROs have a culture that allows for creative and innovative solutions that promote patient safety. One way this gets done is through deference to expertise, which permits bedside nurses to become part of a solution. Educating nurses to become bedside scientists, knowledgeable about the conduct of research, promotes ownership in the profession as well as documenting the evidence about how truly valuable nurses really are.

KEY POINTS

- The nurse at the bedside has critical expertise essential to meet the goals of achieving an HRO.

- Nursing programs must better prepare their students to take on research responsibilities.

- Continuing education in the work setting is necessary to maintain competency in research.

- Numerous committees and activities engage staff, provide motivation to learn, and promote the research agenda, thus bridging the gap between knowledge and action.

- Whether bedside nurse, advanced practice nurse, or nurse scientist, there is an important role for each that propels the healthcare HRO to meet its goals of zero errors.

REFERENCES

Barr, J., Fraser, G. L., Puntillo, K., Ely, E. W., Gélinas, C., Dasta, J. F., ... American College of Critical Care Medicine. (2013). Clinical practice guidelines for the management of pain, agitation, and delirium in adult patients in the intensive care unit. *Critical Care Medicine, 41*(1), pp. 263–306.

Gordon, S., Mendenhall, P., and O'Connor, B. B. (2012). *Beyond the checklist: What else health care can learn from aviation teamwork and safety.* Ithaca, NY: ILR Press.

Grant, H. S., Stuhlmacher, A., and Bonte-Eley, S. (2012). Overcoming barriers to research utilization and evidence-based practice among staff nurses. *Journal for Nurses in Staff Development, 28*(4), pp. 163–165.

Hain, D. J., and Kear, T. M. (2015). Using evidence-based practice to move beyond doing things the way we have always done them. *Nephrology Nursing Journal, 42*(1), pp. 11–21.

Institute of Medicine (IOM). (2010). *The future of nursing: Leading change, advancing health.* Washington, DC: The National Academies Press.

Polit, D., and Beck, C. T. (2012). *Nursing research: Generating and assessing evidence for nursing practice* (9th ed.). Philadelphia, PA: Lippincott Williams & Wilkins.

Robert Wood Johnson Foundation. (2011). Transforming care at the bedside. Retrieved from http://www.rwjf.org/content/dam/farm/reports/program_results_reports/2011/rwjf70624

A

BUILDING A HIGH RELIABILITY HEAD AND NECK OPERATING ROOM TEAM

Kristen A. Oster, MS, APRN, ACNS-BC, CNOR, CNS-CP

The operating room is an interdisciplinary, high-risk health-care setting where potential hazards await each patient. Patients who come to the operating room for treatment of head and neck disorders undergo extensive invasive surgical procedures with unpredictable outcomes. As noted by Sanchez and Barach, "The level of complexity, both in task-oriented and cognitive demands, results in a dynamic, unforgiving environment that can magnify the consequences of even small lapses and errors" (2012, p. 1).

The operating room team is composed of individuals with diversely specialized skills focused on a common task in a defined period of time and space (Sax, 2012). Together, the team of surgeons, anesthesiologists, nurses, and surgical technologists adapt, respond to emergencies, and share responsibility for outcomes. Each healthcare professional brings a set of skills to the operating room environment important to the surgical procedure. The operating room is a fast-paced, high-risk, ever-changing environment requiring multiple team members who must perform with high reliability every time for every procedure. Efficient, open,

> We always hope for the easy fix: the one simple change that will erase a problem in a stroke. But few things in life work this way. Instead, success requires making a hundred small steps go right—one after the other, no slipups, no goofs, everyone pitching in.
>
> —Atul Gawande

and honest communication among the members of the surgical team must occur if the surgical procedure is to conclude safely for the patient. Focus must be on patient safety. This appendix describes one operating room team's journey to a becoming a highly reliable surgical team.

THE PROBLEM

Head and neck cancers can vary in type and treatment options. Treatment options include chemotherapy, radiation, and surgery. Surgical treatment options may require the removal of important functional structures and tissues located within the head and neck region of the body. Consequently, a head and neck patient may require extensive reconstructive surgery involving the using of an autologous graft—tissue transplanted from one part of the body to another that is obtained from the same individual, including but not limited to skin, bone, and tissue (Phillips, 2013). The autologous graft is harvested from another part of the body or donor site and then placed where cancer-affected tissue previously was located in the head and neck region or recipient site. However, a drawback of an autologous graft is the creation of a donor site wound. The donor site is a second wound with its own healing process that may take a long time to mend. The goal of reconstructive surgery is to maximize the best function and aesthetic result possible post reconstructive surgery.

Reconstructive surgery for the head and neck patient population often requires extensive surgical time in the operating room to remove cancerous tissue, harvest the autologous graft, and place the autologous graft in the recipient location. This requires ongoing, continuous communication among surgical staff about the planned surgical procedure, location of the autologous graft, type of autologous graft, and care of the autologous graft.

When communication fails, a critical event can occur. A critical event occurred in our operating room that led us to reevaluate the process and procedure used during reconstructive surgeries requiring the harvest and use of an autologous graft. The critical event occurred during a head and neck reconstructive procedure. A tissue autologous graft was harvested by a team of surgeons and handed to the surgical technologist for placement on the back table for preservation until graft inset later in the procedure. The surgical technologist placed the tissue autologous graft in a fluid warmer with the fluid bath at a temperature greater than 100 degrees Fahrenheit, causing tissue damage to the autologous graft. The surgeons were notified of the tissue damage to the graft. Fortunately, the autologous tissue graft was still viable for inset to the recipient site in the head and neck region of the patient.

The team debrief following this critical event gave rise to many questions related to the handling and management of autologous grafts during reconstructive procedures. It was identified that there were no structures or processes in place for the correct management of an autologous graft during reconstructive surgical procedures.

ASSEMBLING THE TEAM

An interprofessional process improvement team was assembled to emphasize the interdependence of all disciplines in the care of head and neck surgical patients requiring autologous grafts (Sax, 2012). The common goal of the team was to develop standardized structures and processes associated with the management of an autologous graft during reconstructive surgery. This team included the head and neck perioperative assistant nurse manager, head and neck surgeons, perioperative leadership, staff nurses, and surgical technologists.

Each member of the team brought a different perspective specific to his or her role for discussion and contributed to designing a solution to the problem. The assistant nurse manager of the head and neck service line led and facilitated the group. The head and neck surgeons acted as subject matter experts during the development of the structure and process for management of an autologous graft during reconstructive surgical procedures. The perioperative surgical services director and operating room manager demonstrated senior leadership support by providing team members time away from the point of patient care to accomplish assigned tasks. The operating room educator acted as an education strategy subject matter expert. Staff nurses and surgical technologists provided peer review of tools along with point-of-care application to determine workflow impact.

METHOD

A root cause analysis (RCA) is a structured method used to analyze an adverse event (Agency for Healthcare Research and Quality [AHRQ], 2014). An RCA was performed to determine the cause of our critical event. The RCA or learning from defects conducted by the team showed no standardized structures and processes in place for staff to use to reliably manage an autologous graft in the operating room environment. (See Figure A.1.)

After conducting the RCA, the team performed a literature search to gather current best evidence practice about autologous graft management. Team members collected and appraised the available evidence. Surgeons offered their expert opinion and experiential knowledge. The outcome was the development of a policy and procedure focusing on the management of the autologous graft (Fuller, 2013). In addition to the policy and procedure, an algorithm, called the "Management of Autologous Graft for Reconstructive Surgery Algorithm," was developed to illustrate the steps of the management of the autologous graft for the operating room team (Phillips, 2013; Steelman, Blanchard, Denholm, and Conner, 2007). The algorithm addresses informed consent, surgical time-out addressing autologous graft location, preparation of the autologous graft, ischemia times, and debriefing. (See Figure A.2.)

Safety Tip:
The fragility of autologous skin grafts must be recognized by OR staff.

Case: Autologous graft harvested from donor site during a head and neck surgical procedure. Graft placed on OR back table in a preservation fluid bath by a surgical tech for preservation until time for graft inset. Fluid bath greater than 100 degrees Fahrenheit causing some damage to the graft.

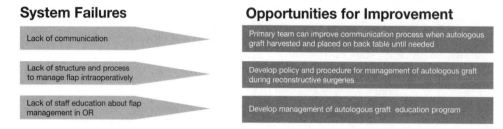

System Failures

- Lack of communication
- Lack of structure and process to manage flap intraoperatively
- Lack of staff education about flap management in OR

Opportunities for Improvement

- Primary team can improve communication process when autologous graft harvested and placed on back table until needed
- Develop policy and procedure for management of autologous graft during reconstructive surgeries
- Develop management of autologous graft education program

Actions Taken to Prevent Harm

Reluctance to simplify	Develop standardized graft algorithm	• Interprofessional team assembled to design autologous graft algorithm
Preoccupation with failure	Develop a surgical checklist for management of autologous graft for reconstruction surgery	• Improve team communication, speak up • Share incident reports and findings with team in non-punitive manner
Sensitivity to operations	Improve communication of the OR team	• Time out: identification and communication about graft being harvested, where from, and how it will be cared for until needed • Team debriefing: did anything happen during care?
Commitment to resilience	Train staff to improve skills and knowledge	• Learning from past errors for patient care improvement • Reviewed surgical checklist, will participate in time out, speak up if needed, and be professionally accountable

Figure A.1 Learning from defects is conducted to determine the cause of the critical event.

After the policy and procedure and surgical algorithm were completed, staff curricula and adherence to protocol checklists were developed with the assistance of the operating room educator to verify staff understanding. A checklist, called the "Management of Autologous Graft for Reconstruction Surgery—Surgical Checklist," was developed for staff to use in the operating room during large reconstructive surgeries requiring an autologous graft. (See Figure A.3.) Staff curricula were created for the surgical checklist and the policy and procedure. A form, called the "Management of Autologous Graft Checklist Compliance" form, was developed and completed by all staff members to evaluate and verify their understanding of the new structures and processes. (See Figure A.4.) Education sessions provided by the educator and assistant nurse manager allowed each staff member to ask questions and seek clarification as needed. The head and neck assistant nurse manager completed surgical safety checklist compliance forms in staff personnel education files for annual performance evaluation purposes.

Management of Autologous Graft for Reconstruction Surgery Algorithm

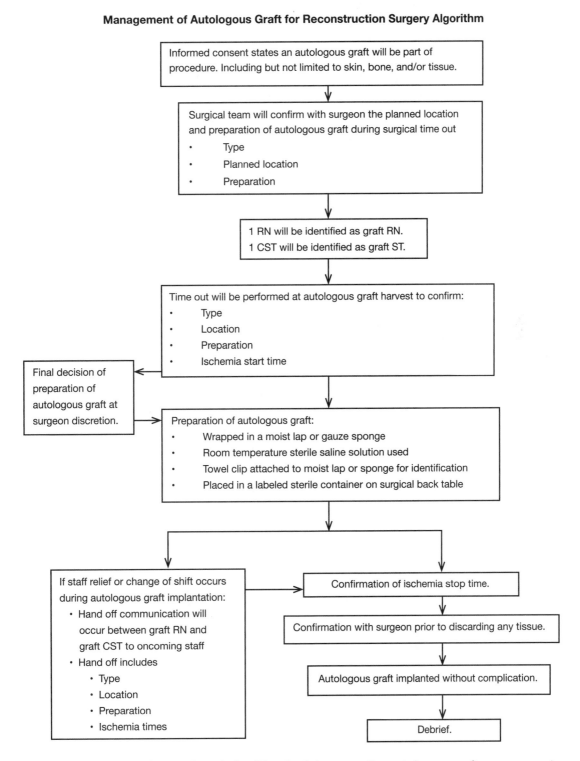

Informed consent states an autologous graft will be part of procedure. Including but not limited to skin, bone, and/or tissue.

Surgical team will confirm with surgeon the planned location and preparation of autologous graft during surgical time out
- Type
- Planned location
- Preparation

1 RN will be identified as graft RN.
1 CST will be identified as graft ST.

Time out will be performed at autologous graft harvest to confirm:
- Type
- Location
- Preparation
- Ischemia start time

Final decision of preparation of autologous graft at surgeon discretion.

Preparation of autologous graft:
- Wrapped in a moist lap or gauze sponge
- Room temperature sterile saline solution used
- Towel clip attached to moist lap or sponge for identification
- Placed in a labeled sterile container on surgical back table

If staff relief or change of shift occurs during autologous graft implantation:
- Hand off communication will occur between graft RN and graft CST to oncoming staff
- Hand off includes
  - Type
  - Location
  - Preparation
  - Ischemia times

Confirmation of ischemia stop time.

Confirmation with surgeon prior to discarding any tissue.

Autologous graft implanted without complication.

Debrief.

Figure A.2   An evidence-based algorithm for intra-operative autologous graft management.

OUTCOMES

The outcome of this process-improvement initiative is encouraging. There has been no injury to an autologous graft critical event since implementation of the algorithm and surgical checklist in October 2014. The surgical checklist was distributed to each surgical team at the start of large reconstructive surgeries during November and December 2014. The checklist continues to be randomly used to assess adherence to structures and processes. A total of 24 surgical checklists have been completed for large reconstructive surgeries with nine team members completing the education activities and surgical safety checklist compliance form. The surgical checklist continues to be distributed to staff periodically to maintain competency and staff compliance with management of the autologous graft.

DISSEMINATION

The weekly team huddle is the primary venue for the dissemination of information for the head and neck surgical service line. It is during this meeting that critical events or occurrences are relayed to the team. These discussions include the rationale for the new processes and procedures for managing autologous grafts during reconstructive surgeries. Dissemination of the policy and procedure, surgery algorithm, surgical safety checklist, and checklist compliance form for new and incumbent staff is done during the huddle to promote understanding and communication among team members. The opportunity to ask questions related to structures and processes is provided, and the operative schedule for the week is discussed. Potential vulnerabilities are identified, and strategies to mitigate risk to patient safety are then implemented. The assistant nurse manager is readily available to assist the team to follow and implement each step outlined in the surgery algorithm. In team huddles, team members provide ongoing feedback about the standardized structures and processes. The team talks about positive patient care happenings, as well as near misses in the management of the autologous graft during reconstructive surgeries. In addition, team members are encouraged to provide ideas on how to improve patient safety for this patient population and decrease the potential for error.

Centura Health.   Management of Autologous Graft for Reconstruction Surgery - Surgical Checklist

Staff Involved: _____   Surgeon: _____

Type: Skin_____   Bone_____   Tissue_____   Date of Procedure: _____

Instructions: Complete on ALL patients when procedure requires autologous graft use	Yes	No	NA	Identified Barriers (If NO, why not?)
Check all activities that apply:				
Surgical Procedure ☐ _____				
Surgical team will **confirm** with surgeon planned location of and preparation of autologous graft in **Surgical Time Out** ☐ 1 RN will be **identified** as graft RN ☐ 1 ST will be **identified** as graft ST				
Team will perform **Time Out** at harvest of autologous graft to confirm ☐ Type ☐ Location of autologous graft ☐ Preparation of autologous graft ☐ Ischemia start time				
Preparation of Autologous Graft ☐ Graft will be wrapped in a moist lap or gauze sponge ☐ Room temperature sterile saline solution used ☐ Towel clip attached to sponge for identification ☐ Graft will be placed in a labeled sterile container ☐ **OR** Surgeon's Preference _____				
Ischemia Time - Start ☐ Surgeon will announce start of ischemia time ☐ RN will confirm start of ischemia time ☐ RN will start timer clock				
Ischemia Time - Stop ☐ Surgeon will announce stop of ischemia time ☐ RN will confirm stop of ischemia time ☐ RN will stop timer clock				
Documentation of Ischemia Time in Meditech and white board includes ☐ Ischemia start time ☐ Ischemia stop time ☐ Total ischemia time in minutes				
Graft RN and CST will **communicate** following information during all staff relief/change of shift hand-off ☐ Type ☐ Autologous graft location ☐ Ischemia start time ☐ Ischemia stop time ☐ Total ischemia time				
Debrief ☐ Team will **discuss** any key concerns				

Checklist should be completed with **ALL** autologous grafts

NOT PART OF THE PERMANENT MEDICAL RECORD

Return to Kristen Oster MS, APRN, ACNS-BC, CNOR

Attach Patient Sticker

10/30/14

Figure A.3   A surgical checklist is used for intra-operative management of autologous graft.

SURGICAL SAFETY CHECKLIST COMPLIANCE

Name (print)	Title	Date

The staff member will be able to:

1. Understand the Surgical Safety Checklist process.

2. Identify critical documentation necessary for Time-Out and Surgical Safety Checklist Audit and Meditech.

3. Correctly perform or participate in the Time-Out and address Surgical Safety Checklist including Briefing and Debriefing.

Check box upon completion	Skill/Function or Role	Associate's initials
	I have read and been informed of the expectations of the Surgical Safety Checklist.	
	I understand and will be held accountable for performing and /or participating in the Time-Out, Briefing and Debriefing.	
	I will speak up during the Time-Out if I have additional concerns (i.e. Implants, instrumentation, equipment)	
	I agree to take responsibility for performing and documenting the Time-Out and Surgical Safety Checklist audit form.	
	I will be accountable to model these standards and will encourage others to do the same.	

Associate's Signature   Date

Evaluator's Signature   Date

Figure A.4   A safety checklist compliance form is completed to verify staff education and under-standing of new structures and processes.

CONCLUSION

The goal of the head and neck surgical service team is to provide highly reliable safe patient care. The concepts of high reliability organizations are relevant to the microsystem of the head and neck surgical service line in the operating room environment (Sanchez and Barach, 2012). The rapid pace of surgical procedures requiring autologous grafts, the expectation of superior performance and patient safety, and the uncertainty inherent in the surgical procedure itself require a team or service line approach. The high complexity level of the head and neck patient requiring surgery that includes autologous grafting can contribute to team failure and critical event occurrence. Our team has become highly reliable as we have created a culture of safety through transparency, building standardized structures and processes into our daily work, designing tools to reduce reliance on memory, and implementing those tools to mitigate errors.

REFERENCES

Agency for Healthcare Research and Quality (AHRQ). (2014). Root cause analysis. Retrieved from http://www.psnet.ahrq.gov/primer.aspx?primerID=10

Fuller, J. K. (2013). *Surgical technology principles and practice* (6th ed.). St. Louis, MO: Elsevier.

Gawande, A. (2008). *Better: A surgeon's notes on performance.* New York, NY: Picador.

Phillips, N. F. (2013). *Berry & Kohn's operating room technique* (12th ed.) (pp. 845–871). St. Louis, MO: Mosby.

Sanchez, J. A., and Barach, P. R. (2012). High reliability organizations and surgical microsystems: Re-engineering surgical care. *Surgical Clinics of North America, 92*(1), pp. 1–14.

Sax, H. C. (2012). Building high-performance teams in the operating room. *Surgical Clinics of North America, 92*(1), pp. 15–19.

Steelman, V., Blanchard, J., Denholm, B., and Conner, R. (2007). Dropping a cranial bone flap; rigid sterilization containers; tourniquet cuffs; OR air exchanges. *AORN Journal, 85*(6), pp. 1225–1230.

CHAMPIONING CAUTI PREVENTION IN THE ICU/SDU: A PROJECT DEMONSTRATING THE CONCEPTS OF HROT

Michelle Norris, BSN, RN, CCRN

Carrie Neyers, BSN, RN, CCRN

When we embarked on our mission to reduce catheter-associated urinary tract infections (CAUTI), we didn't realize the degree of success we would have. Having a large intensive care unit/step-down unit (ICU/SDU) encompassing complex medical, surgical, and neurological patients, we were faced with a challenging proposition to decrease our CAUTI rate. It took a team effort to implement new evidence-based practice (EBP) in our unit that eventually brought our CAUTI rate to zero over 12 months. "Championing CAUTI Prevention in the ICU/SDU" is a project documenting our success. It demonstrates the concepts behind high reliability organizations theory (HROT) (Kemper and Boyle, 2009). HROT concepts—including preoccupation with failure, reluctance to simplify, sensitivity to operations, commitment to resilience, and deference to expertise—were exhibited in this project.

> Our greatest glory is not in never falling, but in rising every time we fall.
>
> —Confucius

PROBLEM

Despite widespread efforts made by hospitals to improve the quality of healthcare, many patients continue to experience preventable harm. One example of such harm is CAUTIs, with 450,000 infections occurring in hospitals each year (Fuchs, Sexton, Thornlow, and Champagne, 2011). More than 25% of patients with an indwelling urinary catheter for anywhere from 2 to 10 days will develop bacteria in their urine, and a quarter of those will go on to develop a CAUTI (Klevens et al., 2007; Rebmann and Greene, 2010; Saint et al., 2008; Saint and Chenowith, 2003). The costs for these hospital-acquired UTIs are staggering, ranging from $1,200 to more than $2,700 per case, costing the healthcare system more than $400 million annually (Fuchs et al., 2011; Pappas, 2008; Scott, 2009; Wald and Kramer, 2007).

Our unit had a significant CAUTI problem. Fiscal and calendar years 2010, 2011, and 2012 showed sporadic CAUTI rates month to month. (See Figure B.1 and Figure B.2.) There were 11 CAUTI occurrences in FY 12 and 4,777 catheter days. Not only did we have a high occurrence rate, we were overutilizing catheters, thus increasing our CAUTI risk. This led us to question what we were doing wrong that resulted in high and varying CAUTI rates on our unit. It was obvious that we needed to improve and sharpen our CAUTI-prevention strategies on our complex 36-bed unit. It was then that unit-based CAUTI-prevention champions came into existence.

2010-2011 ICU/SDU CAUTI Rates

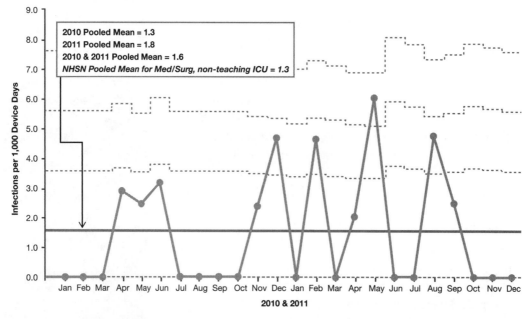

Figure B.1 ICU/SDU CAUTI rates for calendar year 2010–2011. Sporadic CAUTI rates demonstrated from 2010–2011.

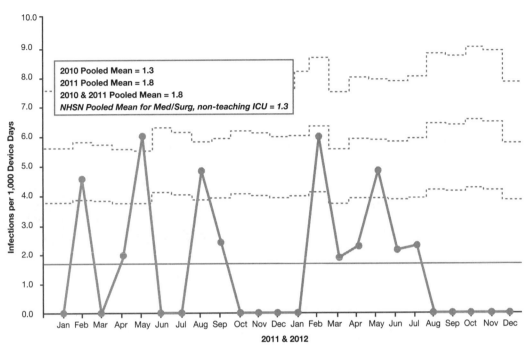

2011-2012 ICU/SDU CAUTI Rates

2010 Pooled Mean = 1.3
2011 Pooled Mean = 1.8
2010 & 2011 Pooled Mean = 1.8
NHSN Pooled Mean for Med/Surg, non-teaching ICU = 1.3

Figure B.2   ICU/SDU CAUTI rates for calendar year 2011–2012. Sporadic CAUTI rates demonstrated from 2011–2012.

METHODS

The idea of unit-based champions originally came from our hospital pressure ulcer prevention (PUP) team. Unit champions performing quarterly National Database of Nursing Quality Indicators (NDNQI) pressure ulcer audits had been in place for more than 8 years. When hospital CAUTI rates began to flare, our hospital nurse scientist approached the PUP team to assist her in auditing catheters in addition to the NDNQI PUP audits. From there, the PUP team evolved into a PUP and CAUTI-prevention team.

In the ICU/SDU, two staff nurses were named unit-based CAUTI champions. They also continued their roles as PUP champions. A hospital-wide CAUTI reduction project took off from there. It was led by our hospital nurse scientist and would not have been as successful without the involvement of the unit-based champions.

After the initiation of the CAUTI-prevention project, it was immediately evident that more unit-based assistance would be needed to make an impact in the ICU/SDU. Management gave approval to bring in more help. Two additional unit-based champions were added to our PUP/CAUTI team. The four nurses who were selected to participate in this project showed interest and commitment in reducing our CAUTI rates in addition to pressure ulcer prevention. They were highly motivated to find ways to eliminate harm to our patients and to promote a culture of safety on our unit (Weick, 1987).

Multiple strategies were implemented to reduce the high CAUTI rate on our unit. By mid-2012, we were up and running with an evidence-based CAUTI-prevention toolkit. The toolkit implementation strategies included the following:

- Focused staff education on guidelines for urinary catheterization and available supplies

- Standardized education for catheter insertion, manipulation, and care

- An infection surveillance program

The toolkit included a CAUTI audit tool and catheter insertion checklist, which are examples of preoccupation with failure and reluctance to simplify. Each month, our CAUTI-prevention champions use the audit tool to assess the ICU/SDU adherence to evidence-based CAUTI-prevention practice guidelines, also known as the *CAUTI bundle* (see Figure B.3).

Our nurse scientist put together an easy-to-read picture guideline that was given to the unit champions to disseminate among the ICU/SDU staff. Each picture represents an intervention in the bundle that we audit. The audit tool shown in Figure B.4 helps the unit-based champions and nurse scientist take a monthly snapshot of CAUTI-prevention adherence on the unit to make sure that best practice is being followed. Additionally, for every catheter that is inserted, the nurse performing the procedure is expected to complete a catheter insertion checklist (see Figure B.5). The checklist takes the nurse through the procedure step-by-step, aiding the nurse to comply to best practice in order to prevent infection. Once the catheter placement is finished, the completed form is turned in to our nurse scientist. Not only does the insertion checklist give the nurse evidence-based guidelines for insertion, the information obtained from the completed checklist allows our nurse scientist to track catheter insertions, reason for insertion, and whether a doctor's order for insertion was obtained. Through these tools, we have demonstrated a reluctance to simplify.

CAUTI PREVENTION BUNDLE

INTERVENTIONS APPLIED TO <u>ALL</u> PATIENTS WITH AN INDWELLING URINARY CATHETER

INSERTION CARE TO PREVENT CAUTI

- Follow Indwelling Urinary Catheter Insertion Checklist

MAINTENANCE CARE TO PREVENT CAUTI

GENERAL CARE ACTIVITIES

- **Assess and document daily for catheter need**
  - Acute urinary retention or bladder outlet obstruction
  - Accurate measurements of urinary output in critically ill patients
  - Perioperative use for selected surgical procedures
    - Urologic surgery/other surgery on contiguous structures of the GU tract
    - Anticipated prolonged duration of surgery (catheters inserted for this reason should be removed in PACU)
    - Anticipated to receive large-volume infusions or diuretics during surgery
    - Need for intraoperative monitoring of urinary output
  - Assist in healing of open sacral or perineal wounds in incontinent patients
  - Requires prolonged immobilization
  - Improve comfort for end of life care if needed
- **Daily perineal hygiene with soap and water – DO NOT use antiseptics for hygiene**
- **Secure catheter to thigh continuously**
- **Identify and manage constipation**
- **Identify and manage fecal incontinence**
- **Keep patient well hydrated**
- **Nutrition consult for malnutrition**
- **Keep system closed – Tamper Evident Seal (TES) intact)**
- **Do NOT perform routine irrigation**

BAG CARE ACTIVITIES

- **Keep below level of bladder at all times**
- **Do NOT let bag touch the floor**
- **Empty bag into clean labeled graduate container**
- **Outlet device (spigot) clamped and in sleeve**

TUBING CARE ACTIVITIES

- **Keep tubing extended**
- **Keep tubing free of dependent loops**
- **Keep below level of bladder**

DOCUMENTATION

Document catheter insertion and removal in "Urinary Catheter Insert & Care" and "DC Urinary Catheter" interventions respectively.

Document catheter care in "Activities of Daily Living ADL Group."

Figure B.3   CAUTI prevention bundle. Evidence-based CAUTI-prevention practice guidelines, including guidelines for urinary catheterization and available supplies; standardized education for catheter insertion, manipulation, and care; and infection surveillance program.

Date: _____   Nursing Unit: _____

URINARY CATHETER MANAGEMENT SURVEILLANCE AUDIT

Instructions: Complete for each patient (whether patient has a urinary catheter or not)

Indicator	Yes	No
Presence of a Urinary Catheter Size: _____ French		
Complete the following _ONLY_ if urinary catheter present:		

1. Catheter secured to patient's:
 	
    abdomen
 	
    leg		

2. Foley system closed – Tamper Evident Seal intact		
3. Drainage tubing extended		
4. NO dependent loops in drainage tubing		
5. Drainage bag and tubing below level of bladder		
6. Drainage system _NOT_ touching floor		
7. Urine meter present		
8. Outlet device (spigot) clamped and in sleeve		
9. Labeled graduated cylinder present		
10. Urine bag contains _____ cc		

Version: CAO 11/22/11

ATTACH PATIENT STICKER

Figure B.4   CAUTI prevention audit tool. Surveillance tool that helps the unit-based champions and nurse scientist take a monthly snapshot of CAUTI-prevention adherence on the unit to make sure that best practice is being followed.

✚
Centura Health.

Indwelling Urinary Catheter Insertion Checklist Form

Insert Nurse: _____

Nursing Unit: _____

Catheter Size: _____

Date of Insertion: _____

Instructions: Complete on __ALL__ patients when inserting an indwelling urinary catheter	Yes	No	NA	Identified Barriers (If NO, why not?)
Insertion Activities				
Assess and **document** catheter need: ☐ Acute urinary retention or bladder outlet obstruction ☐ Measurement of urinary output in critically ill patients ☐ Perioperative use for selected surgical procedures ☐ Surgery:_____ ☐ Open sacral or perineal wound in incontinent patient ☐ Requires prolonged immobilization ☐ Improve comfort for end of life care				
Perform hand hygiene immediately before and after insertion				
Use aseptic technique and sterile equipment				
Use urinary catheter system with **pre-connected and sealed catheter-tubing junctions**				
Perineal Preparation ☐ Cleanse with soap and water or perineal cleanser				
Placement in Bladder ☐ Prep meatus with betadine ☐ Lubricate catheter/urethra with sterile lubricant ☐ DO NOT test inflate balloon ☐ Insert until urine begins to flow ☐ Advance 1 to 3 inches (5 cm) ☐ Inflate 5 mL balloon with 10 mL of sterile water ☐ Gently pull back to seat catheter				
Missed Insertion ☐ **New closed catheter set obtained**				
Obtain urine **sample from sampling port**, if needed				
Secure catheter to leg to prevent movement				
Extend **drainage tubing** with **NO dependent loops**				
Drainage bag and tubing **below level of bladder**				
Drainage bag **NOT on floor**				
Spigot clamped and in sleeve				
Label graduated cylinder				

Checklist should be completed with __ALL__ indwelling urinary catheter insertions

Return completed checklists to Cindy Oster, PhD, MBA, APRN, CNS-BC, ANP, Nurse Scientist

This checklist is NOT PART OF THE PERMANENT MEDICAL RECORD

Attach Patient Sticker

07/10/13

Figure B.5 Indwelling urinary catheter insertion checklist. Checklist provides guidance in best practice for catheter insertion and maintenance.

Taking on the CAUTI-prevention project was a complicated task involving various groups of people. It was clear that a quick and easy fix was not an option for such a project. It was and continues to be a hospital-wide effort to reduce the number of CAUTIs. We do so through a systematic approach of monthly audits, catheter insertion checklists, avoidance of catheter use, and utilization of unit-based CAUTI-prevention champions.

A multidisciplinary approach has been an important factor in CAUTI prevention and is an example of the HROT concept of sensitivity to operations. Our success is due in large part to the flexibility and commitment to excellence of not only the CAUTI-prevention team involved in direct patient care but also our managerial staff and physicians. Furthermore, guidance from our nurse scientist has been essential. The support of managerial staff enabled us to meet the dynamic needs of our unit by bringing in more unit-based experts. The addition of two unit-based champions to help disseminate the CAUTI-prevention bundle and monitor adherence to it was crucial in effectively reducing our CAUTI rate. Daily physician rounds on patients started to include the questions "Why does this patient have a catheter?" and "Can we remove the catheter?" We also advocated for the elimination of catheter use in anuric patients. With all of our extensive prevention strategies in place, our catheter days began to drop, along with our CAUTI rate.

OUTCOMES

Commitment to resilience was demonstrated during the project when we reacted to a spike of three CAUTIs in August of 2013. Just prior to this we had celebrated one year CAUTI-free. Part of the success in the reduction of CAUTI has been to perform a root cause analysis (RCA) for every CAUTI occurrence. RCA helped the CAUTI-prevention team identify specific problems leading to each CAUTI, learn from those problems, and make adjustments in practice accordingly. Our spike in CAUTIs that month was an eye-opener for us. As a learning organization, it prompted us to look closely at our practice to see what may have contributed to this cluster of CAUTIs.

There were multiple factors that we believe contributed to the CAUTI cluster. We identified unintended consequences of a new protocol of chlorhexidine (CHG) bathing that was implemented for central line–associated bloodstream infection (CLABSI) prevention and methicillin-resistant Staphylococcus aureus (MRSA) decolonization. Although it would seem that this intervention might help our CAUTI rates, we believe it actually contributed to the CAUTI spike, with three infections occurring within a matter of a few weeks only 2 months after this major change in our practice.

Upon further analysis, we discovered that this new protocol for bathing was actually creating extra steps for the nursing staff when it came to catheter care. Having previously used a CHG product that could not be used on mucous membranes, nursing was under the false assumption that our new CHG wipes could not be used on mucous membranes either. Nursing staff was expected to provide a separate soap and water bath just for peri-care. We believe this led to missed catheter care. Per nursing documentation, two of the three CAUTIs had episodes of missed catheter care. As it turned out, the preparation of CHG that is used in our prepackaged CHG wipes *is* safe for mucous membranes. Through a group effort by our nurse scientist, educator, and CAUTI champions, we were able to reeducate our staff that the CHG wipes should be used specifically for catheter care, along the catheter tubing, and on mucous membranes.

In addition to the change in practice of CHG bathing, there were insertion checklists that were missing, including one instance that the physician did not document the evidence-based indication for catheter insertion. Perhaps the most enlightening common denominator of our three CAUTI occurrences was the presence of incontinence of stool. At the time of the CAUTI cluster, we were seeing more and more patients with the diagnoses of liver failure in our ICU/ SDU. These immunocompromised patients are frequently incontinent of stool, a likely source of infection for the three CAUTIs. Through our vigilance in surveillance and thorough reeducation of staff, we were once again able to reduce our CAUTI incidence to zero for the remainder of the 2013 calendar year, and we continue to have a low CAUTI rate 2 years later (see Figure B.6). Furthermore, staff is continuously updated on days without a CAUTI occurrence and notified immediately when there is a CAUTI occurrence on the unit. The details around each occurrence are communicated to staff, and any changes that take place as a result of the incident are disseminated.

2012-2013 ICU/SDU CAUTI Rates

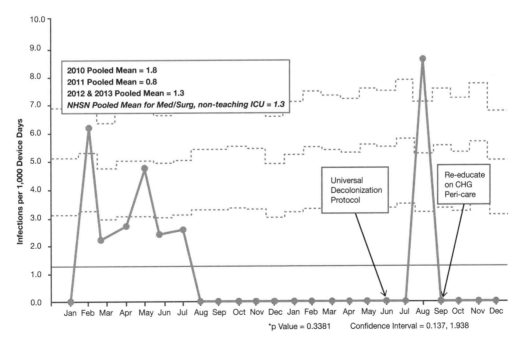

2010 Pooled Mean = 1.8
2011 Pooled Mean = 0.8
2012 & 2013 Pooled Mean = 1.3
NHSN Pooled Mean for Med/Surg, non-teaching ICU = 1.3

Universal Decolonization Protocol

Re-educate on CHG Peri-care

*p Value = 0.3381   Confidence Interval = 0.137, 1.938

Figure B.6   ICU/SDU CAUTI rates for calendar year 2012–2013. Shows low CAUTI rates from 2012–2013, including the cluster of three CAUTIs in August of 2013, with return to baseline.

DISSEMINATION

Deference to expertise is an HROT concept that is demonstrated in this project through the use of unit-based CAUTI-prevention champions. Creating experts on our unit has been a priority for our facility. As mentioned, we currently have four unit-based CAUTI-prevention staff nurses, two of which have been on the team since its inception. As unit-based champions, we ensure adherence to the CAUTI-prevention strategies and provide peer review, education, and recognition for CAUTI prevention. Together with our nurse managers, nurse educator, and nurse scientist, we distribute new information and reinforce current best practice regarding CAUTI prevention to our 96 nurses and 4 nurse assistants.

Our goal is to be approachable regarding CAUTI prevention, and we have found great pride in acting as expert resources for our fellow nurses. During both monthly audits and our scheduled shifts, we provide "just in time" peer review to those not adhering to the CAUTI-prevention bundle. Being removed from management allows us to provide non-punitive feedback to fellow staff to help keep our CAUTI rates low. Additionally, we focus largely on education and have assembled an education board for staff, patients, and family members to use as a reference for best practice. Because the CAUTI champions work alongside fellow staff nurses, we are always available to answer questions and concerns regarding CAUTI prevention. We also work closely with our managerial staff, unit educator, and nurse scientist to reevaluate and make adjustments to the CAUTI-prevention bundle when there is an occurrence on the unit.

CONCLUSION

Harmful, preventable events in our patient population including CAUTIs are no longer acceptable. Our project, "Championing CAUTI Prevention in the ICU/SDU," is an example of how our CAUTI-prevention team significantly lowered the CAUTI rate in our ICU/SDU. It is a prime example of how our hospital strives to be highly reliable.

Numerous CAUTI-prevention strategies were put into place throughout this project. The implementation of monthly audits, systematic processes such as catheter insertion checklists and CAUTI-prevention bundles, close analysis of our CAUTI events, and a multidisciplinary group of approachable experts are representative of a highly reliable organization.

REFERENCES

Fuchs, M. A., Sexton, D. J., Thornlow, D. K., and Champagne, M. T. (2011). Evaluation of an evidence-based, nurse-driven checklist to prevent hospital-acquired catheter-associated urinary tract infections in intensive care units. *Journal of Nursing Care Quality, 26*(2), pp. 101–109.

Kemper, C., and Boyle, D. K. (2009). Leading your organization to high reliability. *Nursing Management, 40*(4), pp. 14–18.

Klevens, R. M., Edwards, J. R., Richards, C. L., Horan, T. C., Gaynes, R. P., Pollock, D. A., and Cardo, D. M. (2007). Estimating health care-associated infections and deaths in U.S. hospitals, 2002. *Public Health Reports, 122*(2), pp. 160–166.

Pappas, S. H. (2008). The cost of nurse-sensitive adverse events. *Journal of Nursing Administration, 38(5)*, pp. 230–236.

Rebmann, T., and Greene, L. R. (2010). Preventing catheter-associated urinary tract infections: An executive summary of the Association for Professionals in Infection Control and Epidemiology, Inc. Elimination Guide. *American Journal of Infection Control, 38*(8), pp. 644–646.

Saint, S., and Chenowith, C. E. (2003). Biofilms and catheter-associated urinary tract infections. *Infectious Disease Clinics of North America, 17(2)*, pp. 411–442.

Saint, S., Kowalski, C. P., Kaufman, S. R., Hofer, T. P., Kauffman, C. A., Olmsted, R. N., … Krein, S. L. (2008). Preventing hospital-acquired urinary tract infection in the United States: A national study. *Clinical Infectious Disease, 46*(2), pp. 243–250.

Scott, R. D. (2009). The direct medical costs of healthcare-associated infections in US hospitals and the benefits of prevention. *Centers for Disease Control and Prevention.* Retrieved from http://www.cdc.gov/HAI/pdfs/hai/Scott_CostPaper.pdf

Wald, H. L., and Kramer A. M. (2007). Nonpayment for harms resulting from medical care: Catheter-associated urinary tract infections. *Journal of the American Medical Association, 298*(23), pp. 2782–2784.

Weick, K. E. (1987). Organizational culture as a source of high reliability. *California Management Review, 29(2)*, pp. 112–127.

OVERSTAYING YOUR WELCOME: DECREASING ED STAY FOR STEMI PATIENTS TO IMPROVE REPERFUSION TIMES

Dianna Ingraham, MS, RN, CNS

REVIEW OF LITERATURE

It is well established that timely reperfusion of the infarct-related coronary artery during ST-segment elevation myocardial infarction (STEMI) improves patient outcomes. Tight, well-defined process metrics are associated with shorter treatment times that ultimately decrease morbidity and mortality (Parikh et al., 2009).

Door-to-balloon (D2B) time is the segment of time between when a patient enters the hospital and the first intervention on the infarcting coronary artery. Hospitals throughout the country have implemented strategies—with guidance from the American College of Cardiology Foundation, American

> We are what we repeatedly do. Excellence, therefore, is not an act but a habit.
>
> —*Aristotle*

Heart Association, and Mission Lifeline—to shorten reperfusion times and ultimately improve the care of patients suffering STEMI (O'Gara et al., 2013).

In a study by Bansal et al., it was noted that walk-in patients had significantly longer D2B times compared to patients arriving by EMS. In fact, mode of hospital entry was the most important influence in predicting longer D2B times. The study also established that prolonged door-to-ECG and cardiac catheterization laboratory (cath lab) activation times contributed to longer D2B times (Bansal et al., 2014).

PROCESS IMPROVEMENT METRICS, PDSA, AND HRO

The Plan, Do, Study, Act (PDSA) model was chosen for its ease of use and feasibility as it showed improvements on a small scale. The tool provided the framework to categorize process steps and identify improvement targets. It allowed for easy measurement and feedback of metrics related to D2B.

Table C.1 is the PDSA worksheet for a process improvement project initiated by the cardiovascular clinical nurse specialist in an acute care hospital. The goal was to decrease door-to-balloon times of STEMI patients presenting to the emergency department by private vehicle.

TABLE C.1   PDSA WORKSHEET

Project Name
Overstaying Your Welcome: Decreasing ED Stay Times for STEMI Patients
Insert Title:

Project Champion
Dianna Ingraham
Insert Name:

Team Members
Dianna Ingraham
Jennifer Brooks
Insert Names:

Reason for Action:

The American College of Cardiology (ACC) and the American Heart Association (AHA) set expectations for reperfusion of an occluded coronary artery during a STEMI at 90 minutes from the time the patient arrives in the emergency department (ED) to the time the coronary artery blood supply is restored. This is commonly known as the *door-to-balloon (D2B)* time. Studies have shown that expedited care to open the blocked artery is crucial to lower morbidity and mortality related to STEMI.

Tight system processes are essential to consistently achieve D2B times of 90 minutes or less. System and non-system factors often affect an institution's ability to be successful. Because non-system delays are very difficult, if not impossible, to control, the focus is shifted to system opportunities to improve the likelihood of obtaining unfailing D2B times of less than 90 minutes.

System delays such as identification of STEMI with an electrocardiogram (ECG) and time in the ED are two metrics commonly measured as system components affecting D2B times. The standard of care is for the patient to receive an ECG within 10 minutes of ED arrival and spend as little time as possible in the ED. The latter is often the biggest challenge, as confounding factors impede the ability to transfer the patient expediently to the cardiac catheterization laboratory (cath lab). It was decided to identify and implement processes for the walk-in STEMI patient that could be improved to lessen their stay in the ED and hopefully decrease D2B times.

Who Is Involved in the Process

Cardiovascular clinical nurse specialist (CV CNS)

Manager of the cardiac catheterization laboratory

Director, manager, and educator of the emergency department

Past State

In 2011, patients arriving via private vehicle (POV) to the ED with STEMI had a mean length of stay of 41 minutes with a median D2B time of 70 minutes. Although D2B times were well under the expected 90 minutes, improvements could still be made to decrease length of stay in the ED and possibly decrease D2B times.

2011 Median STEMI D2B Times in Minutes

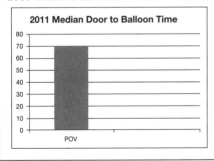

2011 Mean Walk-in ED Length of Stay in Minutes

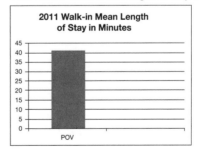

Target State

The target for POV patients is a mean length of stay of 40 minutes, or less 80% of the time.

continues

TABLE C.1   PDSA WORKSHEET   (CONTINUED)

Gap Analysis

Processes evaluated for improvement opportunities:

- Patient arrival to ED through cath lab transfer

- Cath lab staff call in to patient arrival time in cath lab

- Opportunities identified for patient arrival to ED through cath lab transfer

- Less time in triage

- Timely ECG performance (10 minutes or less)

- Immediate interpretation and identification of ECG for STEMI by ED licensed independent practitioner (LIP)

- Timely activation of cath lab (< 5 minutes after ECG interpretation)

- Opportunities identified for cath lab staff call-in time to patient arrival time in cath lab

- Cath lab staff assist with ED transport to cath lab

Solution Approach

ED

- Chest pain patient arrival is announced overhead and taken directly to ED room (when available) instead of triage

- Overhead announcement alerts

    - Performance of 12-lead ECG ASAP by Critical Care technologist or RN

    - Evaluation and ECG interpretation immediately by ED LIP

If a STEMI is identified by the ED LIP a "Cardiac Alert" is called overhead starting a chain of automated events:

- ED unit secretary pages cardiologist and cath lab team via universal pager. This is known as the *STEMI recognition time*

- ED RN implements STEMI treatment protocols

- If present, cath lab team goes to ED to assist with treatment protocols and expedites handoff communication

- Realistic time intervals for each step of the cardiac alert process

- Positive feedback for reaching time interval goals

- Identify, investigate, and adjust processes with unmet time interval goals

Cath Lab

- If during normal business hours, will immediately go to ED to assist with treatment protocols and expedite transfer

- If outside of business hours, will go to ED after second person arrives

What	Who
Reported stats of prolonged ED length of stay for 2011 during acute coronary syndrome monthly meeting	Cardiovascular CNS
Collaborative meeting with ED manager, director, cath lab manager	Cardiovascular CNS
Brainstorm during meeting to identify process steps and set realistic time interval goals	Cardiovascular CNS
Process steps with time interval goals discussed with ED staff	ED director, manager, and educator
Process steps with time interval goals discussed with cath lab staff	Cath lab manager
Monitor process steps and time intervals	Cardiovascular CNS
Provide follow-up on progress of goals to ED and cath lab	Cardiovascular CNS
Provide feedback on progression of goals	Cardiovascular CNS, cath lab manager, ED director, manager, and educator
In-depth review of process steps that did not meet goals	Cardiovascular CNS
Adjust process steps as needed	Cardiovascular CNS

						Follow Up				
Metric	Base-line	2 Mos	6 Mos	9 Mos	12 Mos	18 Mos	24 Mos	30 Mos	36 Mos	Goals
Mean ED length of stay for POV patients	41 min	30 min	30 min	33 min	36 min	35 min	35 min	34 min	34 min	40 min
Percentage of POV ED patients with a length of stay less than 40 minutes	50%	100%	78%	77%	68%	70%	70%	69%	71%	80%
POV median D2B time	70 min	61 min	60 min	58 min	58 min	58 min	59 min	60 min	60 min	60 min or less

continues

TABLE C.1 PDSA WORKSHEET (CONTINUED)

2012 to 2014 ED Mean Length of Stay for POV STEMI Patients

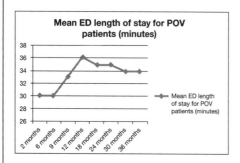

2012 to 2014 Percentage of Benchmark Times Met for POV STEMI ED Length of Stay

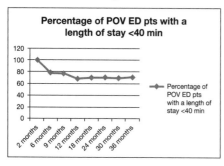

Median D2B Times

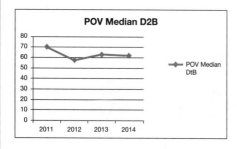

Lessons Learned

Overall the project was considered a success because mean times for ED stay and median D2B times decreased.

The goal of 80% for the percentage of ED POV patient length of stay less than 40 minutes was too ambitious. Given the confounding factors associated with caring for POV patients, the goal should have been set at 75%.

Sustainability is possible when a good process is in place even though our goal of 80% was not achieved.

The aim was to take a systems approach to reduce time in the ED and determine how that affected D2B times. The focus was the process of getting the patient out of the ED quickly and into the cath lab for reperfusion. It needed to be simple and easily reproducible in multiple circumstances. This relates to the HRO concepts of preoccupation with failure and reluctance to simplify.

The cardiovascular clinical nurse specialist (CV CNS)/chest pain coordinator routinely collects D2B times and reports to the monthly heart section meeting. When D2B times appeared to start to become longer, the CV CNS began evaluating process steps affecting this metric. A small group of key stakeholders led by the CV CNS that included ED and cath lab leadership came together to review the results. This relates to the HRO concept of deference to expertise.

The small group appraised the results of the STEMI care processes for walk-in and emergency medical service (EMS) patients. It was determined that patients arriving by EMS had ideal practices and ED length of stay. These metrics would continue to be tracked and reported monthly. The walk-in STEMI patients had less-than-ideal practices, potentially causing prolonged ED and D2B times.

The group identified key factors that affected walk-in ED stay time. They were as follows:

- Time in triage
- Timely 12-lead ECG performance (less than 10 minutes)
- Immediate STEMI ECG identification
- Timely activation of the cath lab

Efforts were already in place to decrease door-to-ECG times, so the team decided to focus on time in triage, immediate STEMI ECG identification, and timely activation of the cath lab.

TIME IN TRIAGE PROCESS CHANGE (HRO CONCEPT: SENSITIVITY TO OPERATIONS)

Current and new practices are outlined here:

1. Current practice for arriving patients complaining of chest pain was the registration staff or triage nurse taking the patient to triage for a full assessment and ECG. There was a practice change to placing the patient in a wheelchair, taking the patiently directly to an ED room (if available) or triage bay (if bed unavailable), and announcing overhead "Chest pain arrival room 3."

2. The ED critical care technician or available nurse performs the 12-lead ECG within 10 minutes.

3. The ED physician arrives immediately to interpret the ECG and perform a targeted chest pain assessment.

4. If a STEMI is identified by the ED physician, the cath lab team and cardiologist are called in for reperfusion therapy within five minutes of ECG performance.

5. If the STEMI is called during normal cath lab hours, at least one cath lab nurse is to go to the ED to assist with treatment protocols, receive the handoff report, and help transport the patient to cath lab. If the STEMI is called after hours, a cath lab nurse is to go the ED after other team members arrive.

This new practice was endorsed by the small group, which also took on the responsibility to inform, coach, and evaluate during the first 3 months of 2012. Metrics collected by the CV CNS related to the change process were shared with the ED and cath lab on a monthly basis. Table C.2 is part of a larger table known as the "Cardiac Alert Summary," which is posted monthly in the ED and cath lab for metric sharing.

TABLE C.2 CARDIAC ALERT SUMMARY EXCERPT

Arrive Type	Date	ED Arrive Time	1st ED EKG	Universal Page for Cath Lab (CL) (EKG Interpretation Time)	Door to EKG	ED EKG to CL Page	Leave ED	CL Page to ED Depart (Min)	Time in ED (Min)
Goals					≤ 10 min	5 min		≤ 35 min	≤ 40 min
Walk-in	11/10	10:17	10:22	10:26	0:05	0:04	10:43	0:17	0:26
	11/23	10:19	10:26	10:26	0:07	0:00	10:38	0:12	0:19
	11/23	11:17	11:22	11:23	0:05	0:01	11:51	0:28	0:34

The CV CNS was the keeper of the PDSA worksheet and metrics. When time intervals were not met, the CV CNS would contact the manager of the ED and/or cath lab so a modified cause analysis could be determined. This also provided the opportunity for real-time feedback and coaching of staff.

The CV CNS reported progress on the metrics and case reviews of unmet goals to staff and at the monthly heart section meeting. This was felt to be very effective in determining cause and effect to improve practice. It also created a culture of accountability as the ED and cath lab staff collaborated with the CV CNS on ways to decrease delays in care related to system and non-system components. This relates to the HRO concept of commitment to resilience.

CONCLUSION

This was a successful implementation of a process change using HRO concepts and PDSA to ensure sustainability. For 3 years, the mean ED length of stay has remained less than 40 minutes for more than half of STEMI patients. The lowest times in the ED, which also correlate to lower D2B times, took place in 2012, immediately following change execution. Our goal of 80% of walk-in length of stay in ED of less than 40 minutes was not met, but the D2B times continue to be lower. It was determined that confounding variables may affect a patient's length of stay irrespective of meeting metric goals.

Several HRO concepts were used during this project that contributed to its success:

- **Preoccupation with failure**
    - The process was an improvement strategy rather than an individual performance evaluation.

- **Reluctance to simplify**
    - For example, process or system delays were not accepted as a standard of care for STEMI patients.
    - All extended times in the ED for system and non-system causes were thoroughly investigated.

- **Sensitivity to operations**
    - There was an awareness of processes that were not functioning for the safety of the patient.
    - Staff were dedicated to improving those processes through improved communication and transparency.
    - There was an openness to adjusting processes to improve performance.

- **Commitment to resilience**
    - A plan was in place to tackle less-than-optimal performance in a non-judgmental manner with coaching and open communication.
    - Real-time feedback and coaching provided the expectation to improve process performance.
    - Metrics were shared.

- **Deference to expertise**
  - Instead of managers and directors leading the process change, the CV CNS, with specialty training in process improvement and program management, led the project.

REFERENCES

Bansal, E., Dhawan, R., Wagman, B., Low, G., Zheng, L., Chan, L., … Shavelle, D. M. (2014). Importance of hospital entry: Walk-in STEMI and primary percutaneous coronary intervention. *Western Journal of Emergency Medicine, 15*(1), pp. 81–87.

O'Gara, P. T., Kushner, F. G., Ascheim, D. D., Casey, D. E., Chung, M. K., de Lemos, J. A., … Zhao, D. X. (2013). 2013 ACCF/AHA guideline for the management of ST-elevation myocardial infarction: A report of the American College of Cardiology Foundation/American Heart Association task force on practice guidelines. *Journal of the American College of Cardiology, 61*(4), pp. e78–e140.

Parikh, S. V., Treichler, D. B., DePaola, S., Sharpe, J., Valdes, M., Addo, T., … Holper, E. M. (2009). Systems-based improvement in door-to-balloon times at a large urban teaching hospital: A follow-up study from Parkland Health and Hospital System. *Circulation, 2*(2), pp. 116–122.

TELEHEALTH: A HIGHLY RELIABLE INTERVENTION TO PREVENT READMISSIONS

Erin Denholm, MSN, RN, RWJENF

A high reliability organization (HRO) can no longer afford to be hospital-centric. With value-based pay (VBP) for performance mechanisms firmly in place for organizations, penalties are now exacted for 30-day readmissions (Medicare.gov, n.d.). A high-performing HRO focuses on safety and quality across the continuum, including the identification of errors after discharge.

As Dr. Berwick notes, lack of care coordination is a key area that contributes to failure in the healthcare system. A trend in the literature points to coordination of care across the continuum and transitions of care as core to process improvement and prevention of errors (Coleman, 2005). When preoccupation with failure is the driving principle for solving 30-day readmission, the fully integrated delivery team is essential. Often, the time lapse that occurs between intervention (discharge planning) and failure (readmission) distances the original caregiver from the error. Thus the HRO characteristic of deference to expertise requires the specialized competencies of the home care team.

> "
> The failure of the healthcare system stems from six main areas of waste: overtreatment, failures to coordinate care, failures in care delivery, excessive administrative costs, excessive healthcare prices and fraud and abuse.
>
> —*Dr. Don Berwick*
> "

The home care team is integral in avoiding readmissions. Collaboratively involving this team is a best practice in achieving highly reliable patient care that decreases the premature return of patients to the acute care setting. More specifically, telehealth is an innovative process that can and has made a difference.

FRAMING THE PROBLEM

The average 30-day re-hospitalization rate for Medicare beneficiaries with chronic conditions has exceeded 23% nationally (Elixhauser and Steiner, 2013; Weiss, Elixhauser, and Steiner, 2013). The average readmission rate varies depending on geographic location and fluctuates between 19 and 25%.

At Centura Health, when readmissions were reviewed, 90% were found to be unplanned and preventable. Preventability was determined by identifying whether home care had been ordered and the admitting diagnosis. Acute care case managers within Centura Health hospitals are responsible for discharge planning and review eligibility criteria for home care before patient discharge. Interestingly, it was determined that close to 50% of patients discharged were done so after hours or on weekends, when case managers were not available. After hours, discharge-planning responsibilities revert to bedside clinical nurses, who are not as familiar with standardized processes and resources the organization has in place for the chronic condition patient population that is prone to readmission within 30 days.

THE INNOVATION: DEFERRING TO THE EXPERTS

Centura Health at Home (CHAH)—the organization's home care experts—confirmed that telehealth could significantly reduce readmission rates to 6% for Medicare beneficiaries admitted to home care post hospitalization. CHAH is the first home health agency in Colorado to have implemented a telehealth system. The agency's integrated telehealth program represents a culmination of efforts that began in 2004 with video-based interventions for a small population of high-acuity chronically ill patients enrolled in a Medicare Advantage plan.

Telehealth has enabled CHAH personnel to virtually visit with patients between scheduled, in-person home visits. These virtual visits allowed pertinent data to be collected, thus enabling the home health nurse to identify when the patient's chronic disease was exacerbating. Early identification and treatment of disease-exacerbation signs and symptoms reduced readmission rates.

Patients with specific conditions who meet the Medicare home health benefit criteria are eligible for the telehealth program. (See Table D.1.) Therefore, there has been no program cost for those who participate. The program extends the continuity of care on a 24/7 basis, more effectively uses healthcare resources, and broadens the reach of limited nursing staff to manage a larger number of patients on a daily basis.

TABLE D.1 CHAH INTEGRATED TELEHEALTH PROGRAM

Telehealth Program Description	
Remote monitoring of patients by registered nurses and augmented with 24/7 clinical call center and telehealth services	
Patients identified for and introduced to the program during a hospital admission or upon enrollment in CHAH	
Real-time patient education, lifestyle management, and medication adjustments	

Who Is Eligible?	Who Is *Not* Eligible?
Patients with chronic disease (for example, congestive heart failure, chronic obstructive pulmonary disease, hypertension, diabetes)	Active substance abusers
Patients with fall risk factors	Patients with an unsafe home environment
Patients age 80 or older	Patients with pest-control problems
Patients with two or more hospitalizations in the past 6 months	Patients with documented violence/aggression
Patients with two or more emergency department visits in the past 6 months	Patients with advanced dementia, unless they have a competent caregiver
Patients taking five or more medications	Patients with low functional vision, unless they have a competent caregiver
Patients with a documented history of non-adherence to prescribed regimen	
Patients with any other indicator that they may return to the hospital in 30 days or less	
Patients who are not qualified for traditional Medicare home care program but meet other eligibility requirements	

ASSEMBLING THE TEAM

There was clear opportunity to apply expertise to a discharge process that was yielding an outcome readmission rate nearing 20%. The decision was made to convene an interdisciplinary team from across the care continuum from the five targeted hospitals. The team included leaders and staff from home care and case management as well as clinical nursing staff from the inpatient setting.

To capture the expertise of home care for a broader patient base, it was necessary to connect the "failure" of readmission to discharge planning in a way that engaged rather than alienated inpatient clinical nursing staff. The inpatient clinical nurses had a substantial home care and telehealth knowledge gap and required intense training and education to close the gap.

A burning platform of a high readmission rate of chronic condition patients led us to use a rapid decision-making team approach to address the problem. The team needed to develop an understanding of the telehealth technology and assessment criteria to identify eligible beneficiaries.

The team wanted to decrease 30-day readmission rates and to increase older adult quality of life by augmenting the current telehealth continuum by merging two successful programs: call center and telehealth. The integration of these two programs would expand the population we serve geographically and also create a deeper level of service by making telehealth monitoring available 24 hours a day, 7 days a week. This is an example of a rapidly formed team that made decisions, engaged in intensive learning together, and then applied this learning to discharge planning done by case managers and by clinical staff nurses. The team has since disbanded, but members continue to share knowledge with colleagues in their practice setting.

THE METHOD: TELEHEALTH PROGRAM

Initially, we sought to enroll at least 200 patients eligible for home care and to increase the number of patients served in the program by a minimum of 200 per year. On average, a home care nurse can see 5 to 7 patients a day during in-person home visits, whereas a telehealth nurse can monitor 60 to 70 patients a day. It is widely held that 40% of Medicare patients are eligible for home care after a hospitalization based on eligibility criteria. However, internal organizational data revealed that less than 25% of Medicare patients were appropriately identified as eligible for a home care episode at discharge, even when case managers provided the discharge planning. The technology component of the telehealth program uses remote patient-monitoring equipment for the daily measurement of patient indicators such as heart rate, blood pressure, weight, and lifestyle behaviors, with registered nurses remotely monitoring individual patient data. The telehealth program was implemented to improve the care of Medicare patients eligible for home care.

Patients were recruited from two hospitals. The typical participant was an older adult (average age 76 years), living in his or her own home, managing comorbid conditions, and having recently experienced a hospitalization related to an exacerbation of a chronic health condition. Among the 200 patients in the initial cohort, 44% were diagnosed with congestive heart failure, 34% had chronic obstructive pulmonary disease, and 17% were diabetic.

Patients participating in the project were divided into two categories:

- The first group used remote patient monitoring (RPM) technologies and had access to the 24/7 clinical call center.

- The second group was not home-bound and thus not eligible for a home care episode. These patients were provided telephonic care through the clinical call center only.

Patients were required to transmit monitoring data on a daily basis or more often if their condition required more meticulous monitoring. Patients using RPM received a base station and a number of peripheral devices. The base station displayed behavioral and general health question prompts, and the patient answered the questions. Vital sign data was collected through peripheral devices, such as a scale, blood-pressure cuff, pulse oximeter, and thermometer. The base station then transmitted data elements via telephone line to the central monitoring station, where data was reviewed by a registered nurse. Baseline parameters were customized for each patient using input from primary care physicians as well as a personalized telehealth algorithm. The algorithm was based on a nursing assessment, identified top health priorities, and patient answers to four questions. This data was entered into the monitor system.

Priorities were determined by the following:

- 2,000 different elements (for example, a specific disease condition might require dyspnea assessment, in which case the patient would be asked to state the number of pillows used at night for sleep)

- Patient health history

- Current health status

- Educational needs

Home care field nurses visited and conducted health and environmental risk assessments within 48 hours of patient discharge. Within 24 hours of risk-assessment completion, a telehealth technician visited the patient at home to install and familiarize him or her with the remote-monitoring technology. Nurses and installers were trained to use the teach-back technique to assess the patient and family's level of understanding and commitment to the program technology.

At the time of install, the participant was asked to initiate a visit and answer the automated questions that were customized for him or her on the remote-monitoring technology device. Primary care physicians wrote PRN orders (that is, "as needed" orders that nurses could modify), which allowed the monitoring registered nurses to react to trending and monitoring data within a specified set of parameters. After the technology was installed and operational, dedicated telehealth nursing staff monitored patient data sent from the remote devices. The nursing staff called the patient if there were significant vital-sign or health-status changes.

Patients could also contact the clinical call center with questions 24/7. When telehealth patients contacted the clinical call center, call center registered nurses reviewed patient data, provided assistance, and elevated the alert to a physician, if needed.

Primary care physicians were closely involved in the program and monitored patients' progress by reviewing weekly reports containing the patients' current medication list, vital-sign and symptom readings, and nursing notes. Clinical call center registered nurses set up a series of weekly follow-up calls after discharge to review care-management plans and issues related to patient self-efficacy for patients using the clinical call center as their telehealth strategy.

The telehealth program prepared patients for eventual program discharge. Nursing staff taught patients how to independently monitor core health indicators and identify red flags so they would know when to contact members of their interdisciplinary care team for assistance in disease management.

MEASURING TELEHEALTH PROGRAM OUTCOMES

The team identified the following measurable outcomes for the telehealth program:

- Enroll a minimum of 200 patients.
- Decrease 30-day readmission rates related to congestive heart failure, chronic obstructive pulmonary failure, and diabetes at two participating hospitals by 2 percentage points.
- Improve participants' quality of life as measured by the Quality of Life SF-36.

Home service coordinators at each of the participating five targeted hospitals were crucial in referring patients to the telehealth program. Two hundred patients participated in the initial project and all completed telehealth monitoring. However, 36 did not complete the post-program Quality of Life SF-36 tool.

The 30-day readmission rates related to congestive heart failure, chronic obstructive pulmonary failure, and diabetes were reduced by 62%, and readmission rates for patients receiving telehealth home care (6.3%) were lower than those for traditional home care patients (18%). Emergency department use decreased from 283 visits in the year preceding the program evaluation to 21 visits during the year-long program evaluation. Over the course of 1 year, there were seven readmissions for 87 patients with congestive heart failure, three for 67 patients with chronic obstructive pulmonary disorder, and no readmissions for the 34 patients with diabetes. (See Table D.2.)

TABLE D.2   PROGRAM READMISSION RATES: CENTURA HEALTH AT HOME REMOTE PATIENT MONITORING

	Pre-Intervention Readmission Rates	Post-Intervention Readmission Rates ($n = 200$)
Hospital 1		
Congestive heart failure	13.8%	4.2%
Chronic obstructive pulmonary disease	14.1%	6.7%
Diabetes	14.7%	0.0%
Hospital 2		
Congestive heart failure	17.7%	9.5%
Chronic obstructive pulmonary disease	12.5%	2.7%
Diabetes	9.5%	0.0%

Quality of life was measured at baseline and at the end of the program evaluation period using the SF-36 health survey questionnaire. The questionnaire measures health on eight multi-item dimensions covering functional status, well-being, and overall evaluation of health with good reliability (Cronbach's $\alpha > 0.85$) (Brazier et al., 1992). An increase of 5 points is considered statistically significant (Pearson, n.d.).

Overall quality of life did not significantly improve. However, quality of life did increase for patients receiving home telehealth care by 4.8 points on average in both the physical functioning and mental health dimensions. (See Figure D.1.) While these results were not statistically significant overall, specific components of the quality-of-life survey demonstrated statistically significant changes (≥ 5 point increase) in all ages and sexes: physical functioning, role limitation due to physical problems, social functioning, and role limitation due to emotional problems. By age with both sexes combined, there were statistically significant improvements pre and post intervention for 45 to 54-year-olds, 65 to 74-year-olds, and individuals 75 and older. In addition, there were greater quality-of-life increases for women compared to men. Women significantly increased their scores in mental health, physical functioning, role limitation due to physical problems, vitality, social functioning, and role limitations due to emotional problems, while men showed improvement in their scores for physical functioning, role limitation due to physical problems, role limitations due to emotional problems, and mental health.

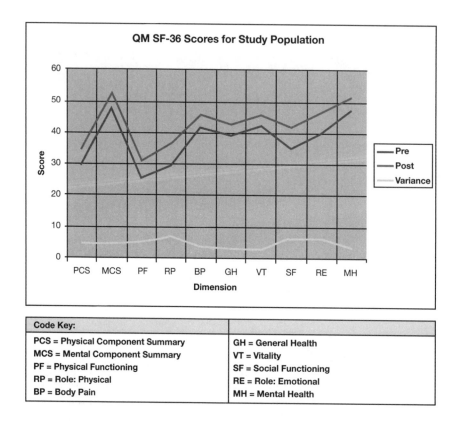

Figure D.1 Pre- and post-intervention Quality of Life SF-36 measures.

Patient satisfaction and self-management were measured with the Centura telehealth patient satisfaction tool. This tool was developed specifically for this project and has received a large uptake of use from subsequent Center for Technology and Aging grantees. The survey addresses several key concepts, such as privacy concerns, time of use, involvement in one's healthcare (patient self-management), and quality of care. The survey was created using a five-point Likert scale, strongly disagree to strongly agree, similar to the Coleman Transitions Measure (Coleman, Mahoney, and Parry, 2005). Satisfaction scores were not assessed for statistical significance; rather, they were viewed in aggregate form only for organizational knowledge (unlike individual patients' pre- and post-intervention scores).

Patient satisfaction and perception of self-management were measured each month during the program evaluation period. The data revealed positive perceptions and beliefs about health technology, patient satisfaction with the technology, and self-management among participants. Figure D.2 is an example of a single month of patient-satisfaction and self-management scores of all patients using telehealth. The frequency of RN visits was reduced from the traditional two to three visits per week over a 60-day episode of care to approximately three visits over the entire 60-day telehealth care-management period. The resulting cost savings was between $1,000 and $1,500 per patient.

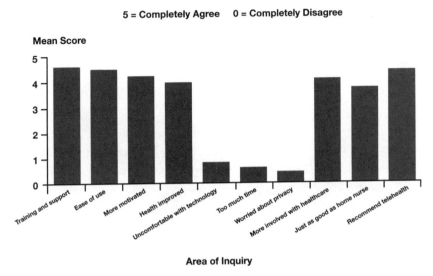

Figure D.2   Telehealth patient satisfaction survey outcome.

KEYS TO SUCCESS

Critical areas for successful implementation of a telehealth program at scale and on a sustained basis include the following:

- Staff engagement
- Training and support
- Streamlining the discharge-planning process
- Having trusted clinicians introduce the telehealth program
- Selecting a technology that will work in the long term
- Establishing physician PRN orders for telehealth patients to maximize efficiency
- Providing real-time education to patients to increase patient self-management

STAFF ENGAGEMENT

For the program to be successful, inpatient and home care nurses and clinicians must see value in the telehealth intervention for patients, nurses, and physicians. One strategy used to accomplish this was to host open houses for nurses to interact with the telehealth technology and ask questions. Key discussion during these events demonstrated the value of the telehealth intervention to patients, nurses, and clinicians by focusing on the following:

- Outcomes
- Visits/episode
- Readmission rate
- Patient-satisfaction data

Discussing how the program could improve chronic disease management by extending the reach of the nursing staff demonstrated the value of the intervention without negatively affecting the workflow of clinicians. As a result of the improved chronic disease management in the program, field nurses were able to focus their time and attention on visits dictated by urgent health circumstances rather than regular assessments, which could be routinely conducted via telehealth equipment. Inpatient nurses were able to provide much more standardized discharge-planning activities after hours and weekends, decreasing cleanup activities for case-management staff upon their return to work on Mondays.

TRAINING AND SUPPORT

Inpatient nurses—the nursing staff who introduced patients to the program during their hospital stays—required additional training for effective communication, particularly to emphasize the value of the program to patients. Remote-monitoring nurses also benefited from effective communication training to bolster confidence in decision-making processes to actively manage patients in response to issues raised during calls. Training focused on key words and phrases that are simple yet effective in describing the program and on the intended outcomes for the patient. Scripting for installers of the technology and the initial RN call to patients (after technology was installed in the patients' home) was a key element for success.

STREAMLINING THE DISCHARGE-PLANNING PROCESS

Centura Health's experience indicates that attention to coordinating home care services is a key factor to program success. As part of the program, the home service coordination discharge-planning process was restructured in the hospital. Case managers and staff nurses were trained to identify patient-eligibility and enrollment criteria for patients discharged without home care. Before discharge, patients are introduced to the telehealth intervention in the hospital. Within 48 hours of discharge, a personalized telehealth algorithm is created, and telehealth technicians install devices and train patients on how to use them. This streamlined process encourages patient and caregiver engagement as they begin to follow their treatment plan at home.

HAVING TRUSTED CLINICIANS INTRODUCE THE TELEHEALTH PROGRAM

Patients were most likely to enroll in the telehealth program when they were introduced to the program during the hospital stay by a nurse or physician or by a primary care physician after discharge. After patients were enrolled, repeat visits from the telehealth device installer were required to train elderly adults on using the technology.

SELECTING A TECHNOLOGY THAT WILL WORK IN THE LONG TERM

The original program design involved the use of either two-way video technology (to meet the needs of patients with a very high acuity level) or remote patient-monitoring technology (to more routinely monitor patients with chronic conditions). Because of the increasing volume of patients served through the integrated telehealth program, our organization decided to change vendors to support more cost-effective scaling of the program while meeting the broader patient population's needs. In particular, the new platform offered the ability to monitor only those patients who fall outside established parameters, thereby placing the emphasis on those patients needing immediate attention. Interestingly, the higher-cost video-technology platform did not produce better outcomes than the non-video componentry.

ESTABLISHING PHYSICIAN PRN ORDERS FOR TELEHEALTH PATIENTS TO MAXIMIZE EFFICIENCY

Monitoring nurses can react to trending and monitoring data more quickly by using physician PRN orders. To operate on a larger scale, physicians should establish the orders when patients are initially enrolled into the program. In fact, standing orders have now been drafted as a straw man to present to primary care physicians. These orders can then be customized and established in the remote-monitoring stations, which allows immediate titration and care-plan modification by the remote-monitoring clinical team.

PROVIDING REAL-TIME EDUCATION TO PATIENTS TO INCREASE PATIENT SELF-MANAGEMENT

Monitoring nurses can connect with patients in real time, helping patients understand the relationship between the cause and effect of lifestyle-related behaviors. For example, if nurses observe data such as missed medications or meals high in salt, they have the opportunity to educate the patient and make the correlation between actions and outcome.

DISCUSSION

As value-based population health best practices continue to evolve, technology-enabled nursing and mobile care will undoubtedly continue to be foundational for HROs in the future. There is no question that nurses will need to expand their definition of quality of care to the post–acute care arena, connecting interventions to time-lapsed outcomes. Additionally, who we identify as key stakeholders in designing improved or new processes will require those who are involved in patient care in the ambulatory setting and in their homes. Implications for nursing curricula are salient and paramount to produce graduates with the kind of competencies that are being deployed in this new landscape. Although the results have been significant and very positive with telehealth for chronically ill patients discharged from inpatient settings, dissemination requires active engagement for each new setting, as new processes need to be vetted with hands-on understanding before adoption is successful.

CONCLUSION

Two key characteristics of HROs—preoccupation with failure and deference to expertise—are evident in the pursuit of decreasing preventable 30-day readmission rates. With the changing healthcare landscape demanding more cohesiveness among providers to produce patient-centric care, acute care–based providers can no longer afford to focus on care episodically. Only by broadening the scope of care planning across the continuum and teaming with home care providers and their resources can we produce the results that truly reflect high reliability.

REFERENCES

Brazier, J. E., Harper, R., Jones, N. M., O'Cathain, A., Thomas, K. J., Usherwood, T., and Westlake, L. (1992). Validating the SF-36 health survey questionnaire: New outcome measure for primary care. *British Medical Journal, 305*(6846), pp. 160–164.

Coleman, E. (2005). Care transitions model. Retrieved from http://www.caretransitions.org/documents/hartford%20report%20 2007.pdf

Coleman, E. A., Mahoney, E., and Parry, C. (2005). Assessing the quality of preparation for posthospital care from the patient's perspective: The care transitions measure. *Medical Care, 43*(3), pp. 246–255.

Elixhauser, A., and Steiner, C. (2013). Readmissions to U.S. hospitals by diagnosis, 2010. HCUP Statistical Brief #153. Agency for Healthcare Research and Quality. Retrieved from http://www.hcup-us.ahrq.gov/reports/statbriefs/sb153.pdf

Medicare.gov. (n.d.). 30-day unplanned readmission and death measures. Retrieved from https://www.medicare.gov/hospitalcompare/ Data/30-day-measures.html

Pearson, L. (n.d.). Medical outcome short form (36) health survey. Retrieved from http://www.clintools.com/victims/resources/ assessment/health/sf36.html

Weiss, A. J., Elixhauser, A., and Steiner, C. (2013). Readmissions to U.S. hospitals by procedure, 2010. HCUP Statistical Brief #154. Agency for Healthcare Research and Quality. Retrieved from http://www.hcup-us.ahrq.gov/reports/statbriefs/sb154.pdf

A

G

H

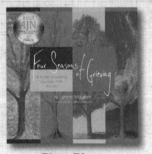
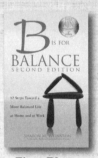
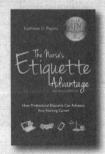
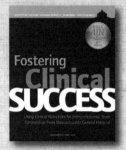
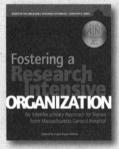
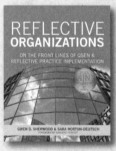
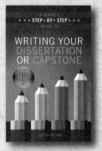

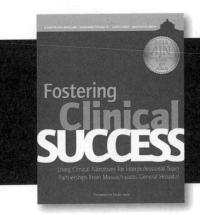
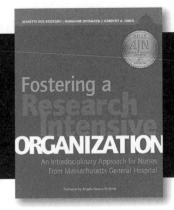
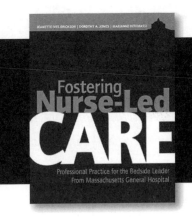

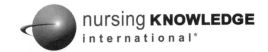

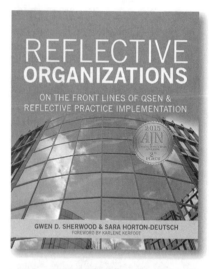
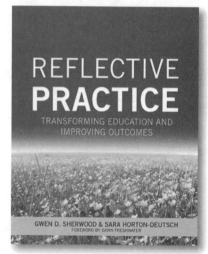
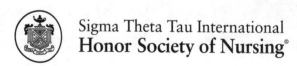
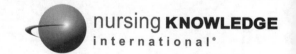